RADSTEP

RADIOLOGY FOR THE USMLE & COMLEX EXAMS

Sensei SLACman, M.D.
Board Certified Musculoskeletal Radiologist

RADSTEP: 1st Edition (2021)

This book is intended to be used as a course companion for: RADSTEP: Radiology for the USMLE & COMLEX exams, which can be found at www.radstepmd.com.

Disclaimer:
This book is to be used as a source of preparation for radiology-related questions on the United States Medical Licensing Exam (USMLE) and Comprehensive Osteopathic Medical Licensing Examination (COMLEX). **This book is not used for clinical decision making.**

To the fullest extent of the law, neither the Publisher, nor the authors, contributors, or editors, assume any liability for any injury and/or damage to persons or property as a matter of products liability, negligence or otherwise, or from any use or operation of any methods, products, instructions, or ideas contained in the material herein. The authors, editors, and publishers therefore disclaim all liability for direct or consequential damages resulting from the use of material contained in this book. Readers are strongly advised to carefully pay attention to information provided by the manufacturers of any drugs or equipment they plan on using

Practitioners and researchers must always rely on their own experience and knowledge in evaluating and using any information, methods, compounds, or experiment described herein. In using such information or methods they should be mindful of their own safety and the safety of others, including parties for whom they have a professional responsibility.

With respect to any drug or pharmaceutical products identified, readers are advised to check the most current information provided. It is the responsibility of practitioners to rely on their own experience and knowledge of their patients, to make diagnoses, to determine dosages, and to determine the best treatment for each individual patient, taking all appropriate safety precautions.

Every effort has been made in preparing this book to provide accurate and up-to-date information, which is in accord with the accepted standards and practices at the time of publication. Every effort has been made to disguise the identities of the individuals involved. Nevertheless, the authors, editors, contributors, and publishers can make no guarantees that the information contained herein is totally free from error, not least because clinical standards are constantly changing through research and regulation.

Published by: K-SPACE, LLC

ISBN-13: 978-0-578-93434-1

CONTRIBUTORS

SHVETA KANSAL, M.D.
Resident in Psychiatry
Ocean Medical Center

AMAR ANAND, M.D.
Neurologist
Integrated Neurology & Pain Management, PC

PRATIK MAVANI, M.D.
Chair, Department of Radiology
Jamestown Radiologists

MOHAMMED OMER MIRZA, M.D.
Resident in Radiology
Ascension Providence Park Hospital

LOUIS FANUCCI, D.O.
Resident in Radiology
University of California, Irvine

ABHAY ANAND, MS 2
Medical Student
Lake Earie College of Osteopathic Medicine

SURAJ PATEL, MS 2
Medical Student
Lake Earie College of Osteopathic Medicine

BEN BRAUN, MS 2
Medical Student
Frank H. Netter School of Medicine at Quinnipiac University

For my daughter, Meera, who was picked up late from school a few too many times, while I was writing this.

&

My wife, Mrs. SLACman, who continues to put up with my shit…

TABLE OF CONTENTS

SECTION 1

CHAPTERS 1 - 8:
USMLE & COMLEX CASES

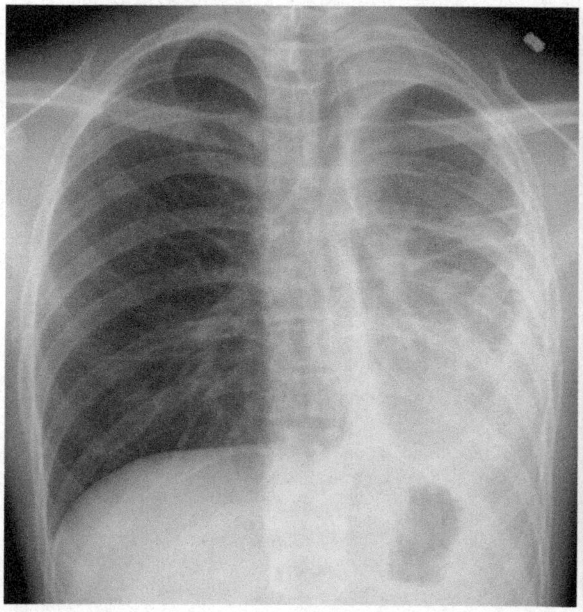

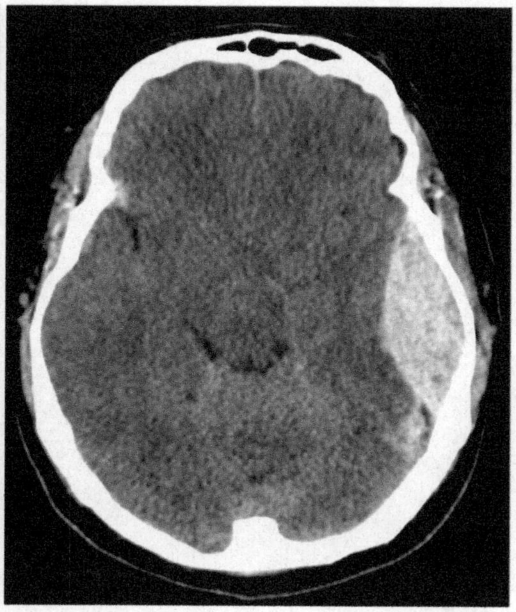

MUSCULOSKELETAL

MUSCULOSKELETAL

JONES FRACTURE

IMAGING: **Located at the metadiaphyseal junction, approximately 2 cm (1.5 - 3 cm) from the tip of the 5th metatarsal,**
Predominantly horizontal course.

USMLE POINTS: **Adduction of forefoot when ankle is plantarflexed**
Prone to non-union
Insertion of **peroneal brevis**
Pain/swelling on outside of foot near base of 5th metatarsal

MODALITIES: XR → MRI

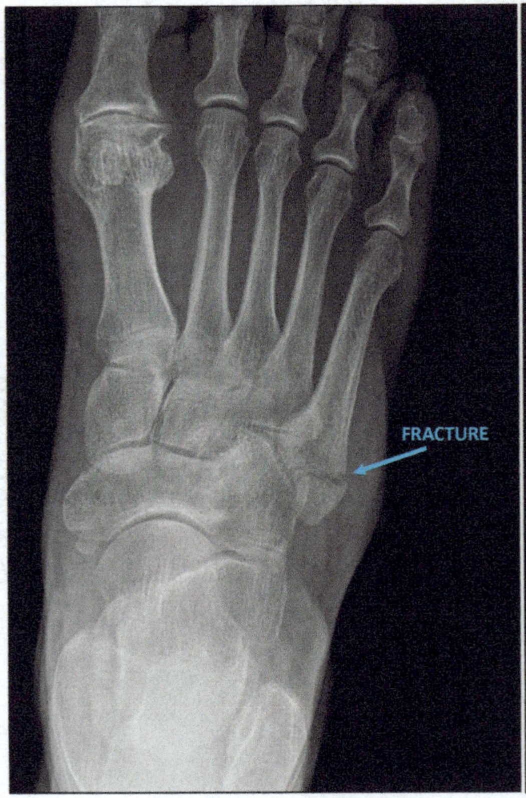

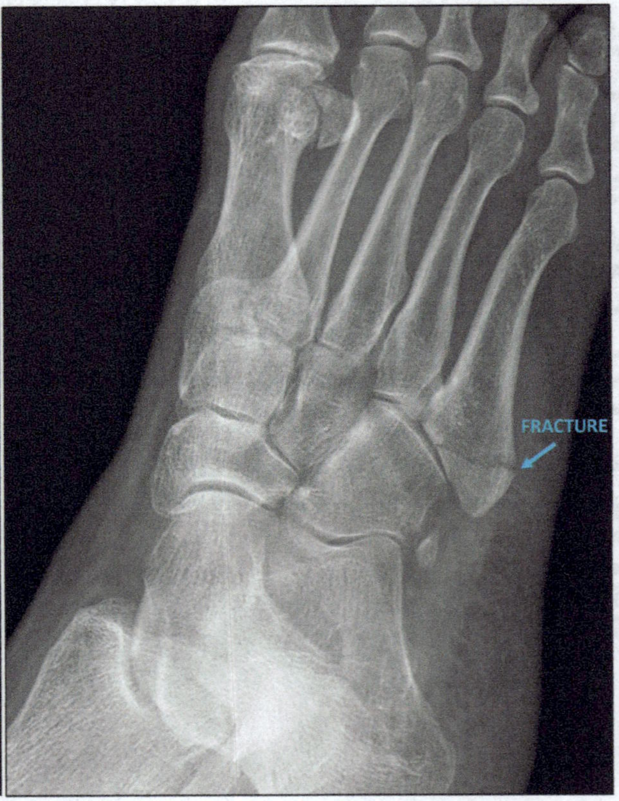

MUSCULOSKELETAL

ACHILLES RUPTURE

IMAGING:

MRI: Tendinous gap filled with edema or blood.
XR: Soft tissue swelling and obliteration of pre-Achilles fat pad

USMLE POINTS:

Achilles reflex tests: Nerve roots S1 and S2 (tibial nerve)
Sudden forced plantarflexion
Tendon is formed from the soleus and gastrocnemius → aids in plantar flexion
Calf squeeze test +

Achilles xanthoma: Shows increased AP diameter of the distal tendon which is often uniform
Loss of the normal anterior concavity of the tendon can also be seen
Familial hypercholesterolemia

MODALITIES: MRI WO

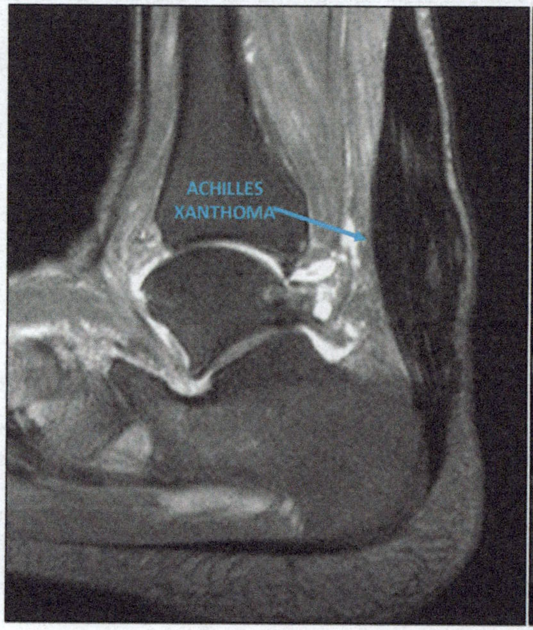

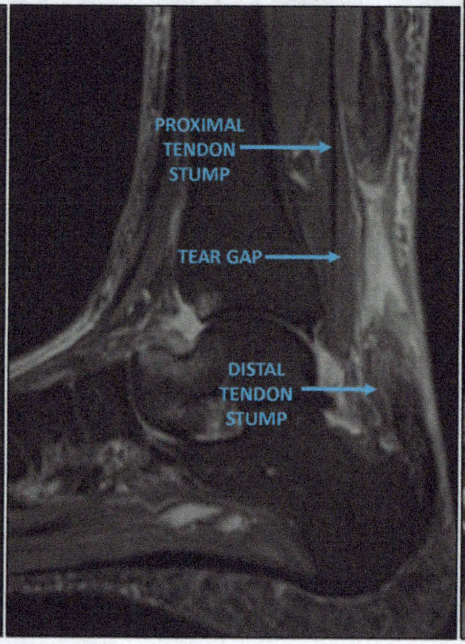

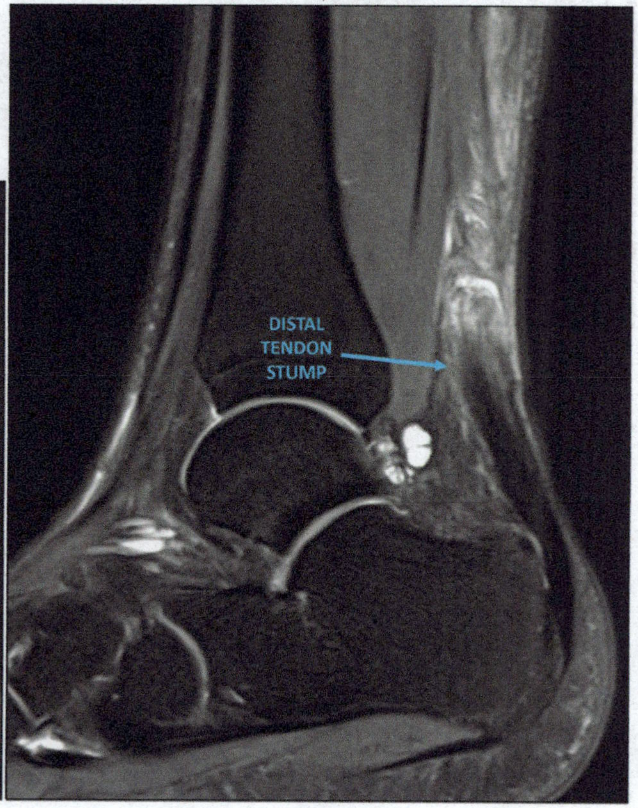

MUSCULOSKELETAL

COMPRESSION FRACTURE AND OSTEOPOROSIS

IMAGING: **Loss of height in the anterior, middle, or posterior dimension of the vertebral body**
Acute fracture signs include **cortical breaking** or impaction of trabeculae

USMLE POINTS: **Osteoporosis**
May be **traumatic**

Osteoporosis: **Lucent bones on radiographs + Loss of cortex**
Osteoblasts lose their biosynthetic and proliferative ability with age
Post-menopausal females → **Decreased estrogen**
DEXA: T-score < -2.5
Age > 65 years old
Poor physical activity + Low Vitamin D
Medications: Warfarin, Lithium, PPI, Steroids
Associations: **Hyperparathyroid, MM, Malabsorption syndrome**
Treatment: Calcium / Vitamin D supplementation + Weight bearing exercises
Labs: **Normal Ca, Phosphorus, PTH, ALP**

MODALITIES: XR → CT WO
DEXA

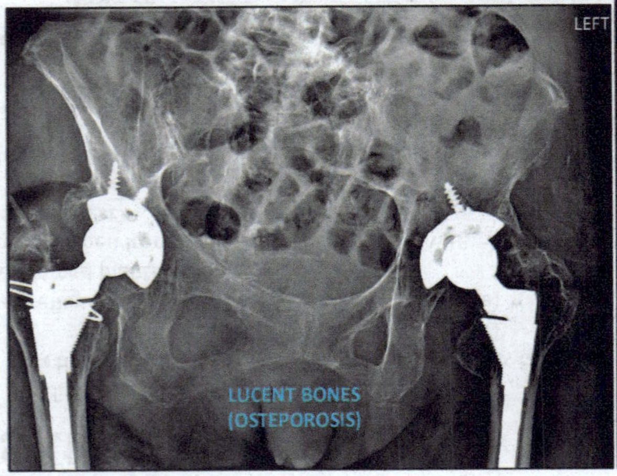

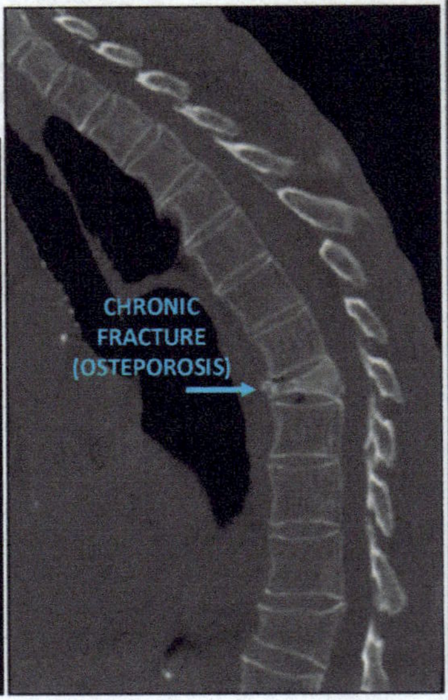

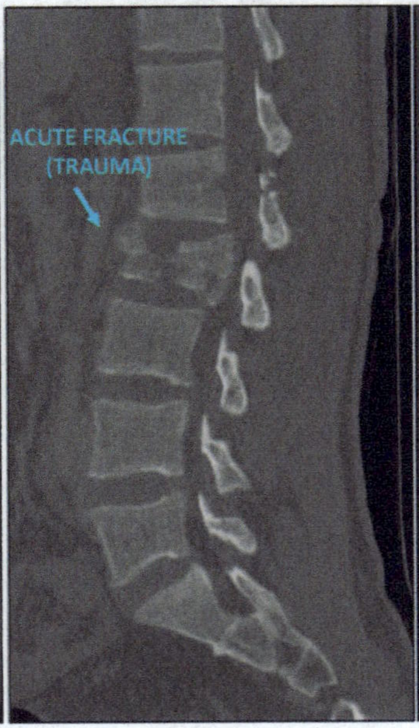

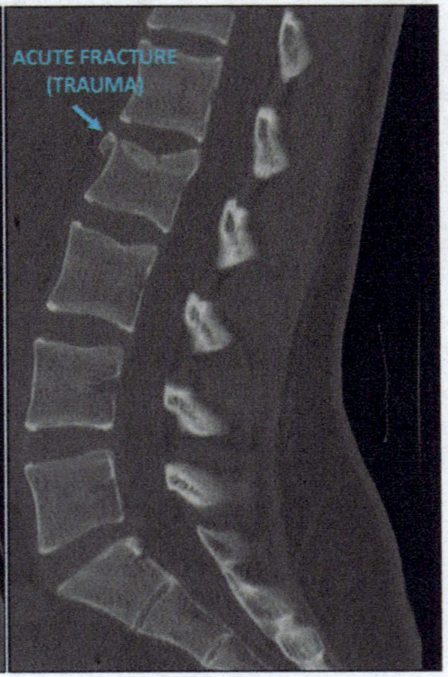

MUSCULOSKELETAL

CALCIUM PYROPHOPHATE DEPOSITION DISEASE

IMAGING: Chondrocalcinosis can occur in many locations

- Knee: **Medial meniscus and patellofemoral joint**
- Wrist: **TFCC & LT**

USMLE POINTS: **Calcium pyrophosphate dihydrate (CPP)**

Due to deposition of pyrophosphate crystals within joint space
Usually affects those >50 years old
Weakly + birefringent rhomboid crystals (vs. gout → negatively birefringent needles)
Blue when parallel to light and yellow when perpendicular to light

Associations: Hemachromatosis
Hyperparathyroidism

Treatment: NSAIDS
Colchicine
Glucocorticoids

MODALITIES: XR → MRI

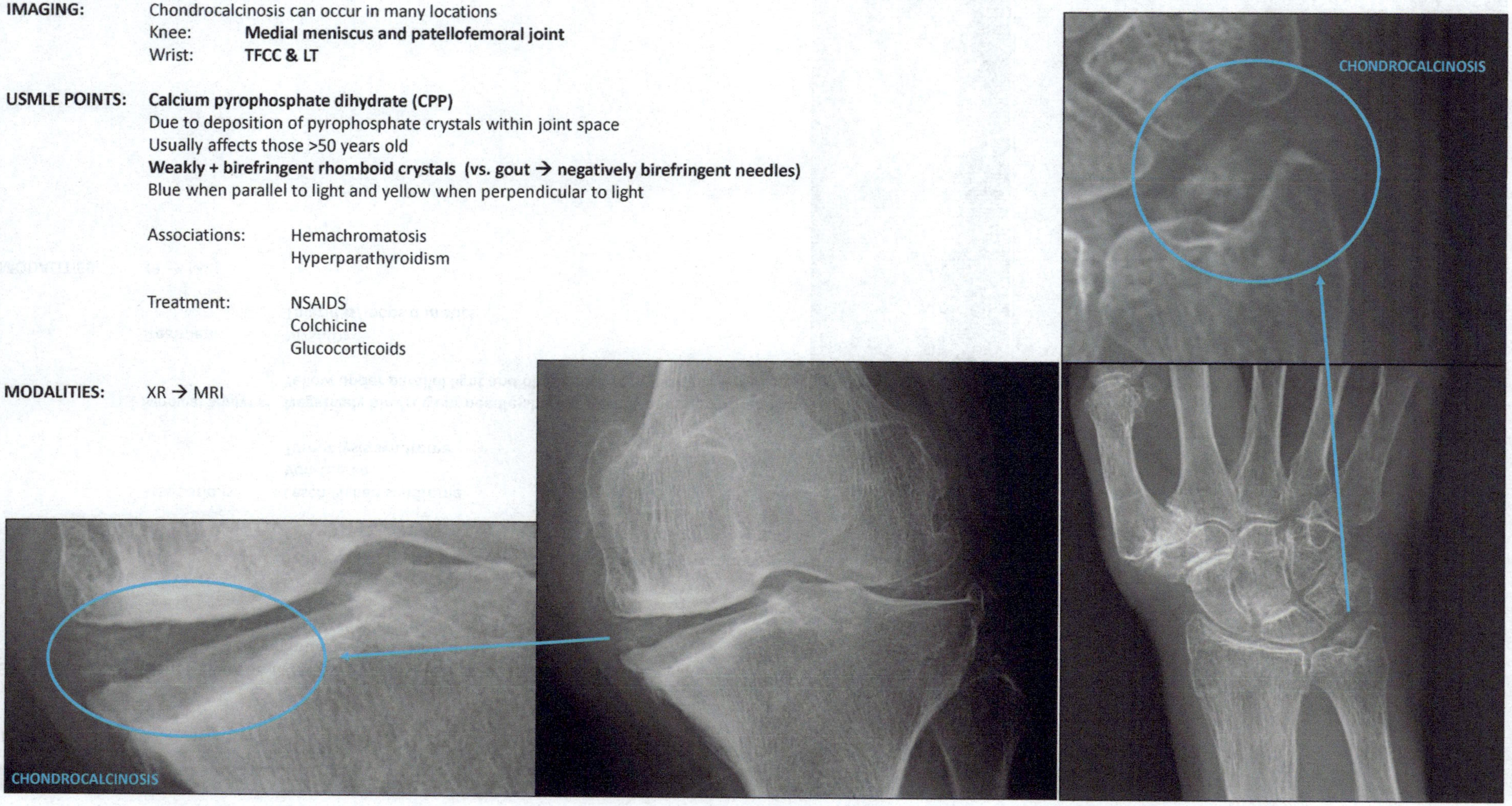

MUSCULOSKELETAL

GOUT

IMAGING: Overhanging edges
Great toe

USMLE POINTS: **Monosodium urate (MSU) crystals leading** to a crystal-induced arthropathy
Defined as a **serum urate level > 6.8 mg/dL**
Extreme pain of the affected joint

Risk Factors: Males
EtOH consumption due to competition for the same excretion site in the kidney as uric acid
Red meat

Associations: **Lesch-Nyhan syndrome**
Von-Gierke
Tumor lysis syndrome

Synovial analysis: **Negatively birefringent needle-shaped crystals under polarized light**
Yellow under parallel light and blue under perpendicular light

Treatment: NDSAIDs
Thiazides/loops diuretics

MODALITIES: XR → MRI

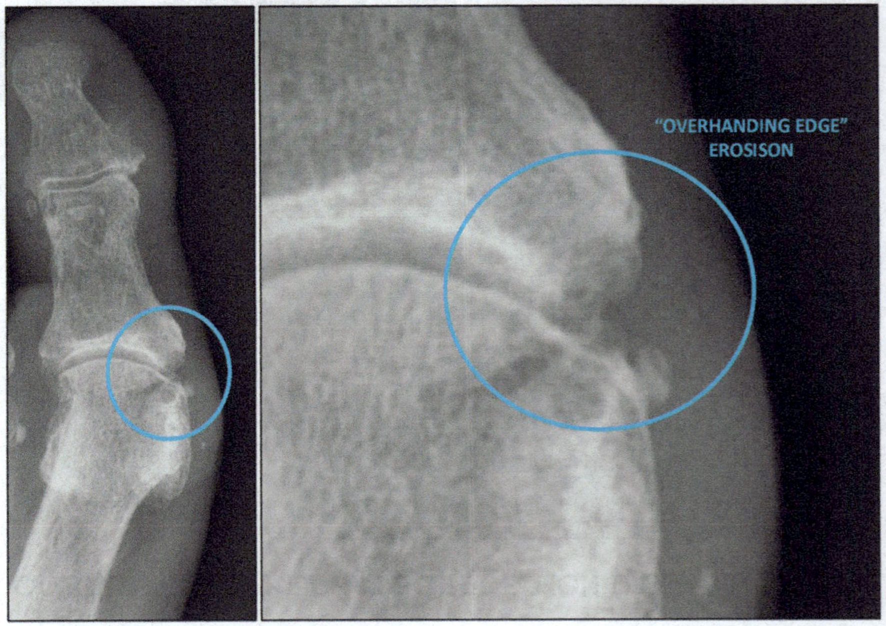

MUSCULOSKELETAL

ORBITAL FLOOR FRACTURE

IMAGING: **Inferior wall most common**
50% of cases, **inferior blowout fractures are associated with fractures of the medial wall**

USMLE POINTS: Damage the **infraorbital nerve (CN5 V2)**
Entrap the inferior rectus muscle → impairing vertical gaze

MODALITIES: CT WO

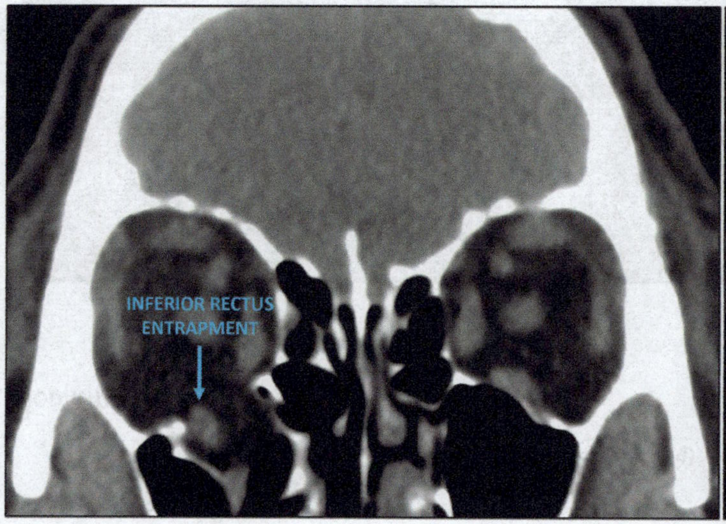

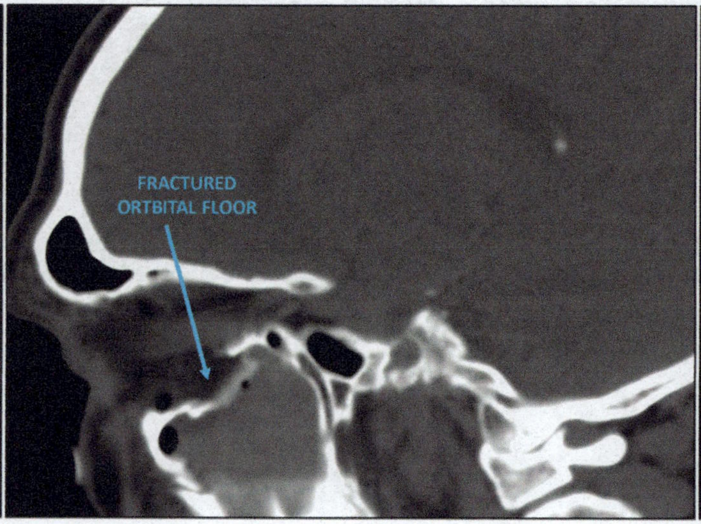

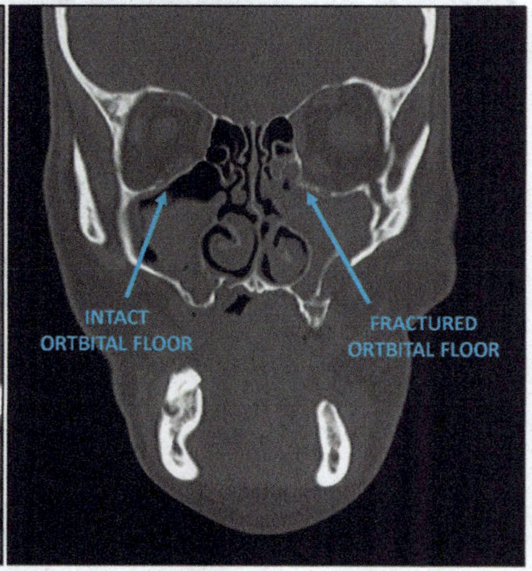

MUSCULOSKELETAL

BOXERS FRACTURE

IMAGING: Fracture appears in the transverse plane through the metacarpal neck
Volar angulation of the distal fragment.

USMLE POINTS: Direct blow with closed fist to an object
4th and 5th metacarpal necks
Often does not require surgery (based on angulation)

MODALITIES: XR

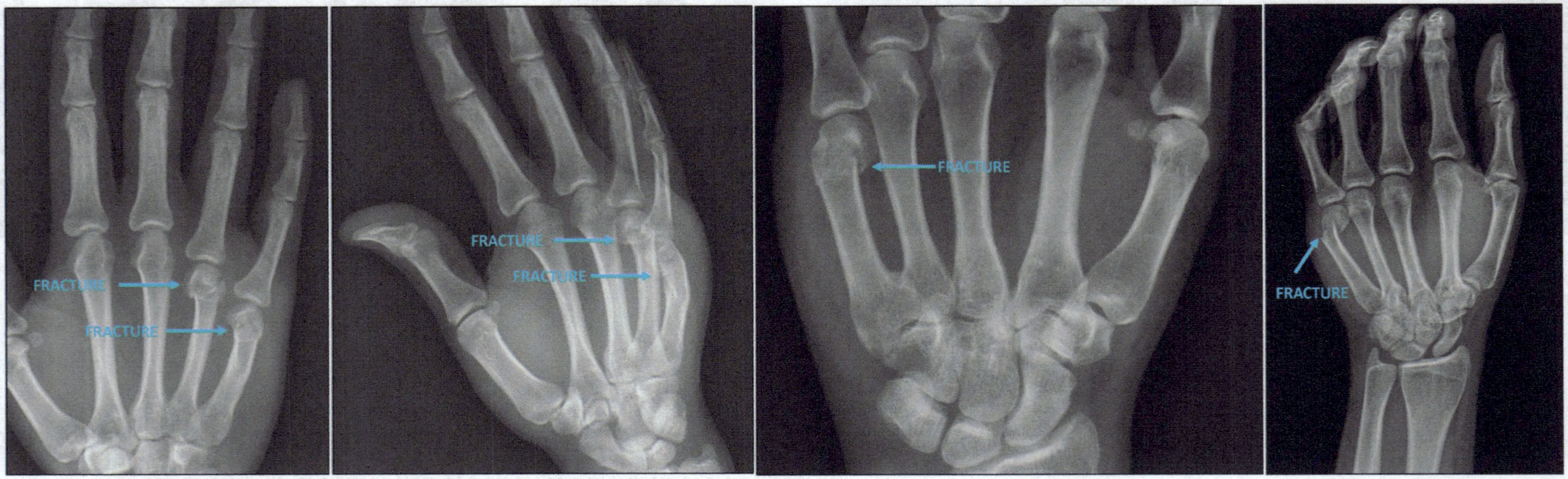

MUSCULOSKELETAL

CHARCOT ARTHROPATHY

IMAGING:

Density change	→	Subchondral osteopenia or sclerosis
Destruction	→	**Osseous fragmentation and resorption**
Debris	→	**Intra-articular loose bodies**
Distension	→	**Joint effusion**
Disorganization and Dislocation	→	Ligamentous laxity

USMLE POINTS:

Diabetics – most common
Lack of sensation allows you to destroy your joints
Tabes dorsalis due to **loss of proprioception**
Associated with **spinal cord pathology** (syrinx, Vit B12 / SCD, myelomeningocele)
Non-painful swelling
Normal WBC, ESR, CRP

If in the **shoulder** → **Spinal cord syrinx**
If in the **knee** → **Syphilis**

MODALITIES: XR → MR WO

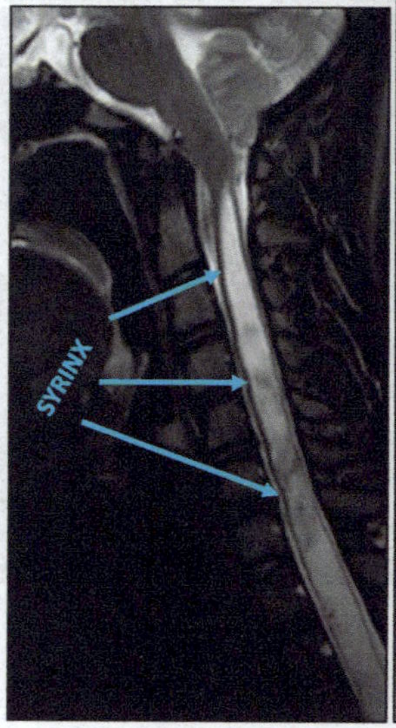

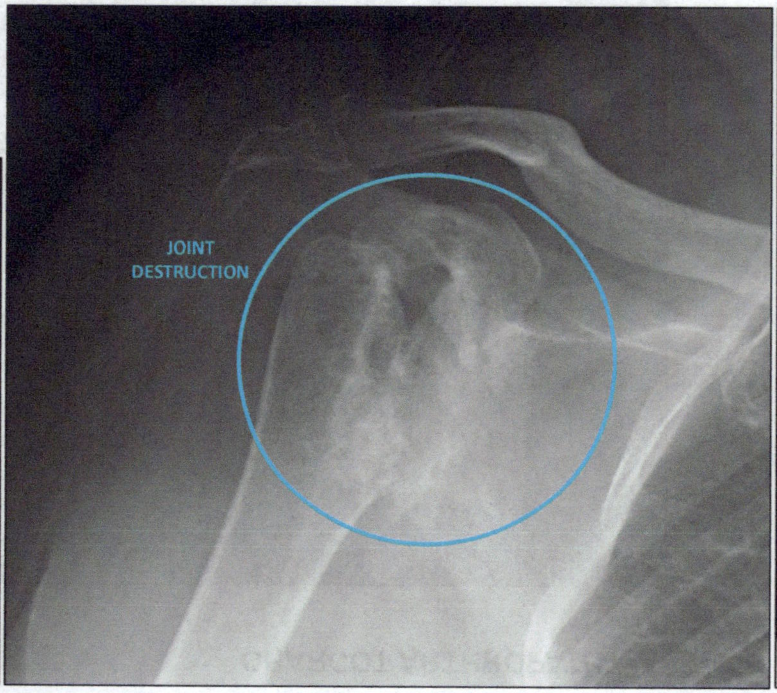

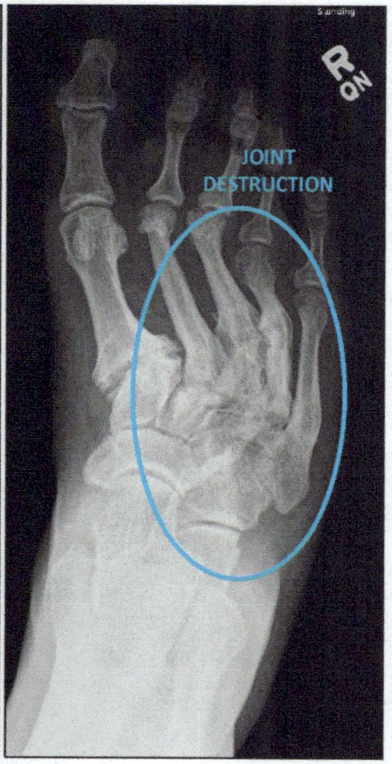

CHARCOT ARTHROPATHY

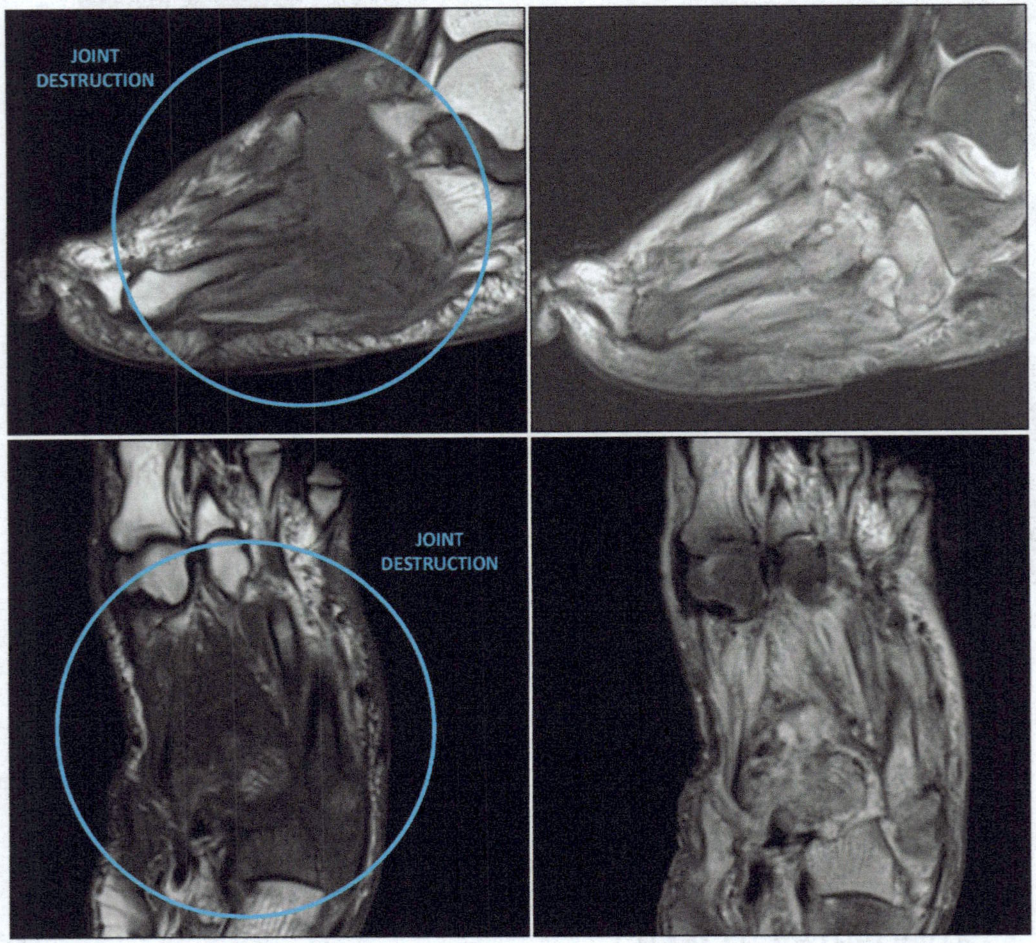

MUSCULOSKELETAL

OSTEOARTHRITIS

IMAGING:
- **Joint space narrowing**
- **Osteophytic spurring**
- **Subchondral sclerosis/cystic changes**

USMLE POINTS:
Due to **overuse** (chondral disease) → Worst in **weightbearing** joints (Knees, lower lumbar spine, hips)
OA improves with REST unlike rheumatoid arthritis which improves with USE
Asymmetric joint involvement
Normal ESR / CRP / RF

Hands: **DIP + 1st CMC (MCP not affected)**
Knees: **Medial compartment often worse**

Erosive OA: "Gull-wing" deformity of DIP / PIP

MODALITIES: XR → MRI WO

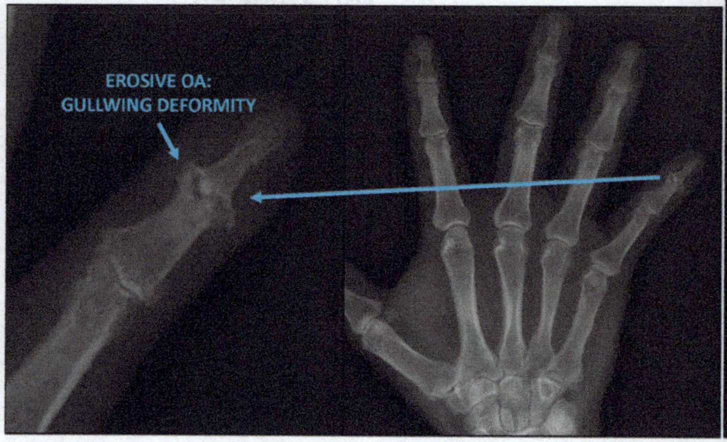

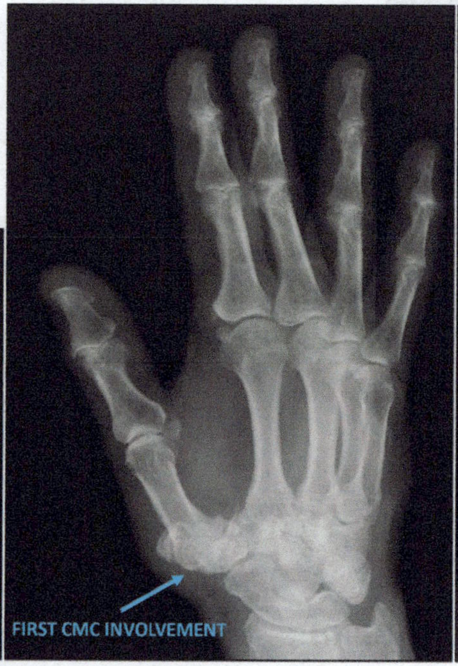

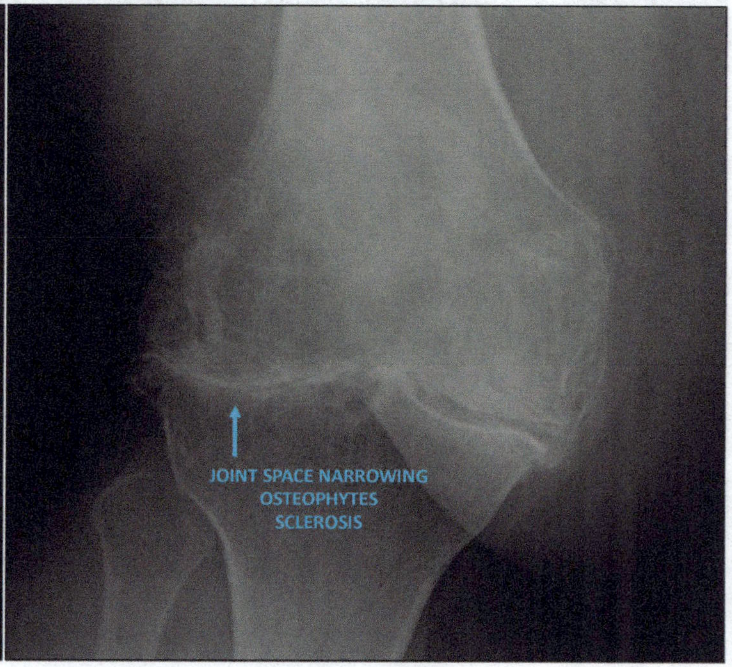

MUSCULOSKELETAL

RHEUMATOID ARTHRITIS

IMAGING:
- **Joint destruction**
- **Erosions**
- **Subluxations**
- **Synovial hypertrophy / Pannus formation on MRI**

USMLE POINTS:
- Synovitis leading to formation of pannus
- HLA-DR4 predisposes to RA
- **PIP, MCP, MTP, Carpal articulations**
- **Symmetric involvement along with systemic symptoms (fever, fatigue)**
- Swan neck and boutonniere deformity
- Can have **subluxation of cervical spine**
- Histology: Rheumatoid nodules with areas of fibrinoid necrosis + palisading histiocytes
- RF + and **Anti-CCP specific**
- **Elevated ESR / CRP**

Associations:
- **Sjogren syndrome**
- **Felty syndrome (RA + neutropenia + Splenomegaly)**
- **Caplan syndrome (RA + pneumoconiosis)**

Treatment:
- **NSAIDs**
- **DMARDS** → **MTX**, **TNF Inhibitors (etanercept and adalimumab)**, **Sulfasalazine**, **Hydroxychloroquine**

MODALITIES: XR → MRI WO

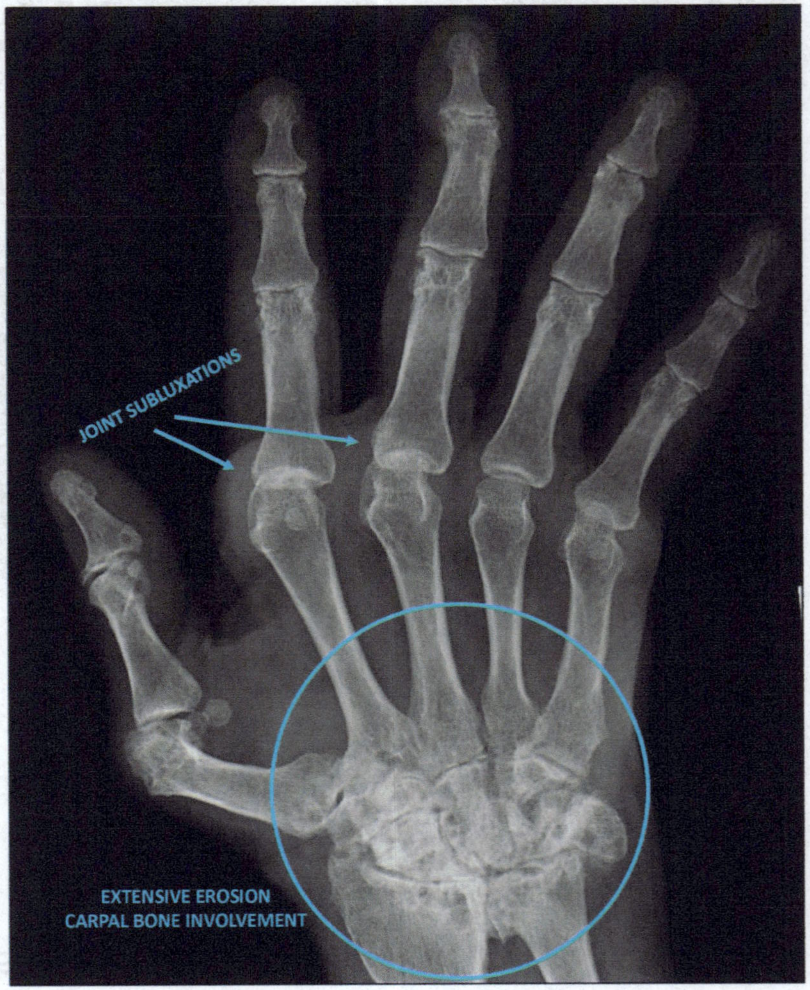

MUSCULOSKELETAL

DENS AND HANGMAN FRACTURES

IMAGING:

Dense fracture: Fracture through **the odontoid process of C2**

Hangman fracture: Bilateral **pars interarticularis** fractures of C2 vertebra.

USMLE POINTS:

Dens fracture: **Low energy falls in elderly patients**

Type 2: Fracture at the base of the dens → **Unstable**
Fracture through waist (**high nonunion rate** → Interruption of blood supply)
Immobilization and often surgery

Hangman fracture: Motor vehicle accident most common → sudden **deceleration and forcible hyperextension**

MODALITIES: CT WO

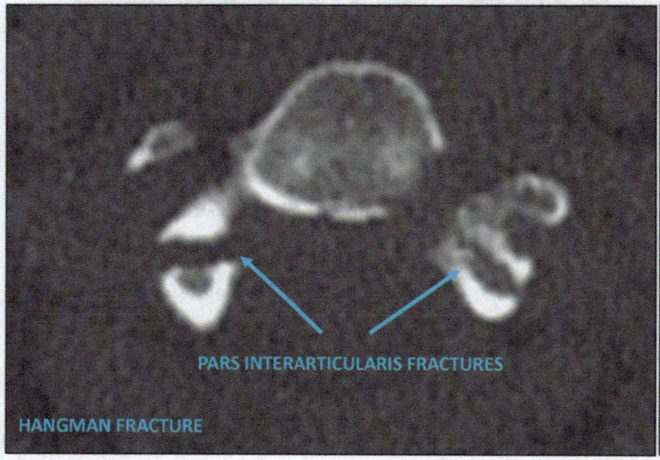

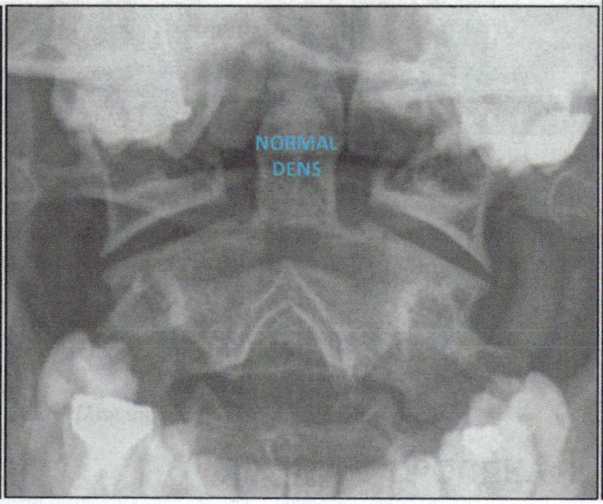

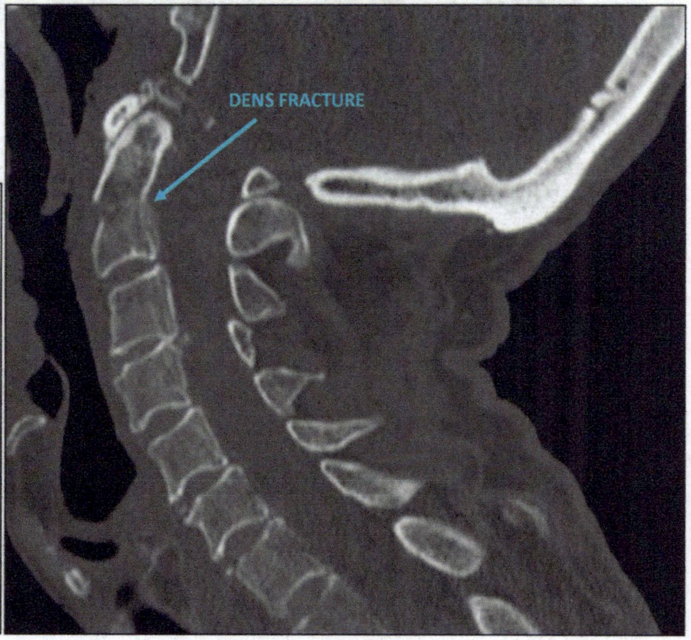

MUSCULOSKELETAL

DeQUERVAIN'S TENOSYNOVITIS

IMAGING: **First extensor (dorsal) tendon compartment of the wrist (typically at the radial styloid)**
APL / EPB **(snuffbox tendons)**

USMLE POINTS: **Radial-sided wrist pain**
APL / EPB (first extensor compartment)
Finkelstein test → ulnar deviation of the hand while thumb is flexed in palm
New mothers (holding baby with first webspace under baby's axilla) and patients who type on small handheld devices

MODALITIES: US / MRI WO

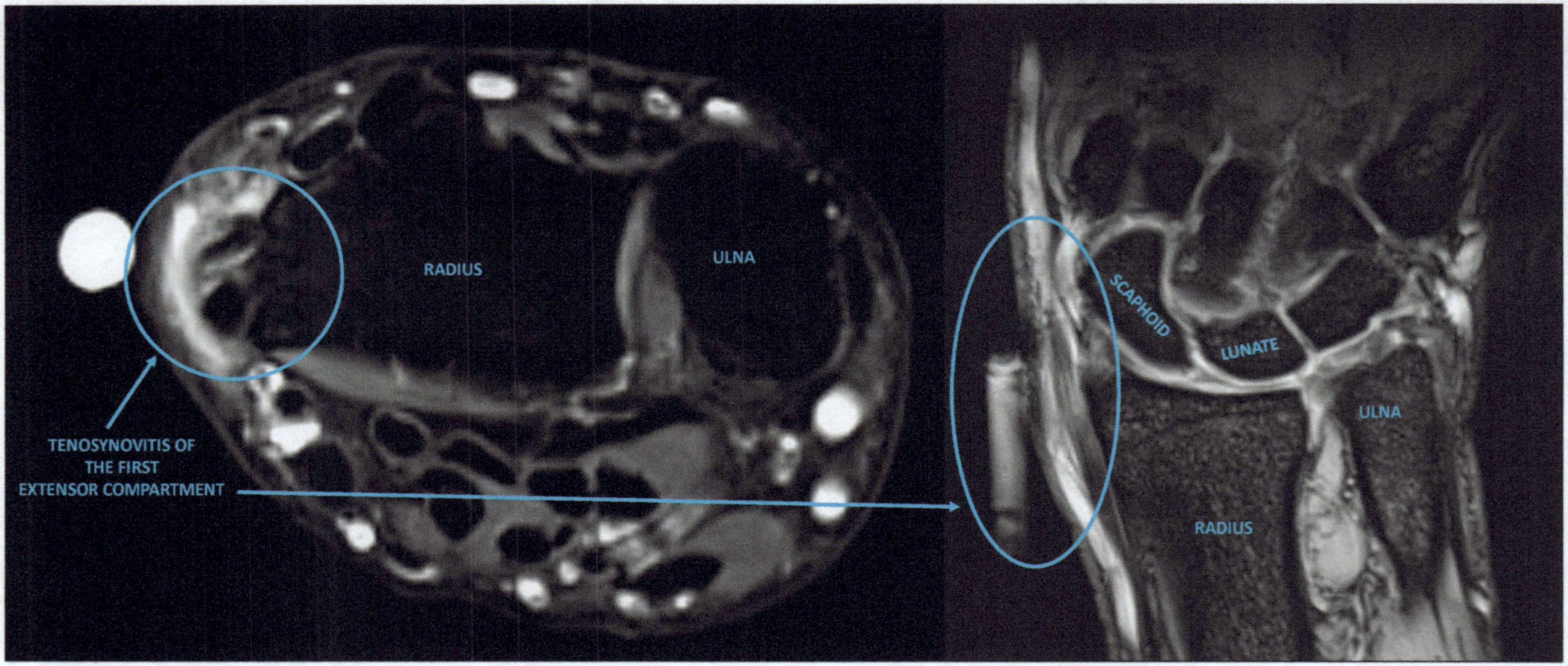

MUSCULOSKELETAL

DISC HERNIATION

IMAGING: Displacement of intervertebral disc material beyond the normal confines of the disc
Involves less than 25% of the circumference (more than 25% = bulge)

USMLE POINTS: Herniation of **nucleus pulposis** → annulus fibrosis
Posterolateral at the level of L4-L5 or L5-S1 most common
Manual labor, heavy lifting, sports
Positive straight leg raise and bowstring test

L5 Radiculopathy:	Affects ankle dorsiflexion and hip abduction	**Normal Achilles reflex**
S1 Radiculopathy:	Affects ankle plantarflexion diminished	**Impaired Achilles reflex**

CERVICAL SPINE
Posterolateral & central disc herniations: Affects the same nerve root
Posterolateral or central disc herniation at C6-C7 impinges C7

LUMBAR SPINE
Posterolateral disc herniations: Affects the **higher** nerve root
Posterolateral disc herniation at L4-L5 impinges **L4** nerve root

Central disc herniations: Affects the **lower** nerve root
Central disc herniation at L4-L5 impinges **L5** nerve root

MODALITIES: MRI WO

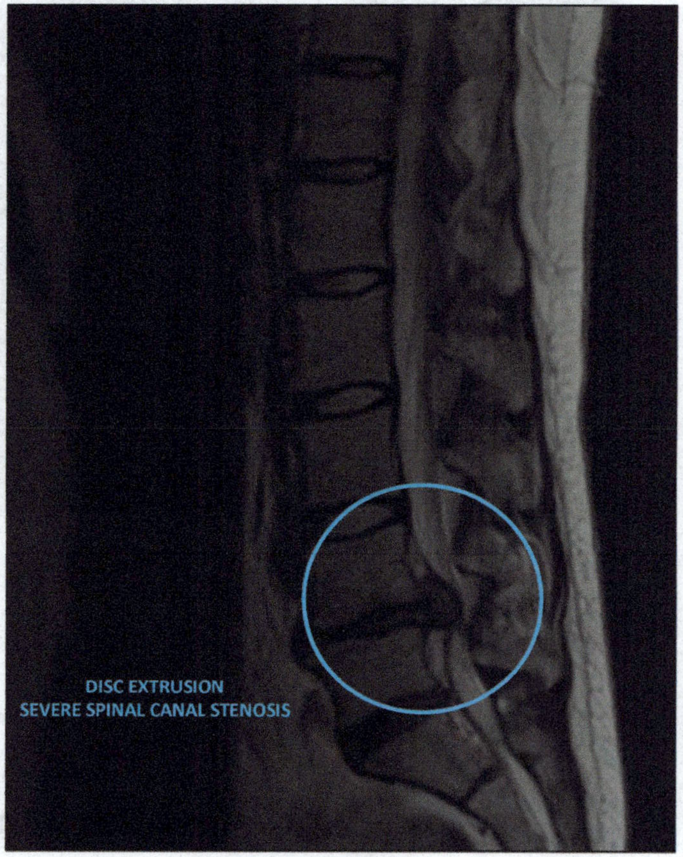

MUSCULOSKELETAL

DISTAL RADIUS FRACTURE

IMAGING: **Colles, Smith, Barton, Chauffeur. Transverse** metaphyseal fractures.
Often extra-articular, but some may extend into the joint, and when they do, it is important to recognize.
The degree of displacement (usually dorsal) is important because it will be a determining factor for treatment

USMLE POINTS: FOOSH
Osteoporosis
Surgical repair depends on **radial tilt, radial inclination, radial height, degree of dorsal displacement**

MODALITIES: XR → CT

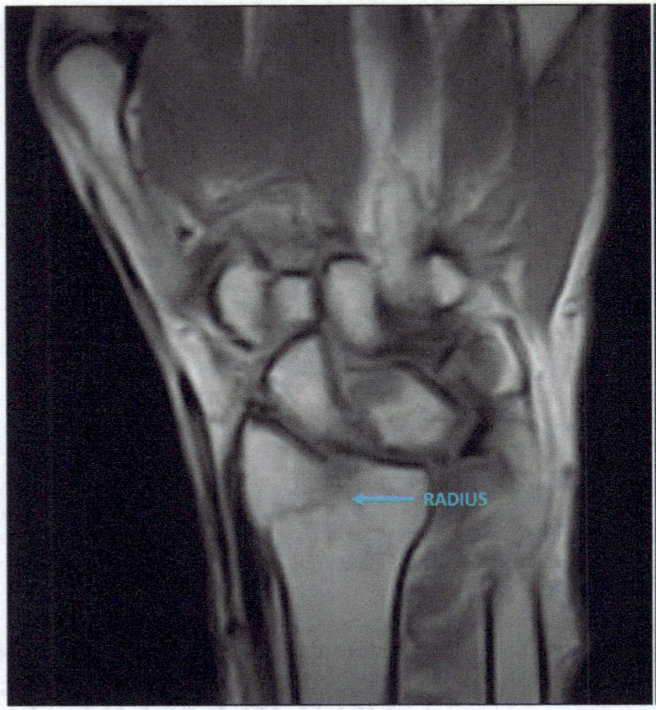

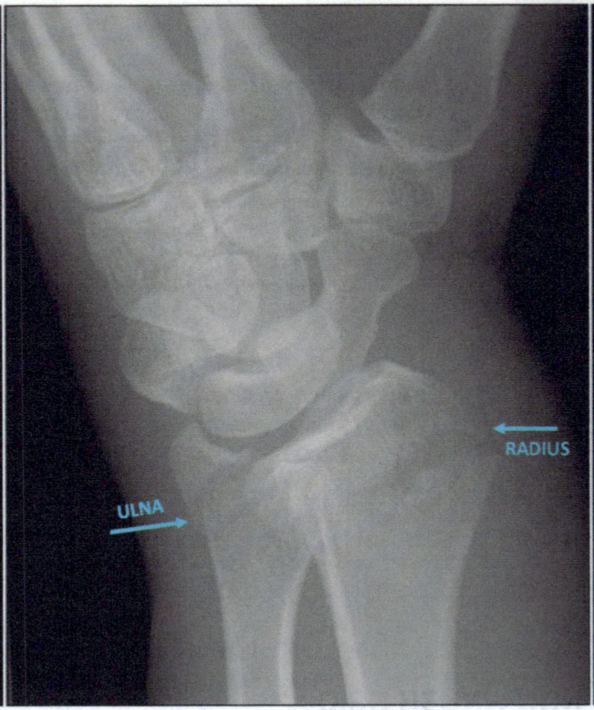

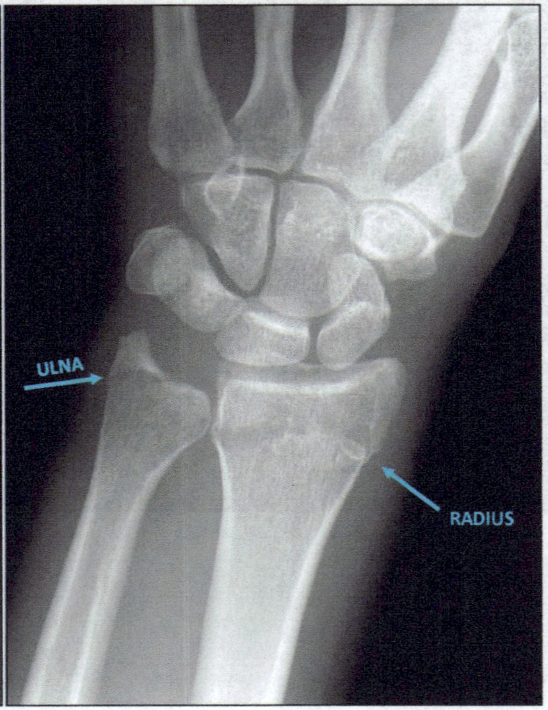

MUSCULOSKELETAL

MONTEGGIA AND GALEAZZI FRACTURES

IMAGING:

Monteggia: **Fracture of proximal 1/3rd of ulnar shaft**
Dislocation of radial head (proximal)

Galeazzi: **Fracture of the radius**
Dislocated distal ulna (DRUJ)

USMLE POINTS: **"MUGR" / "GFR"**

Monteggia: Mostly occur in children, rare in adults
Fall on an outstretched hand (FOOSH) or **direct blow** (night-stick)
Posterior Interosseous Nerve (PIN) palsy

Galeazzi: Fracture of distal part of radius with dislocation of distal radioulnar joint (DRUJ) and intact ulna
Usually seen in children, less common in adults
Fall on an outstretched hand (FOOSH)

MODALITIES: XR

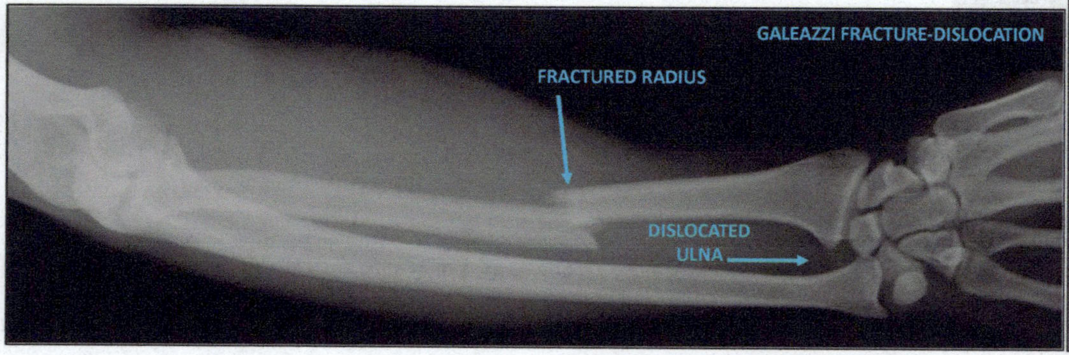

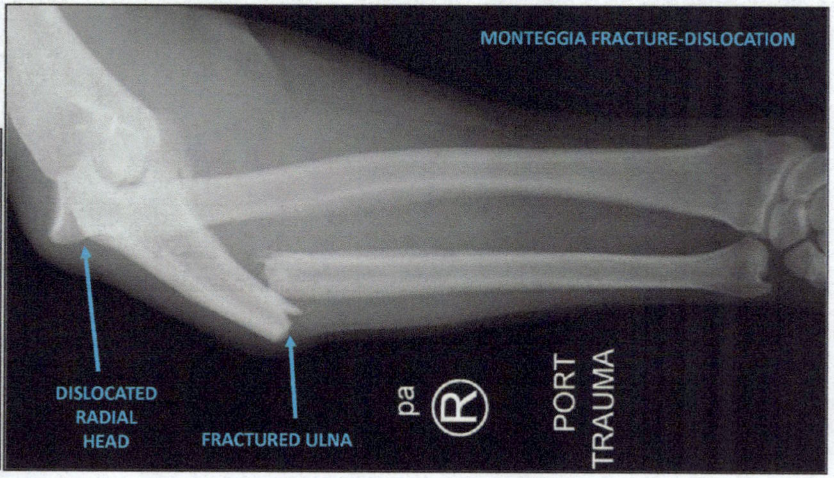

MUSCULOSKELETAL

MULTIPLE MYELOMA

IMAGING: Multiple "punched out" lytic lesions within the calvarium

USMLE POINTS: Neoplastic **plasma cells** → **IL-1** → stimulates osteoclast maturation → **bone resorption** → lytic lesions
Neoplastic proliferation of plasma cells within the bone marrow → production of monoclonal immunoglobulin (Mostly IgG)

Associations: Fanconi anemia
RTA 2

SPEP: **Monoclonal immunoglobulin spike (M protein)**
UPEP: Bence Jones protein

Blood smear: Rouleaux formation of RBC

DDx **MGUS:** **Serum M-protein is low**
Waldenstrom: **No hypercalcemia or renal involvement**

MODALITIES: XR

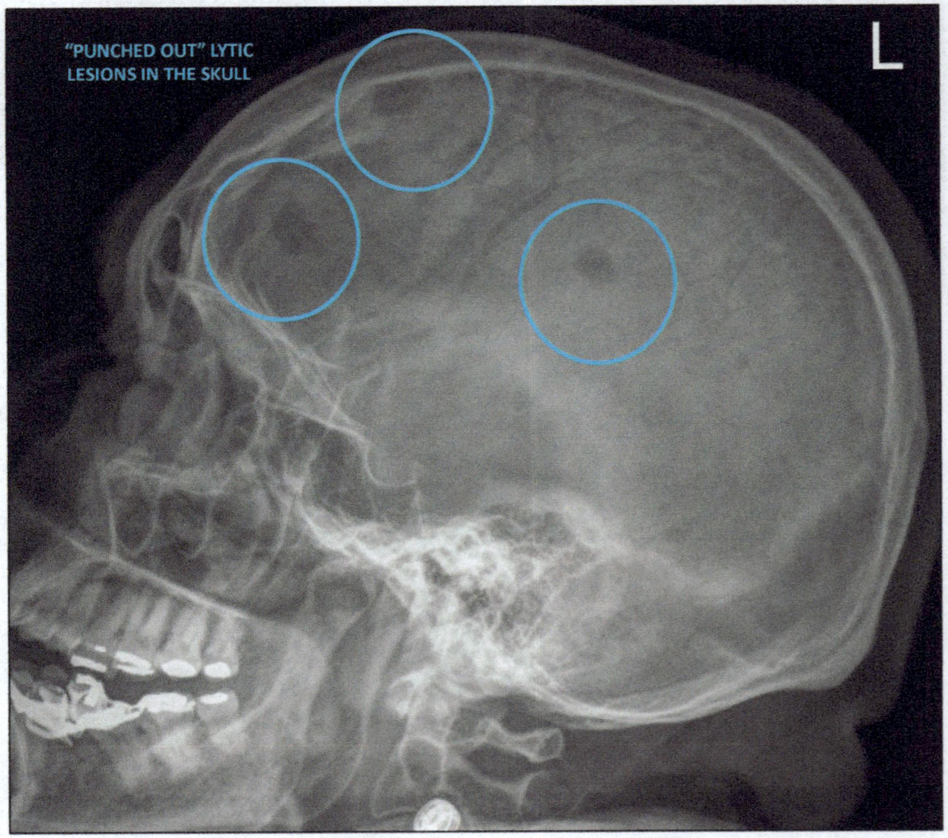

MUSCULOSKELETAL

OSTEOMYELITIS

IMAGING:

MRI: **Edema + Low T1SI + Overlying soft-tissue ulcer**
XR: **Osseous erosion, focal osteopenia + Overlying soft-tissue ulcer**
Periosteal reaction and elevation "Codman triangle"

USMLE POINTS:

Osteomyelitis:

Risk factors: Diabetes, Peripheral vascular disease, IVDA, Surgery
Labs: Elevated **CRP, ESR,** WBC

Pasteurella multocida: **Cat and dog bites**
Pseudomonas & Candida: **IVDA**
Staphylococcus aureus: Most common (including children)
Sickle cell disease
Prosthetic joint replacement

Osteomyelitis-Discitis:

Contiguous involving the intervertebral disc and adjacent vertebrae
Takes 10-14 days post infection for findings to appear
Hematogenous seeding of bone → Transient bacteremia that seeds the metaphysis (children) or epiphysis (adults)
Contiguous spread of infection from adjacent structures

MODALITIES: XR → MRI WO

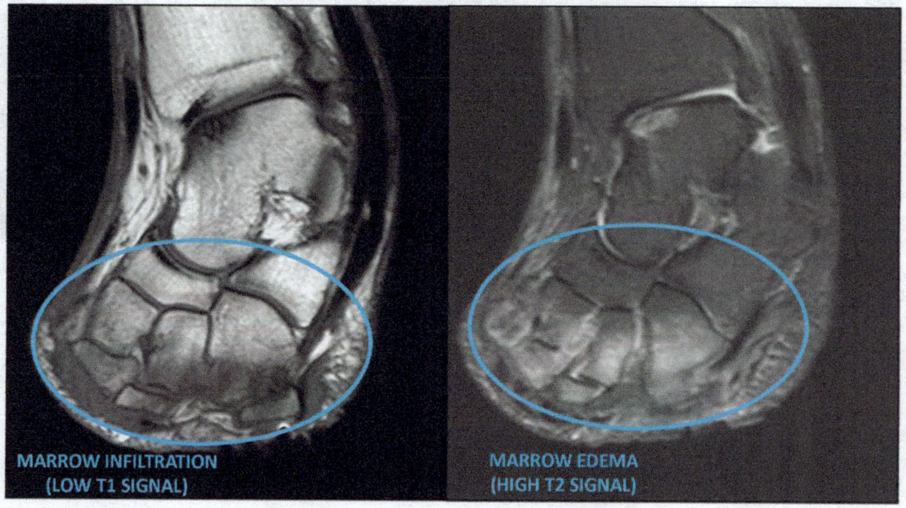

MUSCULOSKELETAL

OSTEOMYELITIS

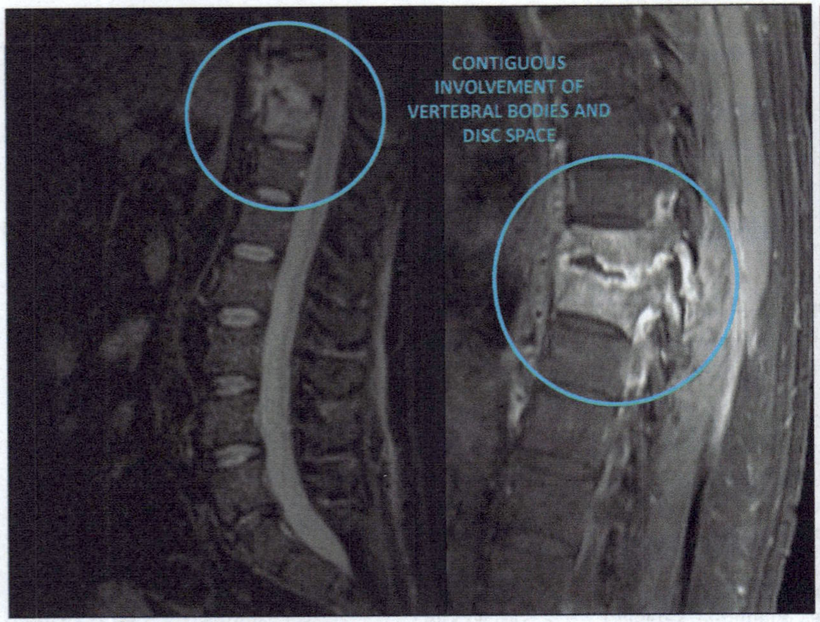

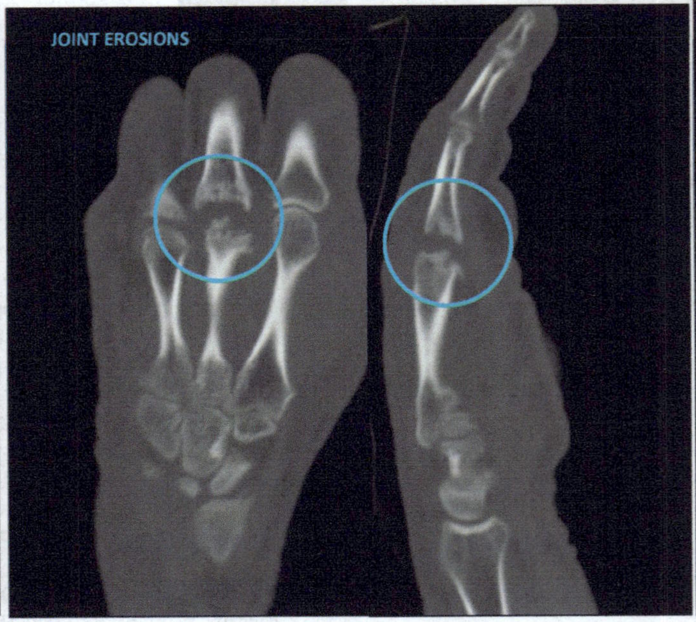

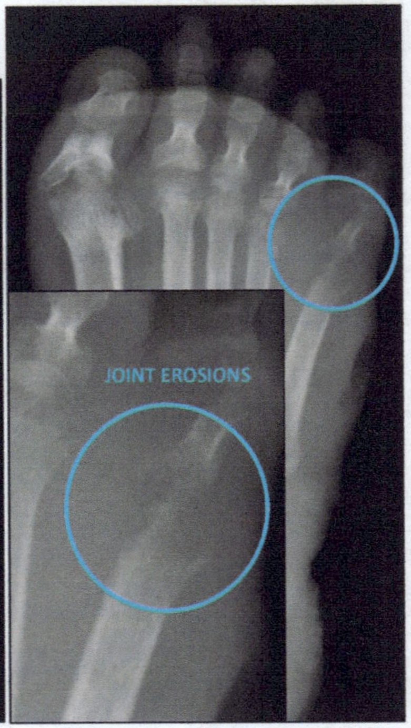

MUSCULOSKELETAL

NECROTIZING FASCIITIS

IMAGING: **Subcutaneous air**
Cellulitis

USMLE POINTS: **Crepitus** in cases of **gas forming** (CO_2 / methane) organisms → **Clostridium & anaerobic organisms**
Direct inoculation

Polymicrobial most common: **Streptococcus spp. (most common)**
Bacteroides spp.
Peptostreptococcus spp.

Risk factors: **Diabetes mellitus**
Chronic corticosteroid use

Treatment: Prompt **surgical** debridement

MODALITIES: XR → CT W

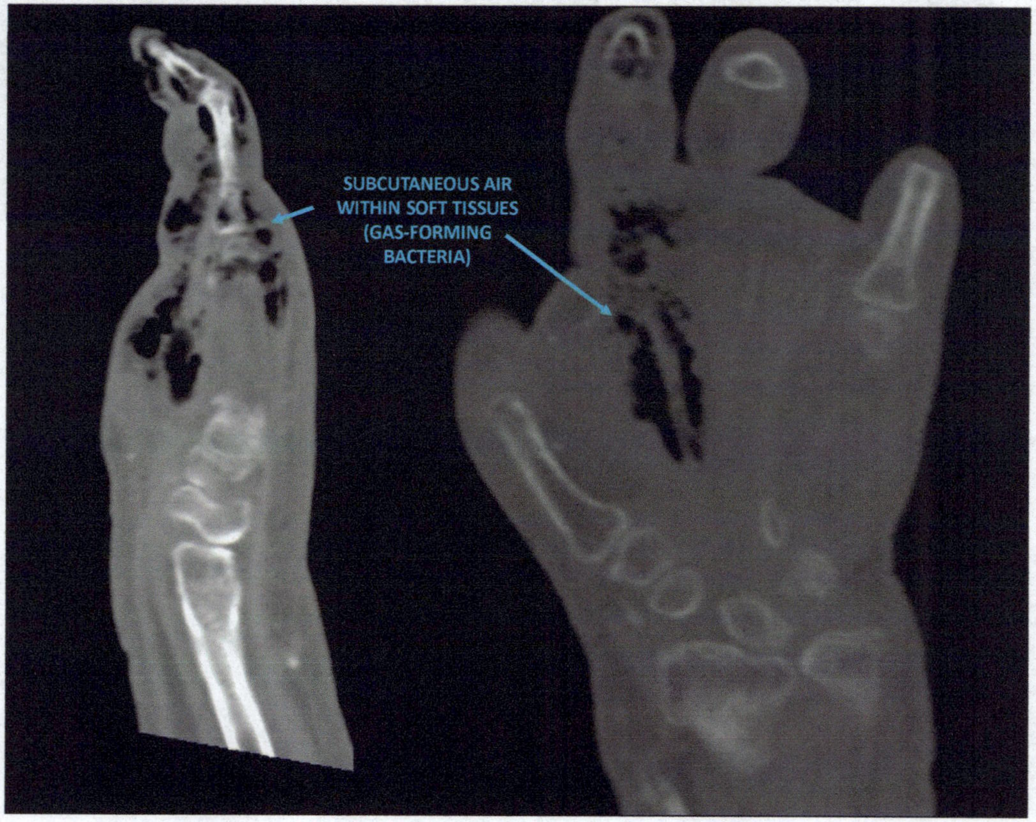

MUSCULOSKELETAL

OSTEOSARCOMA

IMAGING:

Medullary and cortical bone destruction
Wide zone of transition
Aggressive periosteal reaction: Sunburst appearance. **Tumor matrix ossification/calcification**
Metaphysis of long bones, often around the **knee**

USMLE POINTS:

Malignant proliferation of osteoblasts

Risk factors: **Paget** disease
Prior **radiation**
Familial **retinoblastoma (RB suppressor gene)**
Li-Fraumeni syndrome

Treatment: Surgical resection / Amputation, Chemotherapy, Radiation

Primary: **Teenagers**

Secondary: Pagets disease, prior radiation

MODALITIES: XR → MRI WWO

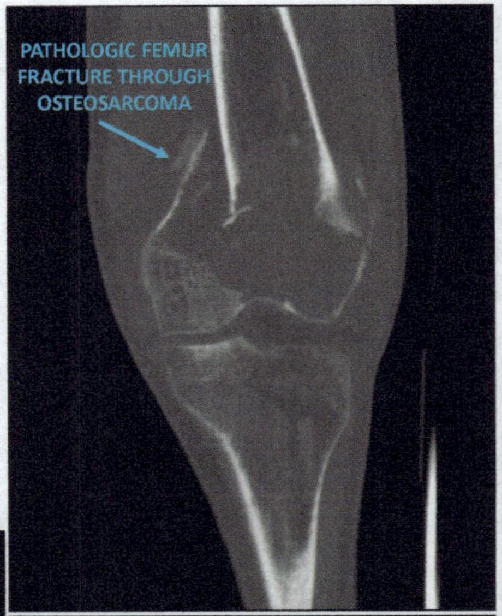

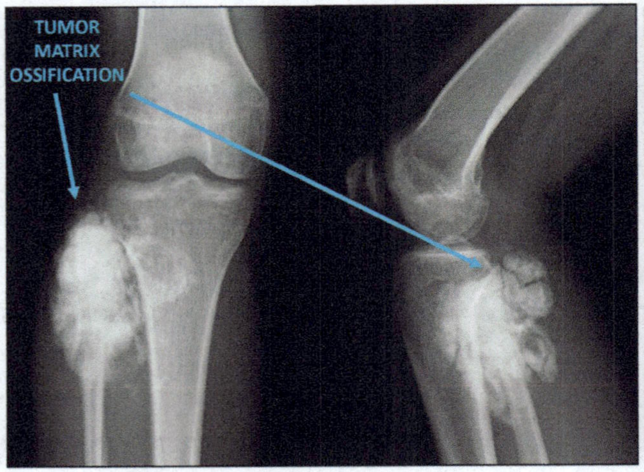

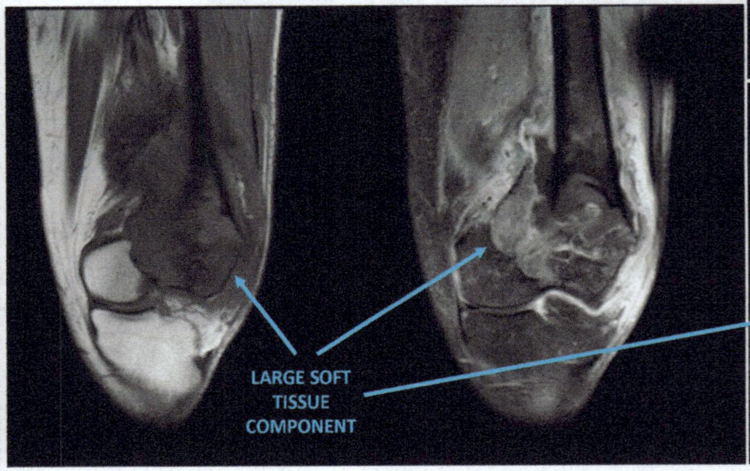

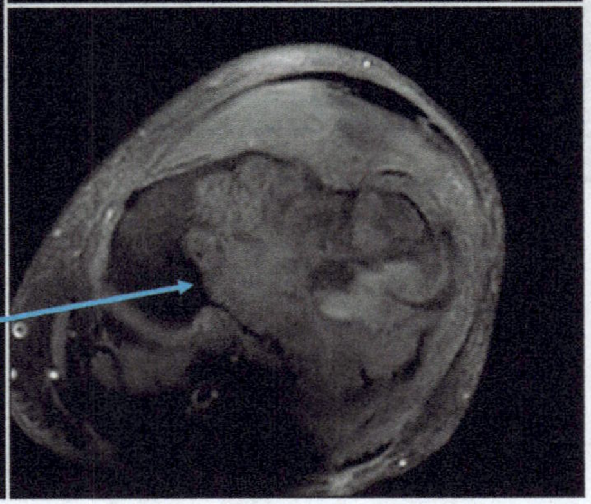

MUSCULOSKELETAL

PAGET'S DISEASE

IMAGING:
Coarsened trabeculae and bony enlargement
Sclerotic changes occur much later in the disease process
Can degenerate into osteosarcoma

USMLE POINTS:
Osteoclastic (lytic) → mixed osteoblastic-osteoclastic → osteoblastic (sclerotic) → Quiescent
Mosaic pattern of woven and lamellar bone
Chalk stick fracture
Increased hat size and lion-like facies
Hearing problems due to nerve impingement
Isolated elevation of alkaline ALP

MODALITIES: XR → NUC / CT

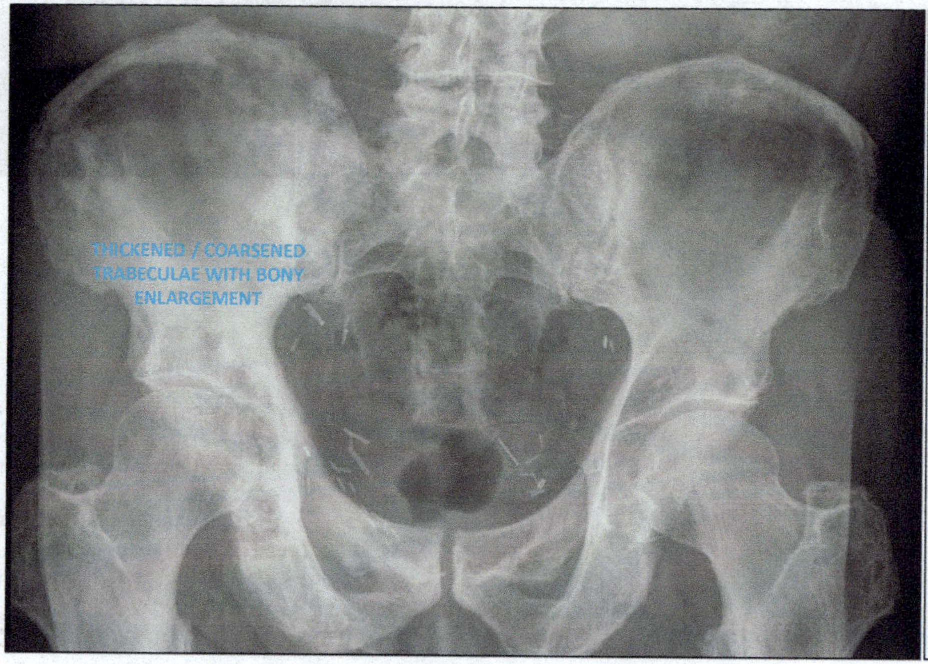

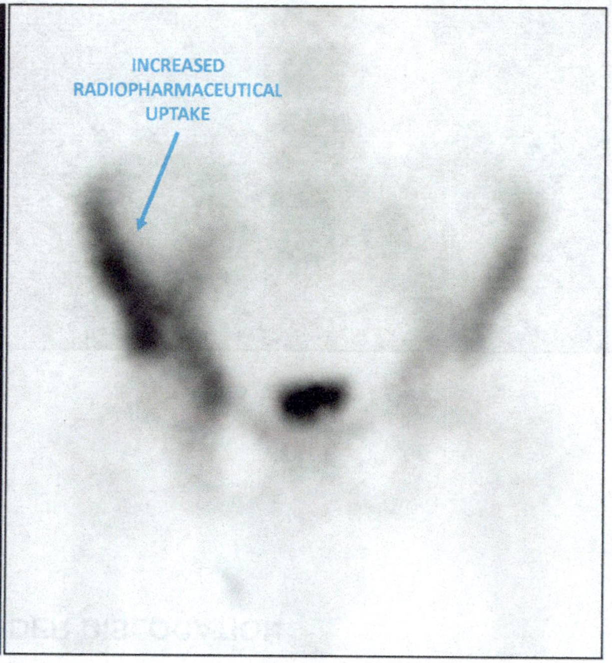

MUSCULOSKELETAL

ANTERIOR SHOULDER DISLOCATION

IMAGING:
Humeral head anterior and inferior to the glenoid
Hill-Sachs Fracture (posterior-super humeral head)
Bankart Fracture (anterior-inferior glenoid)

USMLE POINTS:
Posterior-superior humeral head hits anterior-inferior glenoid
Bankart fracture associated with labral tear → Surgery
May cause damage to **Axillary nerve (C5-C6)**

MODALITIES:
XR → MR W ARTH

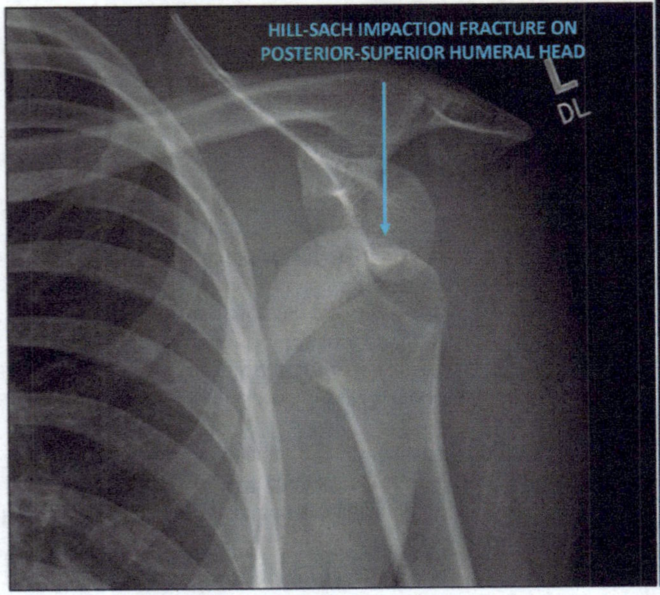

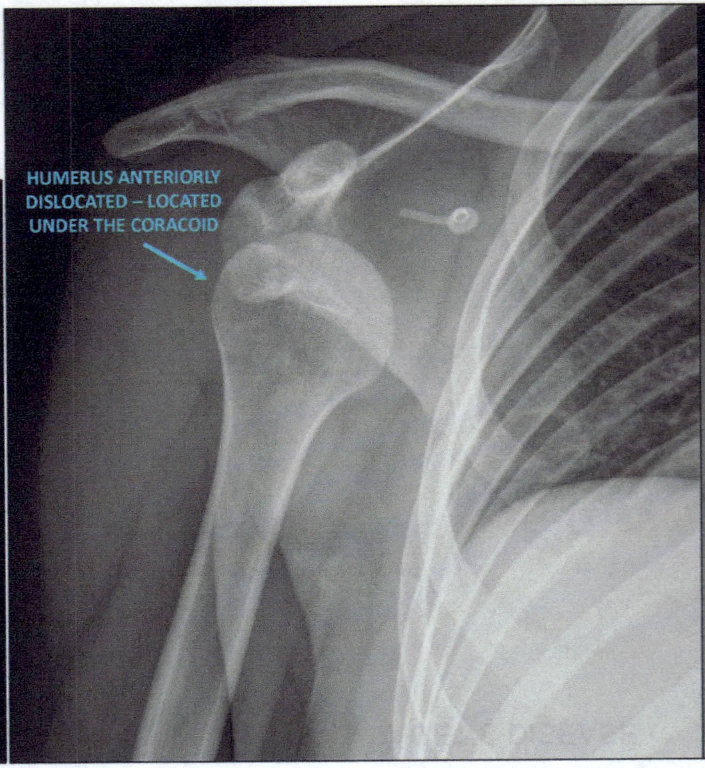

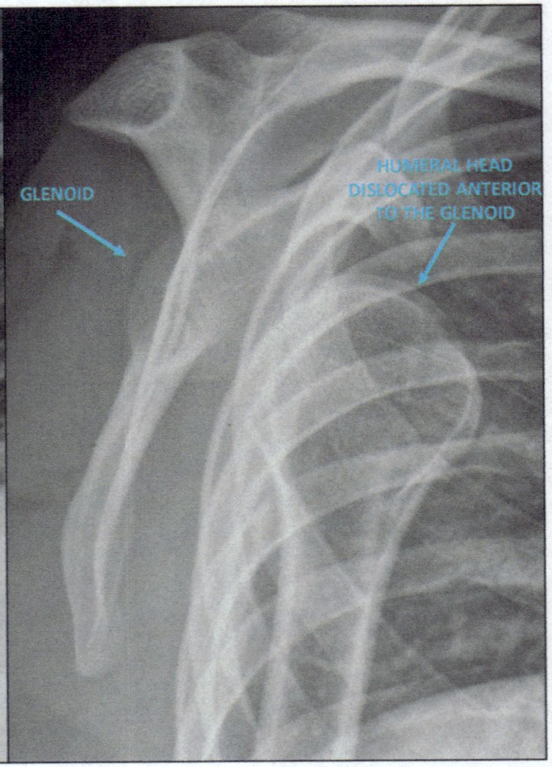

ANTERIOR SHOULDER DISLOCATION

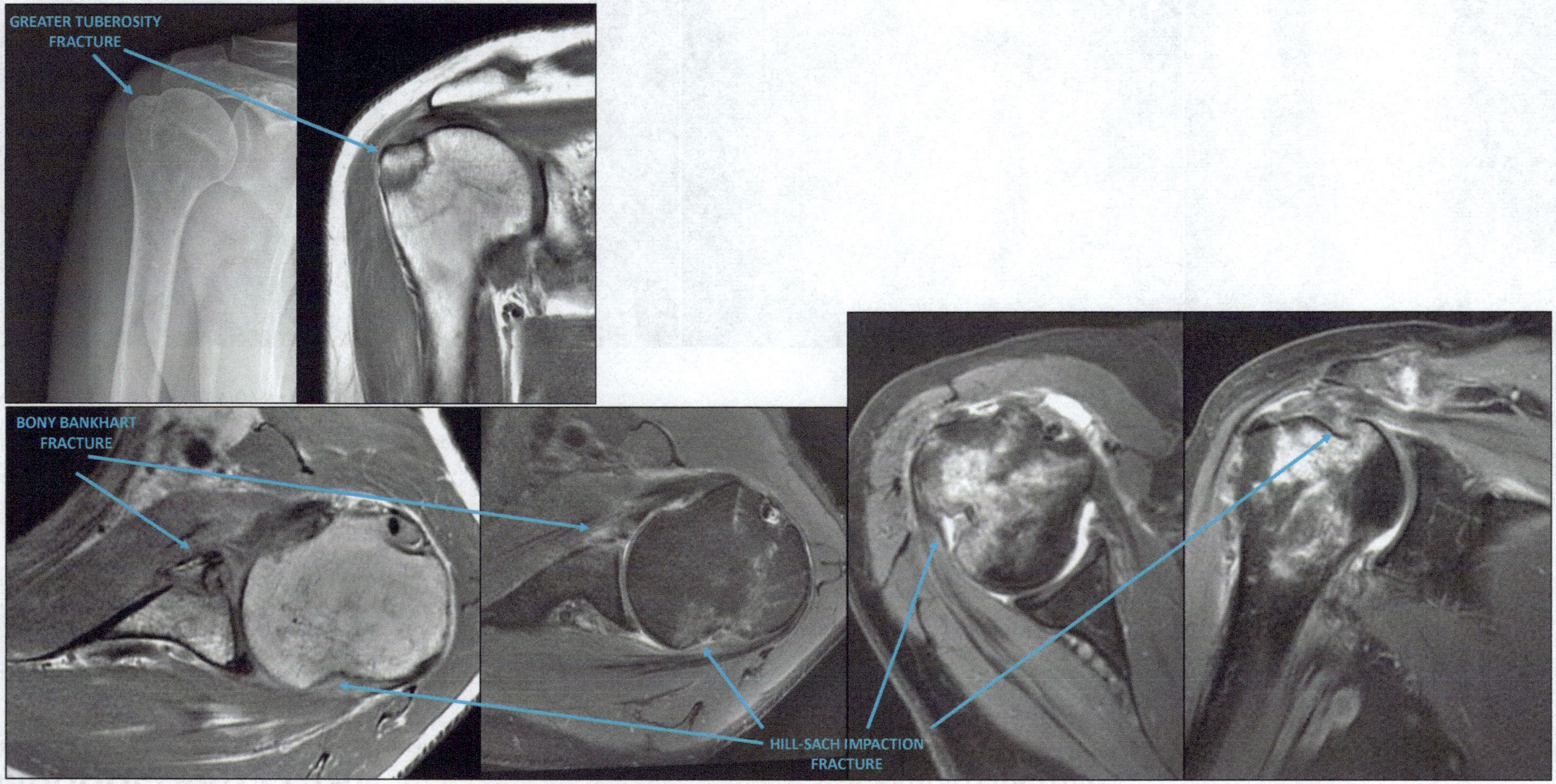

MUSCULOSKELETAL

SCAPHOID FRACTURE

IMAGING: Fracture of **mid-waist most common**
Fractures of the distal pole have worse outcomes due to blood supply

USMLE POINTS: Most commonly fractured hand bone (FOOSH)
Anatomic **snuffbox tenderness**
Proximal scaphoid fracture can result in **avascular necrosis/nonunion due to retrograde blood supply from distal fragment**

Fracture location: **65% scaphoid waist**
25% proximal third
10% distal third

Scapholunate ligament tear: Widening of the SL interval
DISI vs. VISI.
Predisposes to SLAC arthritis

MODALITIES: XR → CT WO / MR WO

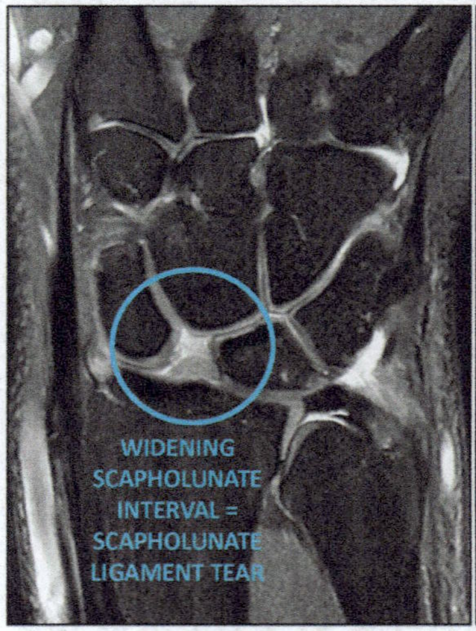

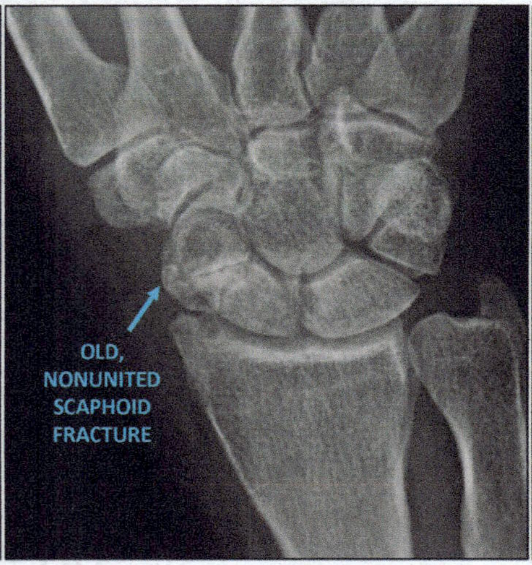

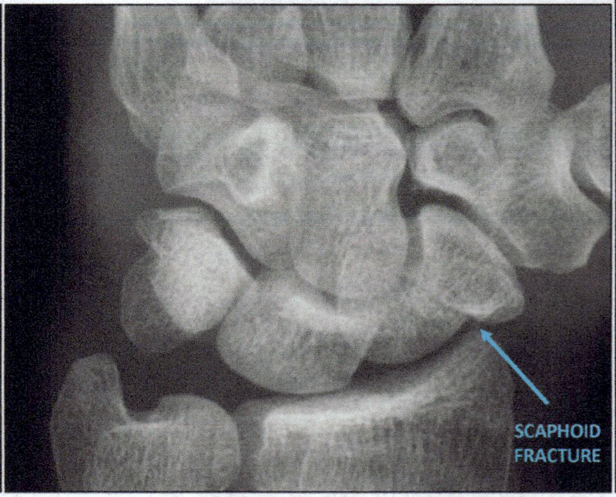

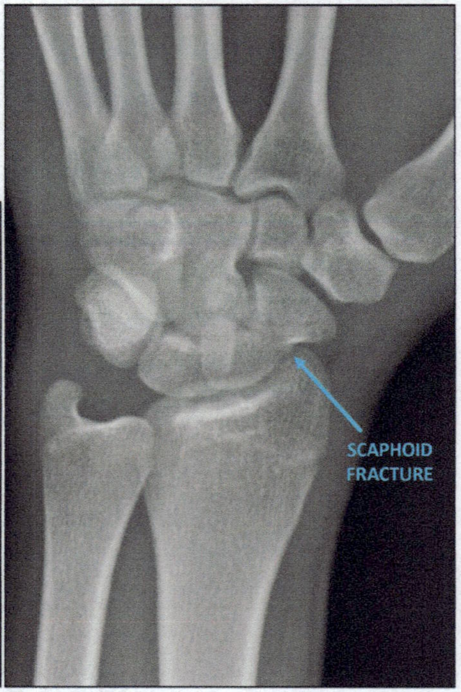

MUSCULOSKELETAL

SEPTIC ARTHRITIS

IMAGING: Joint effusion were severe synovitis and synovial enhancement

USMLE POINTS: Risk factors:
- Increasing age
- Diabetes mellitus
- **Prosthetic joints**
- **IVDA**

Staphylococcus aureus: Most common cause
Streptococci: Second most common cause of nongonococcal arthritis
Neisseria gonorrhoeae: Suspect in healthy and **sexually active patient**

Hematogenous vs. Direction inoculation

Arthrocentesis: **Best initial test for the evaluation**
Synovial fluid culture: **Most accurate test (performed before antibiotic administration)**

MODALITIES: MR WWO

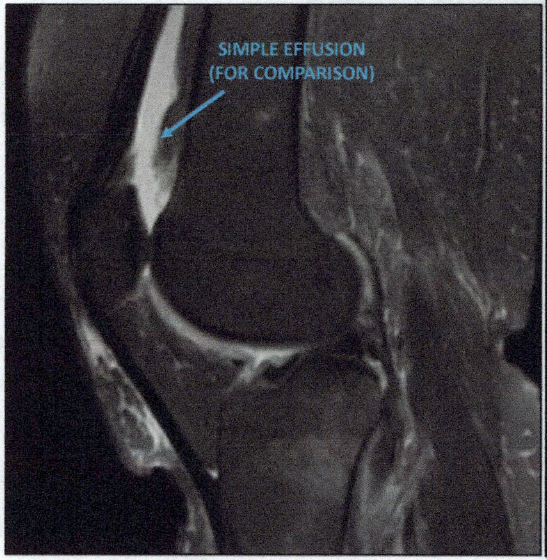

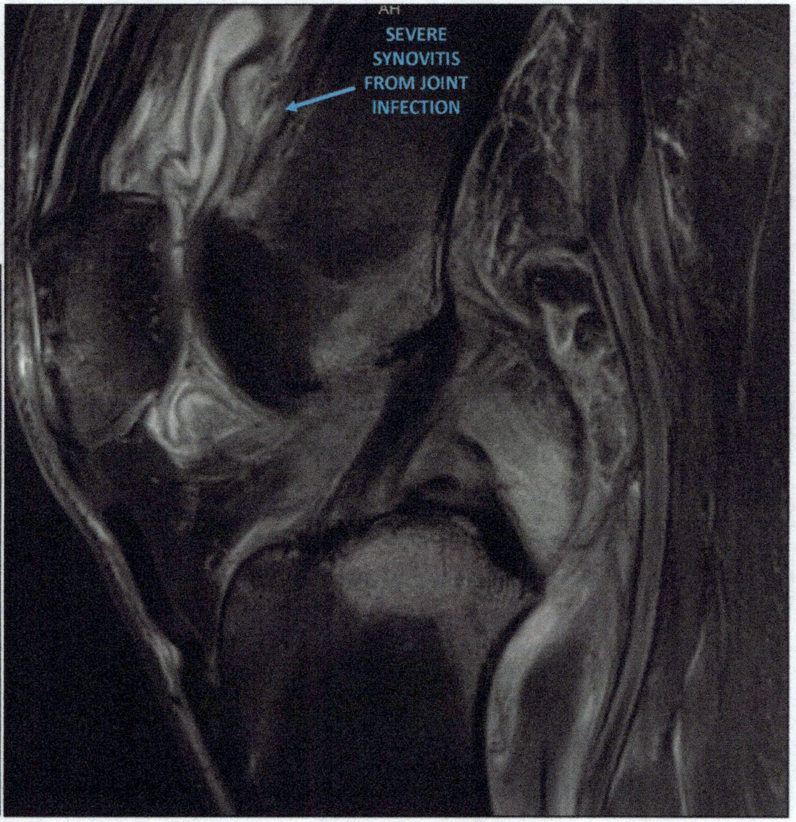

MUSCULOSKELETAL

ANKYLOSING SPONDYLITIS

IMAGING: Diffuse syndesmophytic ankylosis → "Bamboo spine"

USMLE POINTS:
HLA-B27 gene
Involves the spine and **sacroiliac joints**
Young adult males most predisposed
Limited chest wall expansion → Restrictive lung disease
Enthesopathy

Associations:
Psoriatic arthritis
Inflammatory bowel disease
Anterior uveitis
Aortic regurgitation

Treatment: NSAIDs / TNF Inhibitors (Adalimumab, Etanercept)

MODALITIES: XR (gold standard)

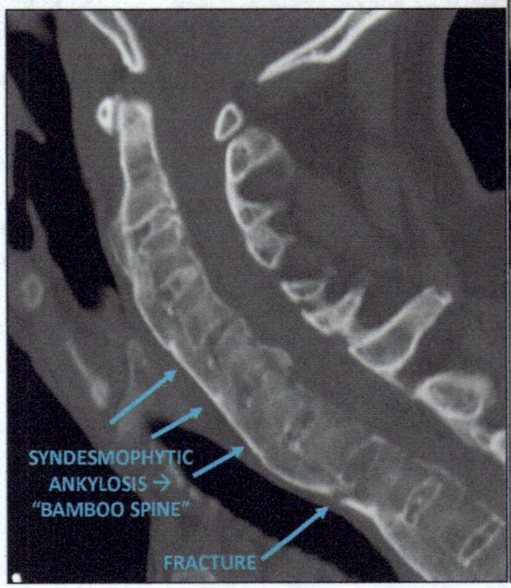

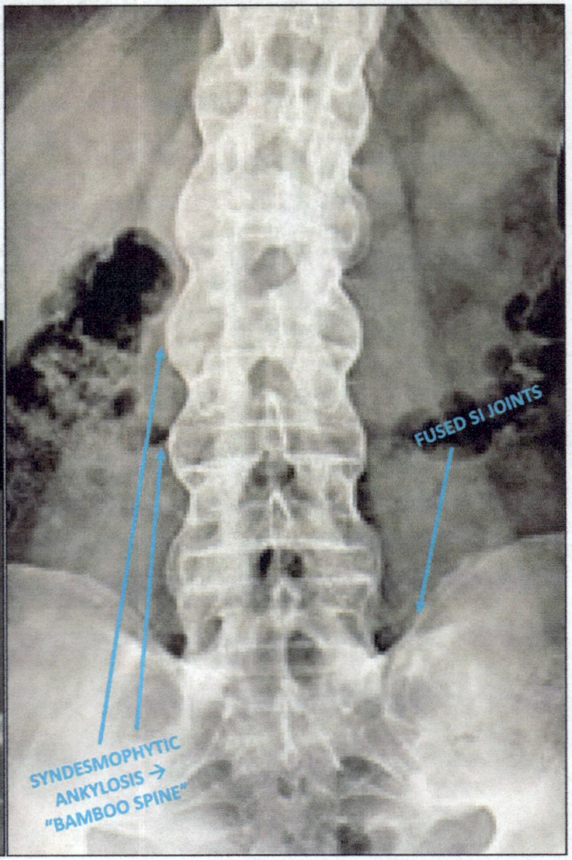

MUSCULOSKELETAL

AVN / BONE INFARCT

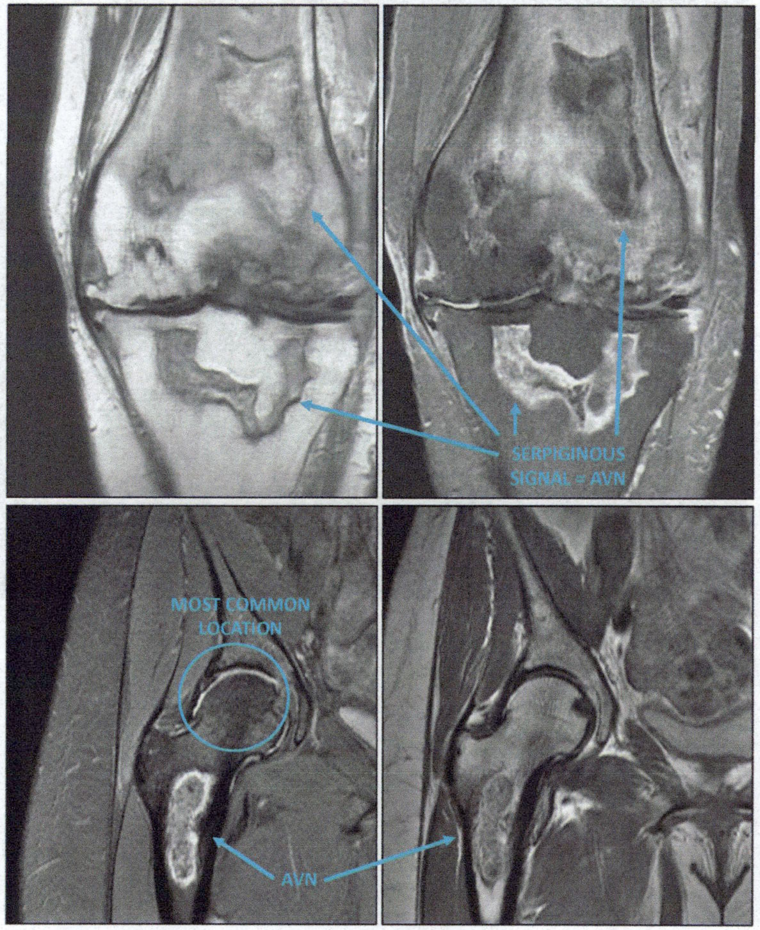

IMAGING: **Serpiginous peripheral low signal due to granulation tissue & sclerosis**
Double-line sign: Hyperintense inner ring of granulation tissue
Hypointense outer ring of sclerosis

USMLE POINTS: Osteonecrosis within metaphysis or diaphysis of bone
Impaired blood supply → Infarction of the bone and bone marrow
Avascular necrosis specifically refers to **subchondral osteonecrosis**
Most commonly affects **hip**
Risk factors:
- Bone fractures
- Joint dislocations
- Alcoholism
- **High-dose corticosteroids or anabolic steroids (SLE / transplant pts)**

Associations:
- SLE
- Gaucher disease
- **Sickle cell anemia**
- Caisson disease

MODALITIES: XR → MRI WO (gold standard)

MUSCULOSKELETAL

CARPAL TUNNEL SYNDROME

IMAGING: Severe synovial noninflammatory fibrosis / thickening within the carpal tunnel (volar) → Compresses median nerve
Enlargement + Increased signal intensity of the median nerve

USMLE POINTS: Entrapment of median nerve between transverse carpal ligament and the carpal bones

Tinel Test: **Percussion over median nerve**
Phalen sign: **Pain during flexion of the wrist**

Median nerve distribution: First 3 digits and radial half of 4th digit

Carpal tunnel contents:
- 4 FDS
- 4 FDP
- 1 FPL
- 1 Median nerve

Surgical release for severe median nerve injury (needle EMG)

MODALITIES: MRI WO

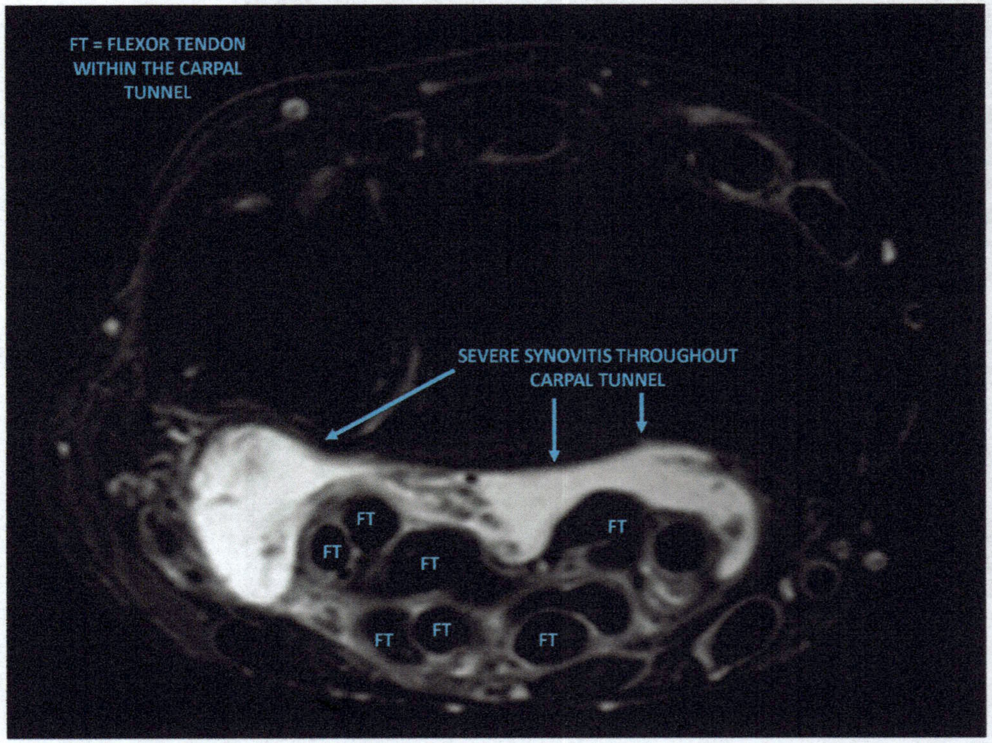

MUSCULOSKELETAL

LUNATE DISLOCATION

IMAGING: Lunate is displaced and rotated volarly
The rest of the carpal bones are in a normal anatomic position in relation to the radius
'Spilled teacup' appearance

USMLE POINTS: Can compress median nerve → acute carpal tunnel syndrome
Fall on an outstretched hand (FOOSH)
MVA → Forceful dorsiflexion of the wrist

MODALITIES: XR → CT WO

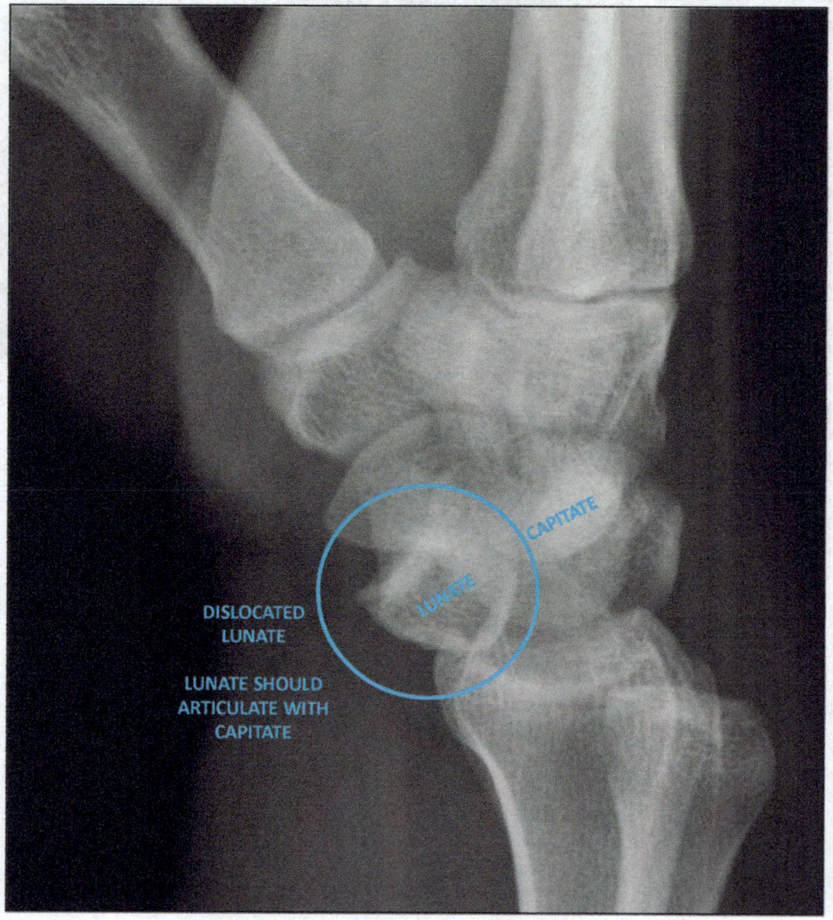

MUSCULOSKELETAL

ACL TEAR

IMAGING: Fiber discontinuity → Grade 1, 2, 3
Lateral contusion pattern

USMLE POINTS: **Pivot-shift mechanism**
Anterior drawer test can diagnose

"Unhappy-Triad": **ACL Tear, MCL sprain, MM tear**

Mucoid: Thickened and ill-defined with a "celery stalk" appearance
Intact fibers are best seen on T2WI.

"Cyclops": **Arthrofibrosis** status-post ACL reconstruction

Lipohemarthrosis: Hemorrhage – Fat level → Must be underlying fracture.

MODALITIES: MRI WO

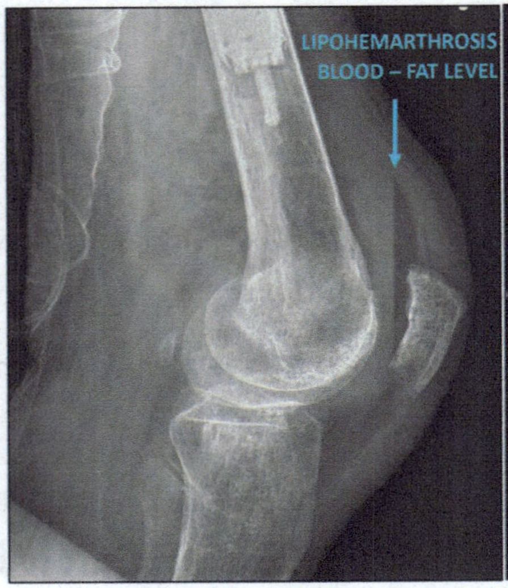

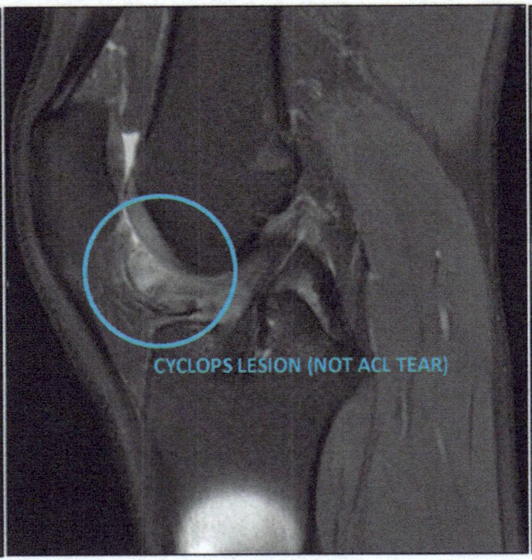

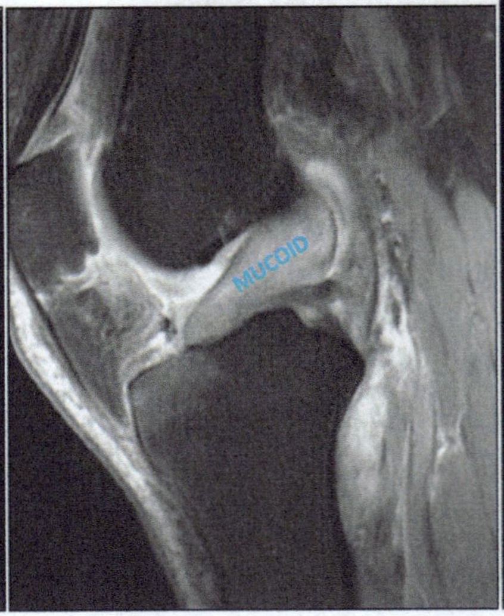

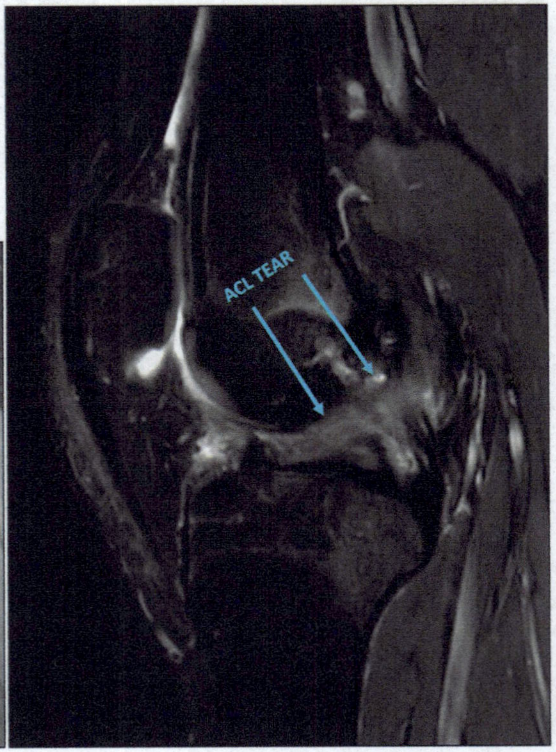

MUSCULOSKELETAL

BAKER'S CYST

IMAGING: Collection of synovial fluid in the **gastrocnemius-semimembranosus bursa**

USMLE POINTS: Posterior knee stiffness with proximal tibial nerve lesions
May form in the setting of chronic degenerative or inflammatory joint disease

MODALITIES: US / MRI WO

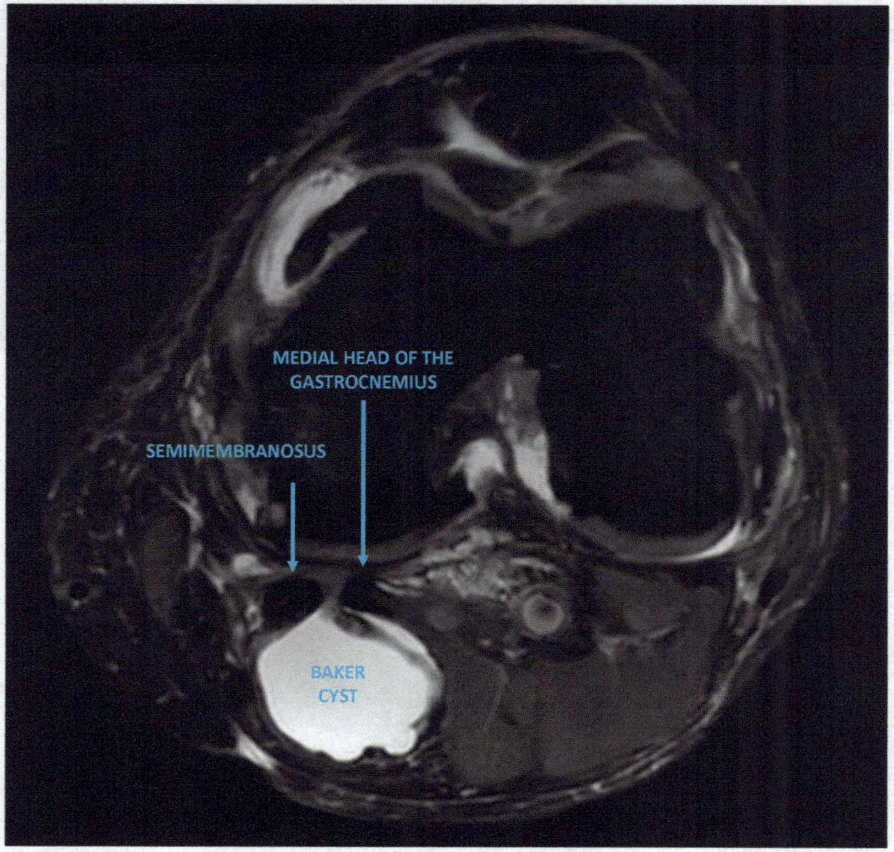

MUSCULOSKELETAL

BICEPS RUPTURE

IMAGING: **Avulsion from radial tuberosity of the proximal radius**

USMLE POINTS:
Extension of a flexed elbow while contracting the biceps
Rupture of biceps at either **superior (BLC / Coracoid) or inferior attachment (radial tuberosity)**
Usually involves long head at proximal origin
Main causes are **injury and overuse**

Presentation: Sudden, sharp pain at elbow or shoulder

Treatment: **Surgical reattachment of tendon to radial tuberosity**

MODALITIES: MRI WO

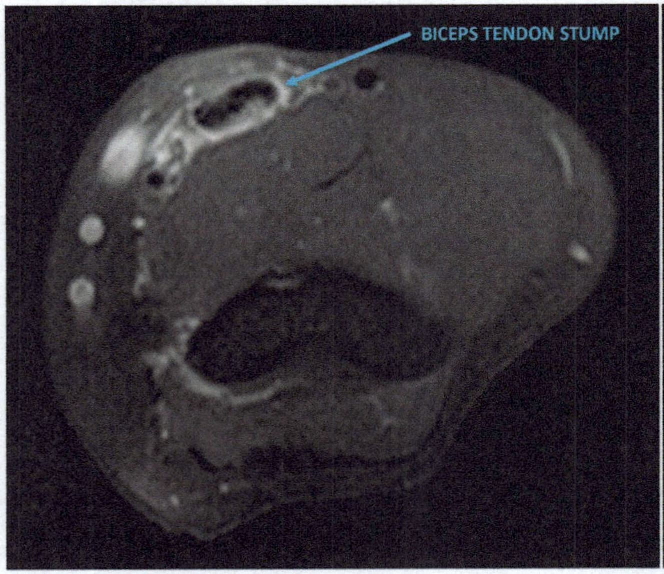

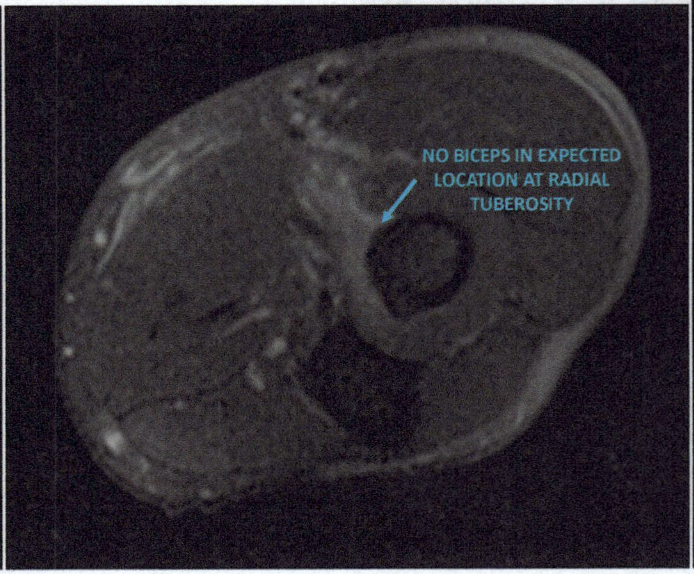

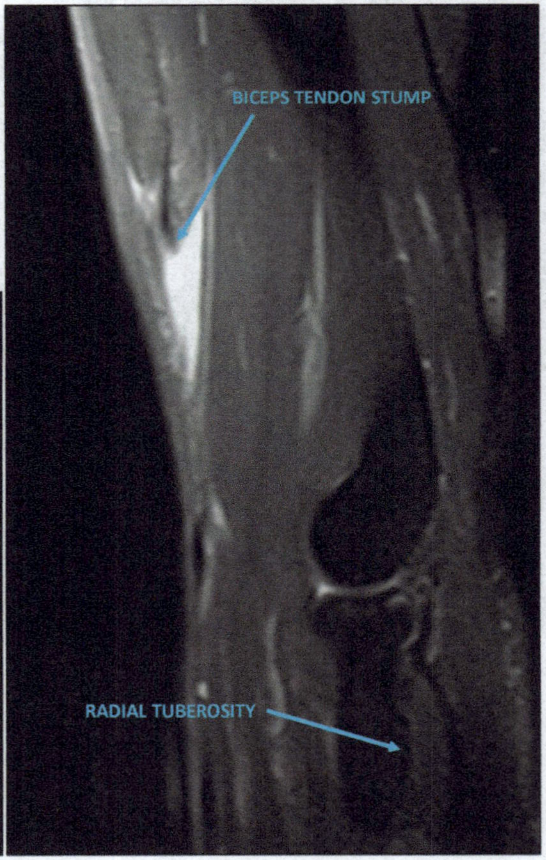

MUSCULOSKELETAL

CALCIFIC TENDONITIS

IMAGING: Hydroxyapatite deposition (calcifications) within the supraspinatus
Globular/amorphous with smooth or ill-defined margins

USMLE POINTS: **Often self limiting**
Usually affects rotator cuff of shoulder (supraspinatus – 80%) in middle-age patients
Due to decreased oxygen tension, leading to fibrocartilaginous metaplasia and secondary mineralization
Treatment: Lavage (aspiration of mineralized component)
NSAIDs

MODALITIES: XR → MRI WO

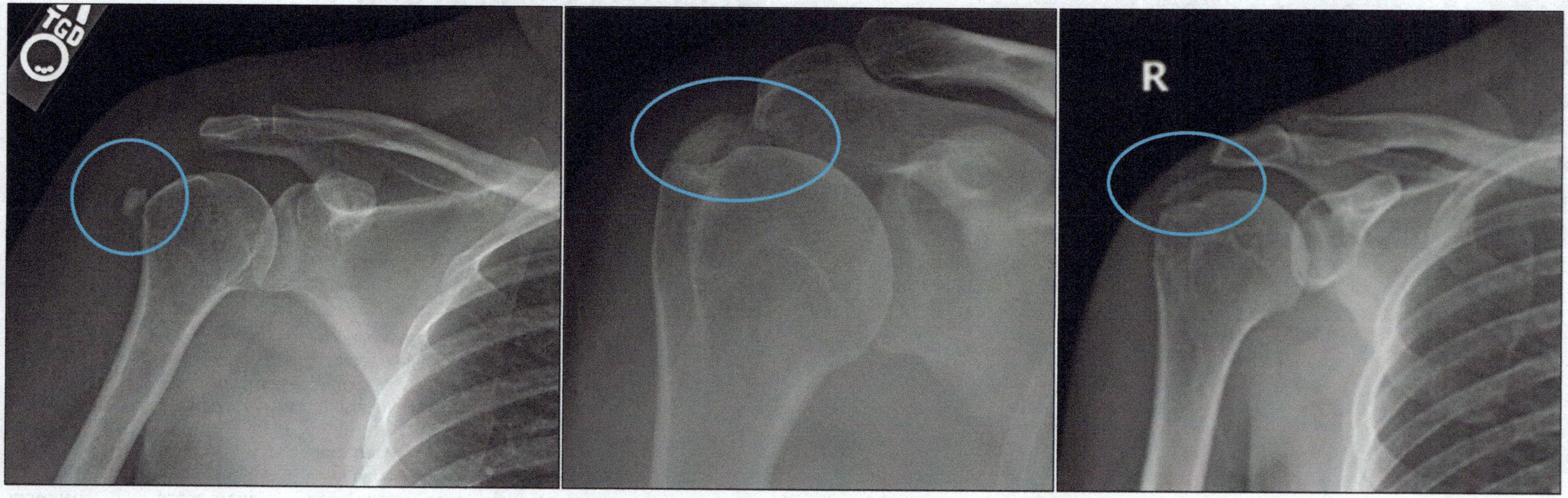

MUSCULOSKELETAL

CHRONIC OSTEOMYELITIS

IMAGING:

Sequestrum:	**Dead, infected bone fragment separates from healthy bone (sequestrum)**
Involucrum:	**Layer of new bone through outside existing bone**
Cloaca:	**Sinus tract**

USMLE POINTS:

Symptoms persists **months - years after infection**

Often no increased WBC

Risk factors: **Diabetes mellitus**

Peripheral vascular disease

MODALITIES: XR → MRI WWO

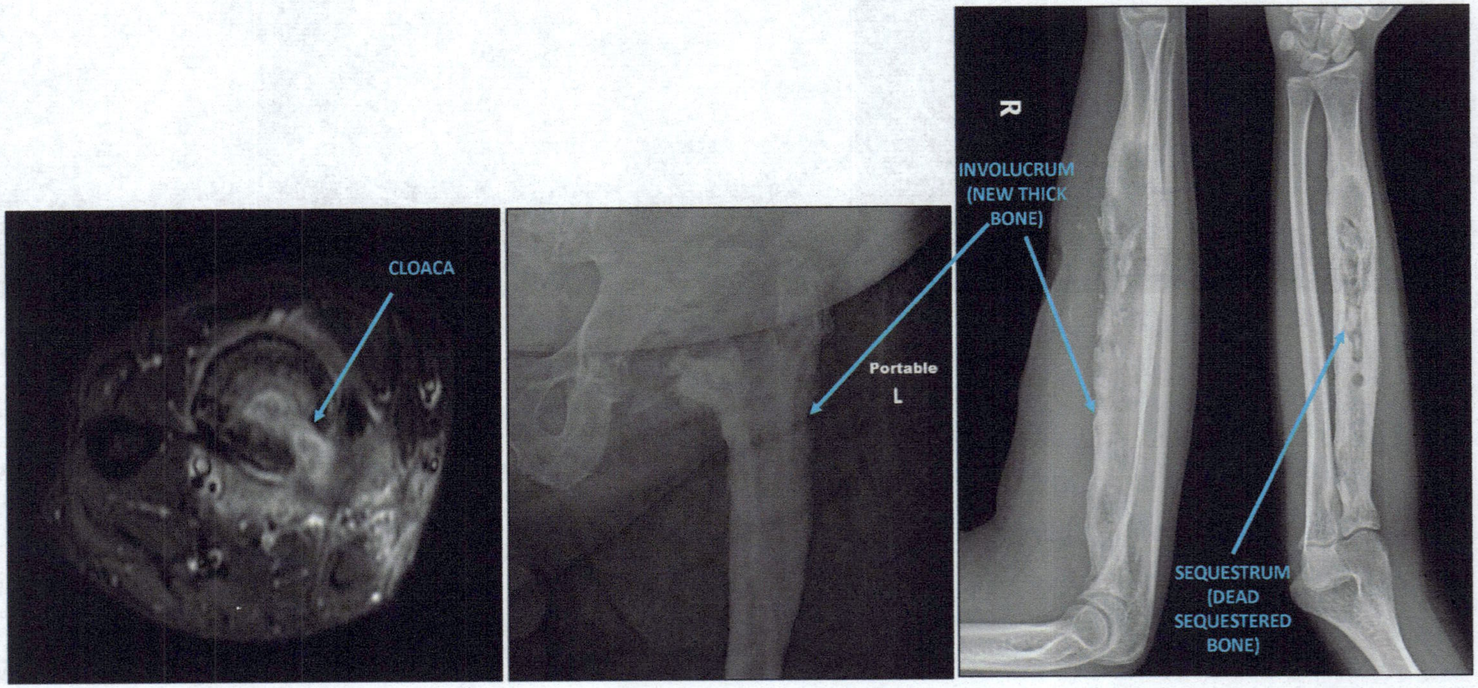

MUSCULOSKELETAL

PSORIATIC ARTHRITIS

IMAGING:

Dactylitis
"Pencil-in-cup" deformity of DIP

USMLE POINTS:

Seronegative spondyloarthritis associated with skin psoriasis
Inflammatory molecules in the psoriatic joint → osteoclast activation → causing **osteolysis**
Hands > Feet
Inflammatory arthritis associated with psoriasis of skin and nail lesions
Negative Rheumatoid Factor

Associations:
- **Psoriasis**
- **Uveitis**
- **Sacroiliitis**
- Insulin resistance
- Hyperlipidemia

Treatment:
- **NSAIDs**
- DMARDS:
  - **MTX**
  - **Sulfasalazine**
  - **TNF alpha inhibitors**
  - Anti-IL agents

MODALITIES: XR → MRI WO

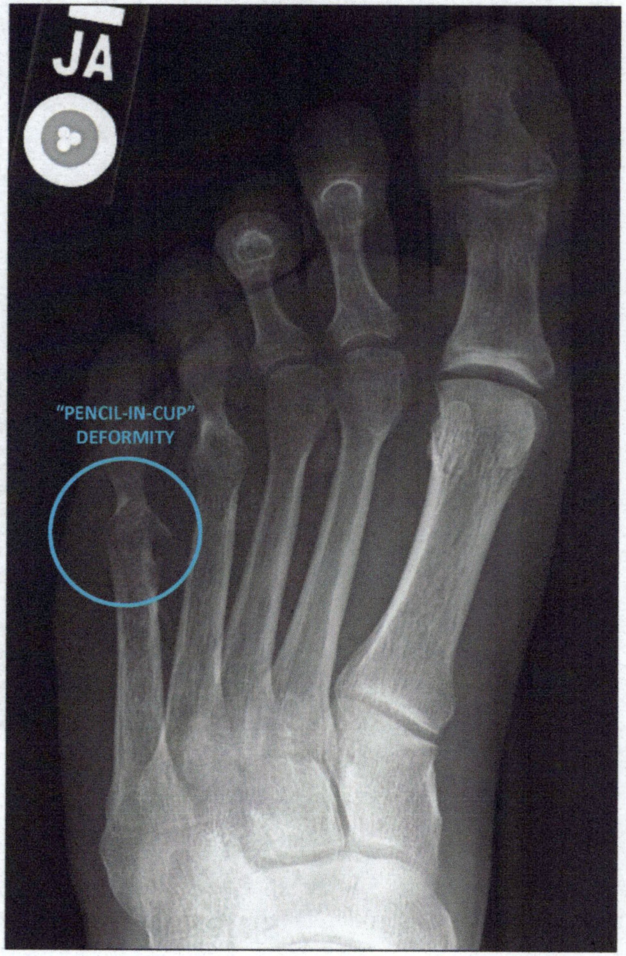

MUSCULOSKELETAL

GREATER TROCHANTERIC BURSITIS

IMAGING: **Bursitis overlying the greater trochanter**

USMLE POINTS: Common cause of lateral hip pain
Gluteus medius (hip abductors)

Presentation: **Lateral hip pain that radiates down thigh**
Tenderness of greater trochanter
Worsens with activity and exercise → Repetitive motions lead to inflammation

Treatment: Conservative / NSAIDs / Corticosteroids

MODALITIES: US / MRI WO

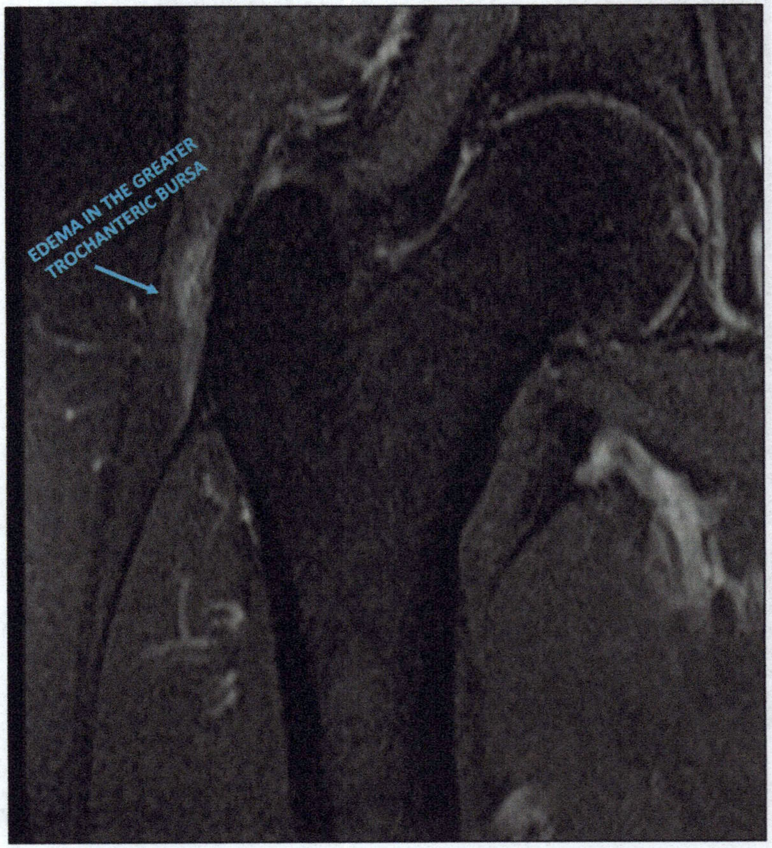

MUSCULOSKELETAL

IT BAND FRICTION SYNDROME

IMAGING: **Edema along the distal IT band (attaches at Gerdy's Tubercle)**
Soft tissues lateral to the lateral femoral condyle

USMLE POINTS: Overuse injury of lateral knee primarily seen in running
Fibrous band originates from the iliac crest to the proximal tibia and provides **lateral knee stability**

Associations: **Runners**
Cyclists
Military personnel

Treatment: Conservative / NSAIDs / Corticosteroids

DDx Pes-anserine bursitis → Medial aspect of the knee (SGT)

MODALITIES: MRI WO

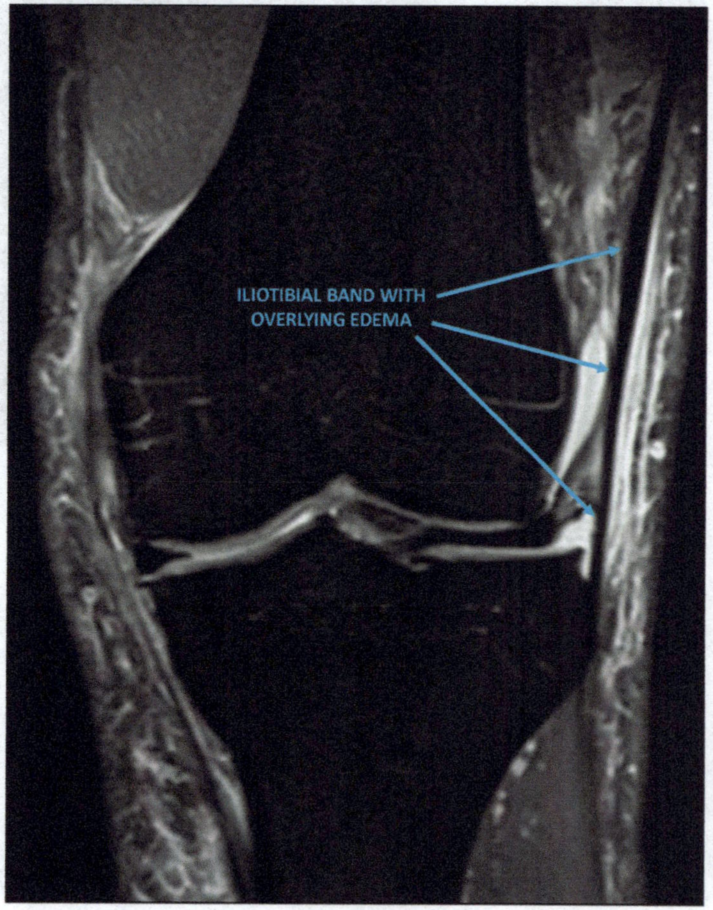

MUSCULOSKELETAL

LIPOSARCOMA

IMAGING:
Aggressive fat signal intensity lesion
Thickened septa
Enhancement
Evidence of local invasion

USMLE POINTS:
Heterogenous class of sarcomas (differentiation towards adipocytes)
Lipomas do not predispose a patient to a liposarcoma
Require resection (wide resection for intermediate and high grade)

MODALITIES: MRI WWO

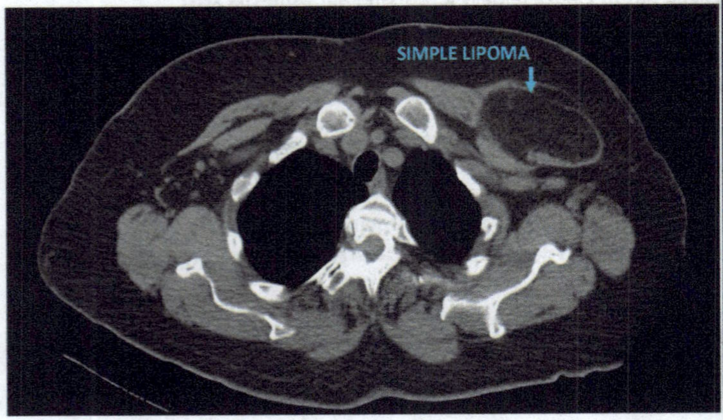

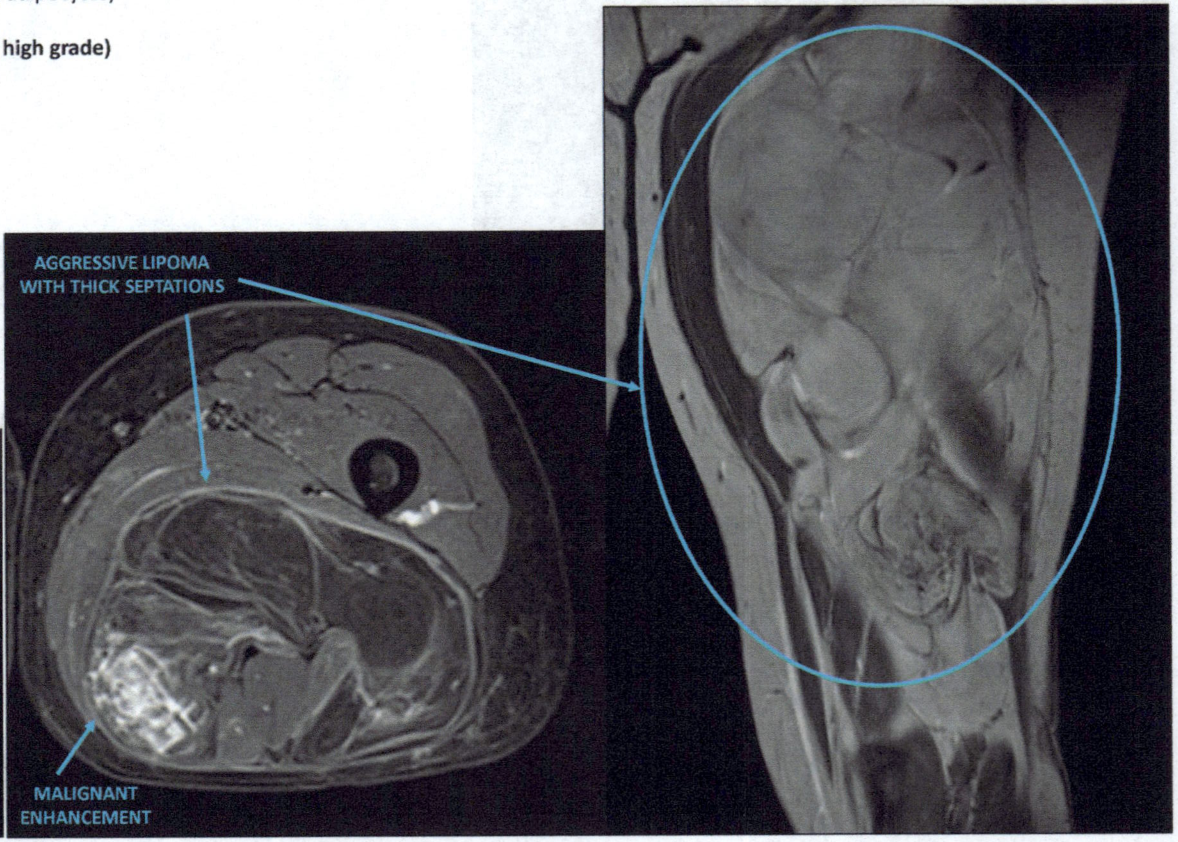

MUSCULOSKELETAL

LISFRANC FRACTURE-DISLOCATION

IMAGING:

Ligament attaching the medial cuneiform to the 2nd metatarsal base
Homolateral, divergent, isolated

USMLE POINTS:

Most common foot dislocation
Integrity is crucial to the stability of the Lisfranc joint
Etiology: Direct crush injury
Indirect load on plantarflexed foot
Commonly seen in football and soccer players

Treatment: Surgery if unstable

MODALITIES:

XR → CT WO / MRI WO

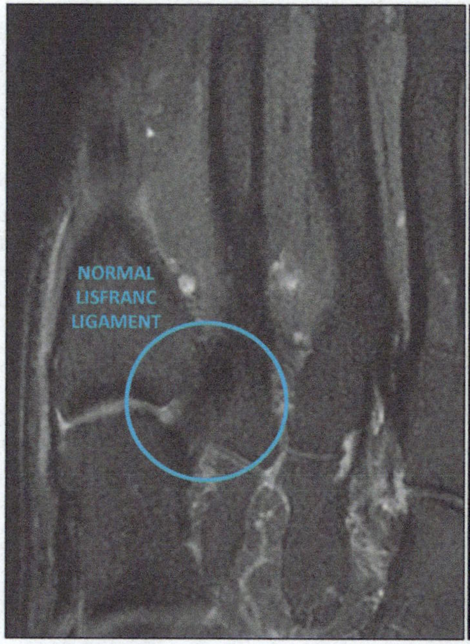

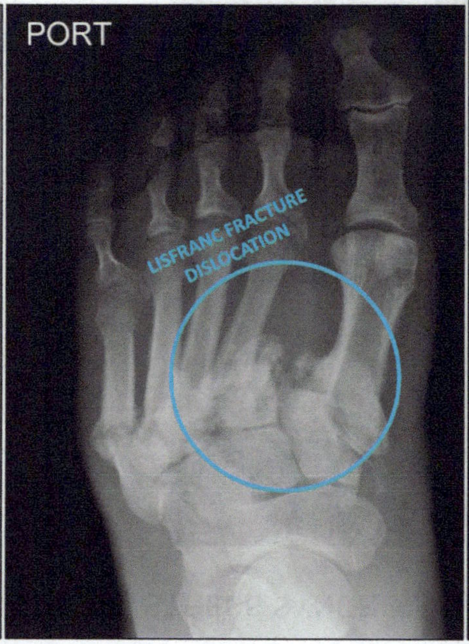

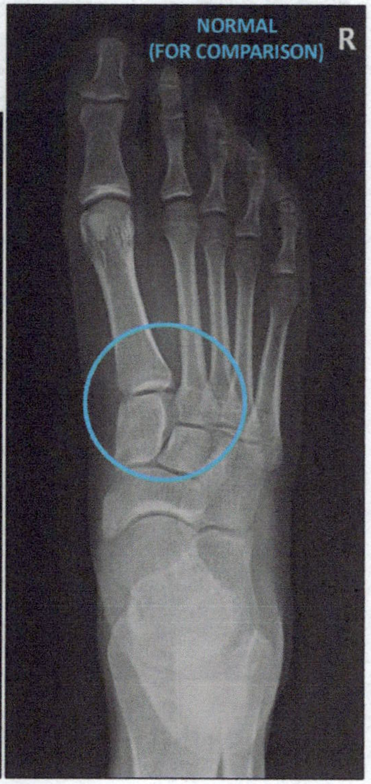

MUSCULOSKELETAL

MEDIAL TIBIAL STRESS SYNDROME (MTSS) – SHIN SPLINTS

IMAGING: **Periosteal edema along the anterior tibia**

USMLE POINTS:
"Shin splints"
Tenderness along posteromedial border of tibia
Common cause of **localized shin pain** and diffuse tenderness
Exercise-induced stress injury
Risk Factors: **Runners**
Military recruits

Results from bone resorption that supercedes bone formation in tibial cortex

"One-leg hop test" → DDx medial tibial stress syndrome (MTSS) from stress fracture
In MTSS, patient can hop on affected leg at least 10 times without severe pain

MODALITIES: XR → MRI WO

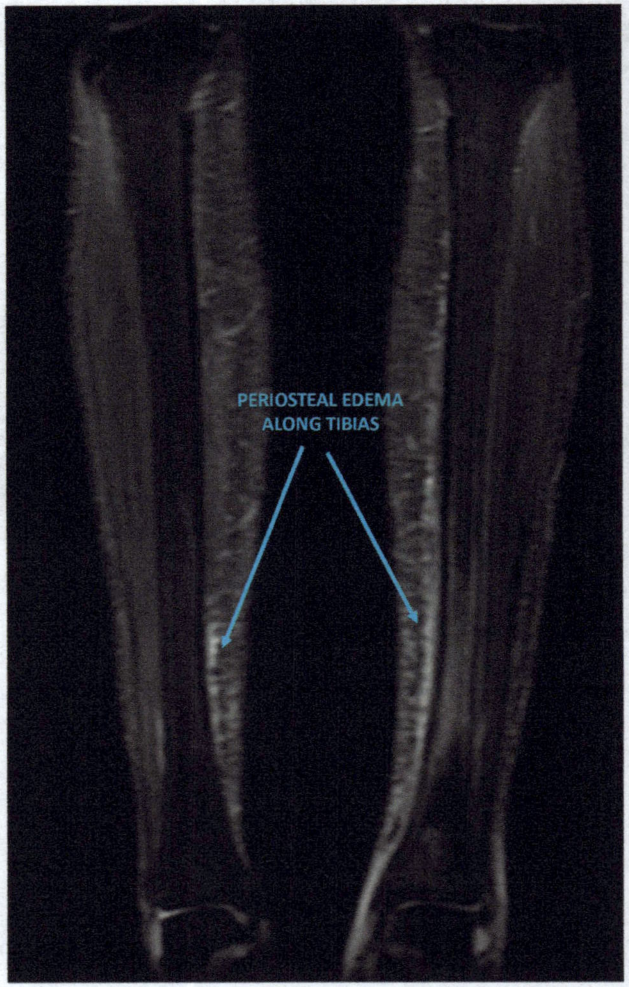

MUSCULOSKELETAL

PERIPHERAL NERVE SHEATH TUMOR

IMAGING:
Fusiform-shaped mass with tapered ends
Nerve seen leading into and out of the mass
Split-fat sign
Denervation changes in muscles supplied by the involved nerve

USMLE POINTS: Etiology: **Schwannoma**
Neurofibroma

Associations: **Charcot-Marie-Tooth** disease most common (peripheral nerves or myelin sheath affected)
Neurofibromatosis type 1 (NF1)

MODALITIES: MRI WWO

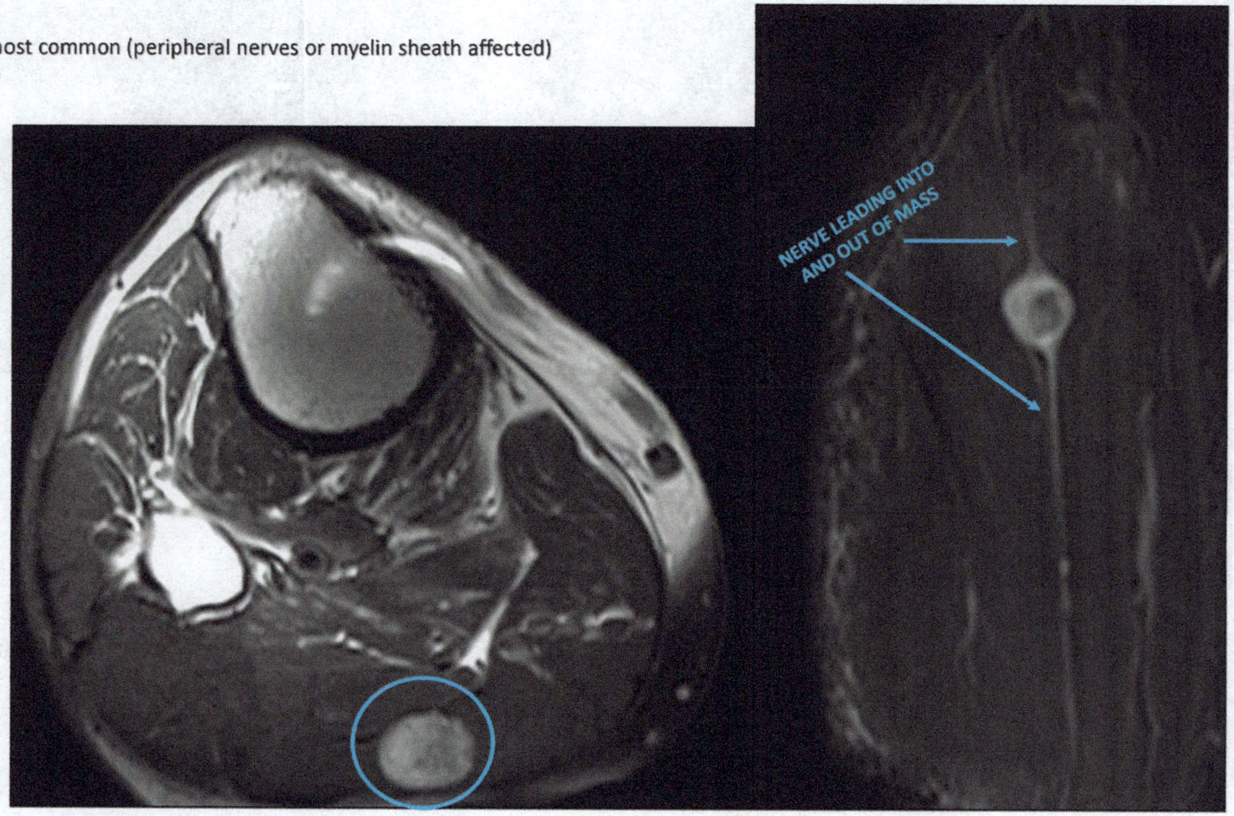

MUSCULOSKELETAL

OSTEOCHONDROMA

IMAGING:
- Bone lesion **points away from the joint**
- **Marrow cavity is contiguous**
- Cartilaginous cap → Malignant transformation
- Sessile (broad base) or pedunculated (narrow stalk) lesions found on the surface of bones

USMLE POINTS:
- Benign tumor with an **overlying cartilage cap**
- **Most common benign tumor of bone**
- Arises as lateral projection of growth plate
- Osseocartilaginous exostosis
- **Hereditary multiple exostosis**

MODALITIES: XR → MRI WO

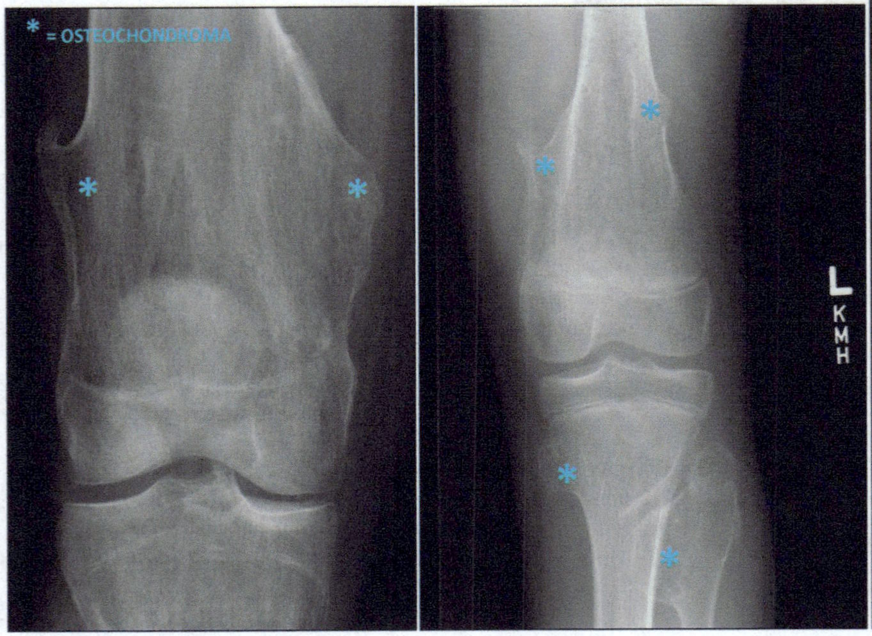

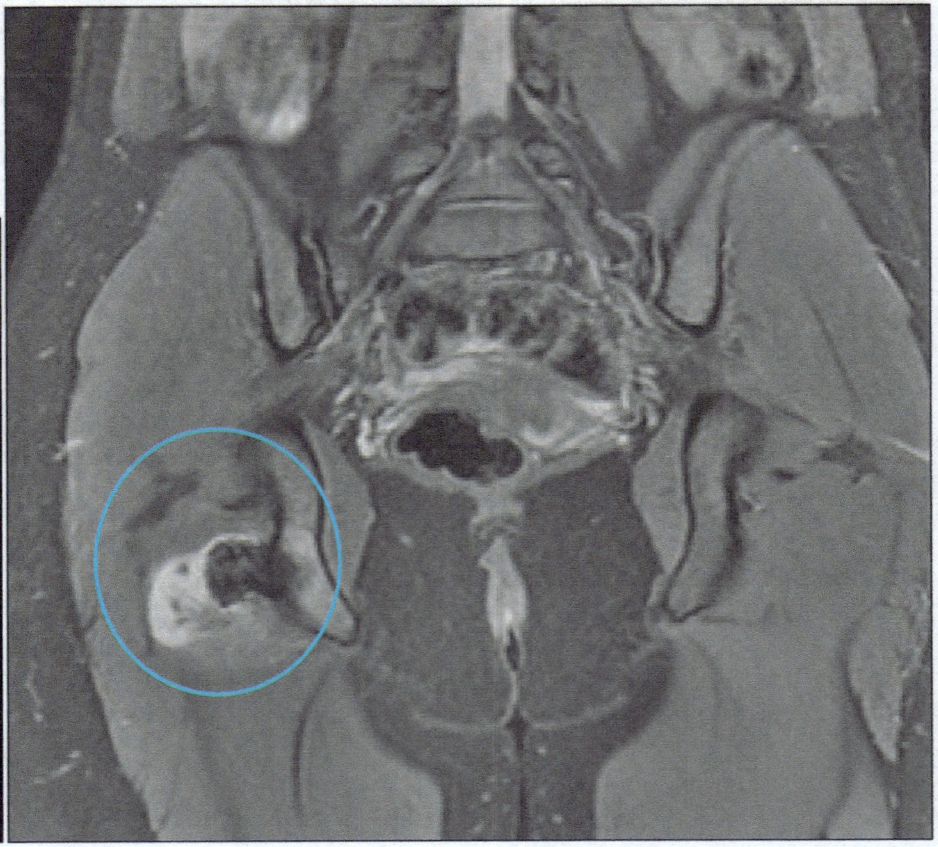

MUSCULOSKELETAL

OSTEOID OSTEOMA

IMAGING: Nidus, representing the neoplastic process.
Focally lucent nidus within surrounding sclerotic reactive bone
A central sclerotic dot may also be seen

USMLE POINTS: **Bone pain that is worse at night and resolve with aspirin**
Painful scoliosis
Benign tumor of osteoblasts surrounded by rim of reactive bone
Cortex of the diaphysis of long bones
Less than < 2 cm with a radiolucent core
Can be ablated with RF ablation

MODALITIES: XR → CT WO

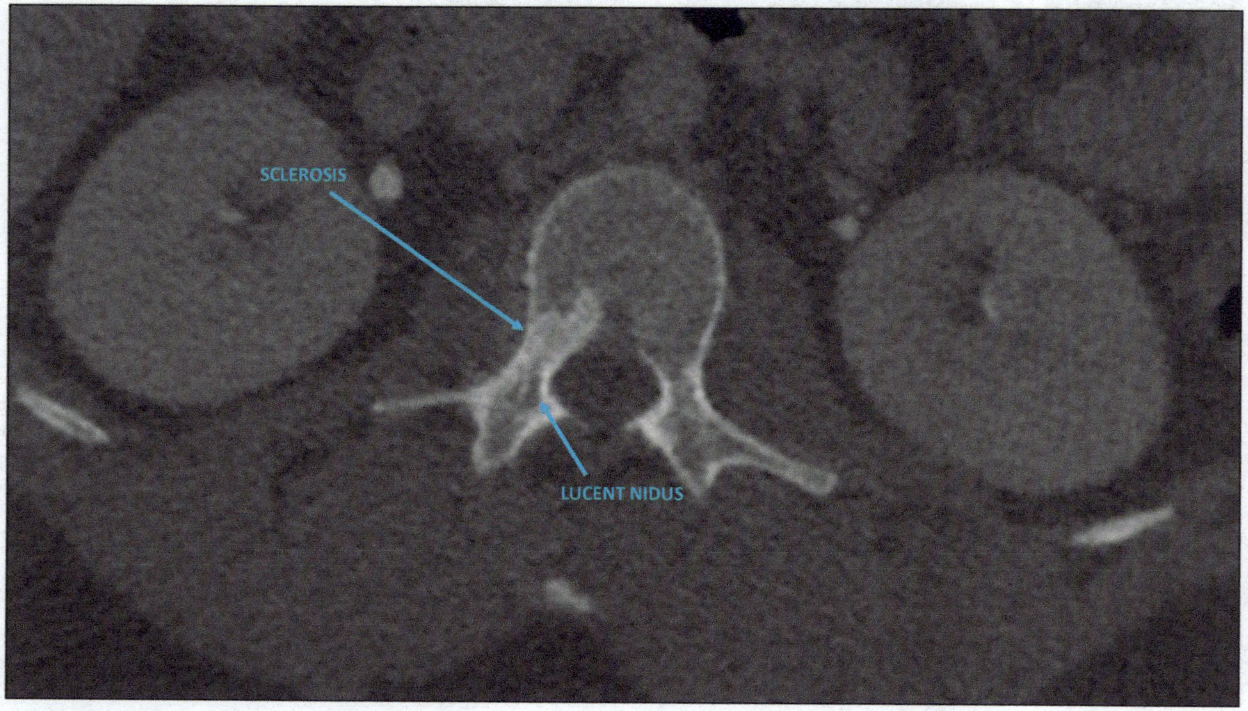

MUSCULOSKELETAL

OSTEOPETROSIS

IMAGING:

Diffuse osseous sclerosis
"Bone-within-bone" appearance
Erlenmeyer flask (under-tubulation)
loss of medullary canal diameter

USMLE POINTS:

Inherited defect in bone resorption **(poor osteoclast function)**
Thick, heavy bone that fractures easily ("Chalk-stick" fracture)
Carbonic anhydrase II mutations → loss of the acidic environment necessary for bone resorption
Hydrocephalus (narrowing of the foramen magnum) → vision/hearing impairment **(cranial nerve impingement)**
Pancytopenia

MODALITIES: XR

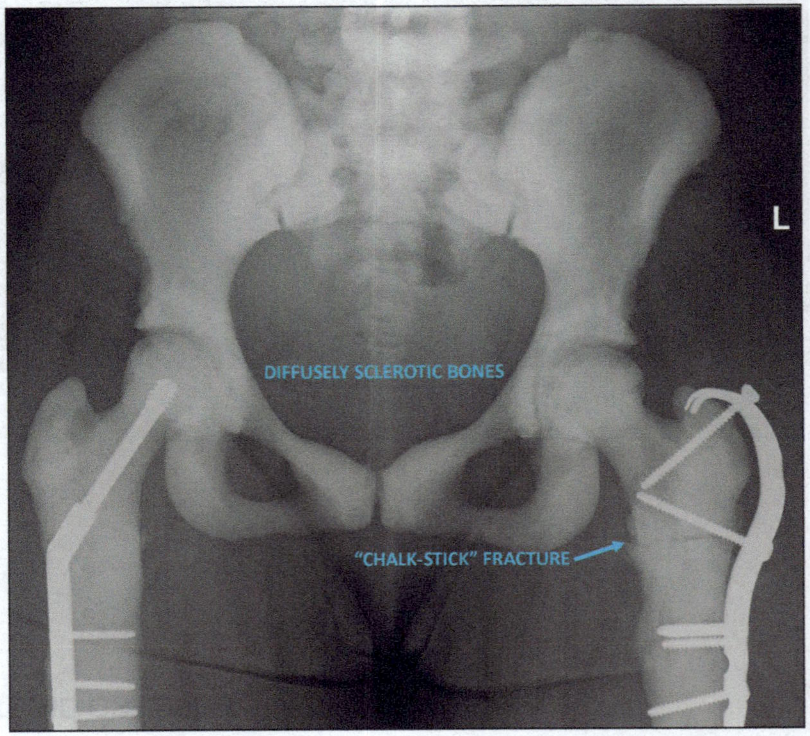

MUSCULOSKELETAL

PLANTAR FASCIITIS

IMAGING: **Plantar fascial thickening → Extends to the calcaneal insertion**
Heel spur, often with edema

USMLE POINTS: **Sharp heel pain → Worse in the morning**
Improves with walking (UNLIKE tarsal tunnel syndrome)
Worse with first step in the morning or after a period of rest

Females & obese patients
Flexor digitorum brevis
Pes planus predisposes

Treatment: Conservative
Stretching
Orthotics
NSAIDs
Corticosteroid injection

MODALITIES: XR → MRI WO

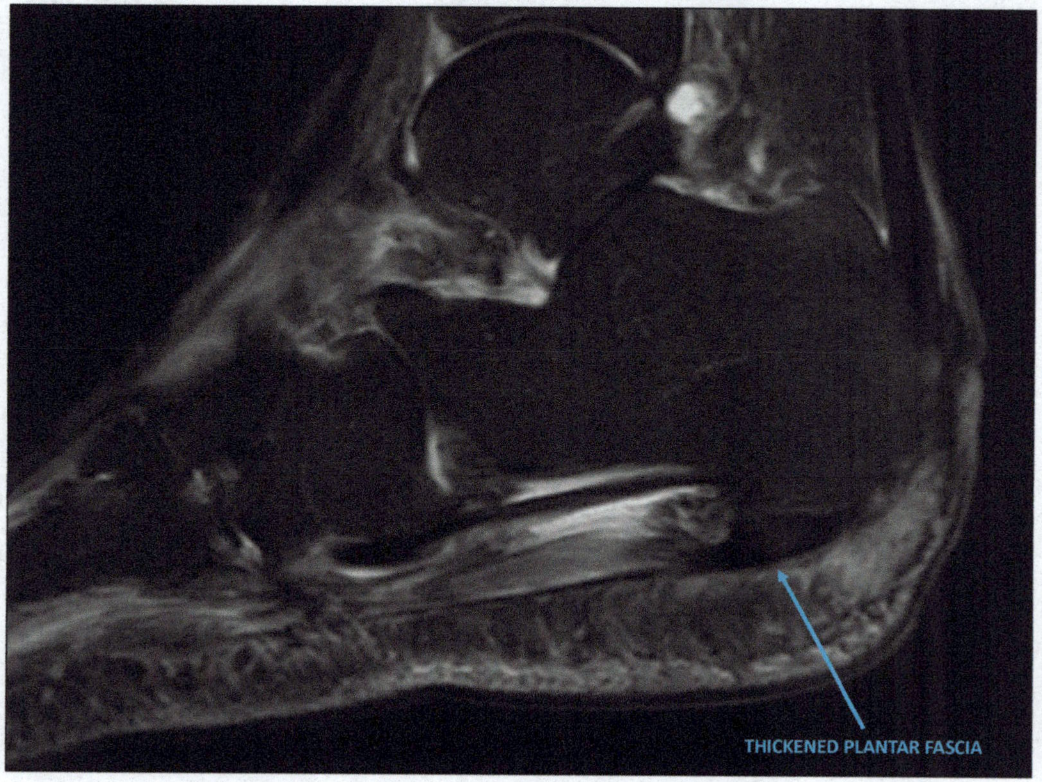

MUSCULOSKELETAL

IMAGING:
Stuck in internal rotation
Look at transcapular Y-View
Overlap between the humeral head and glenoid

USMLE POINTS:
Electrocution / Seizures
Infrequent type of shoulder dislocation (vast majority are anterior-inferior)
Humeral head is posteriorly displaced (relative to glenoid)
Presentation: **Arm is held adducted and stuck in internal rotation**

MODALITIES:
XR → CT WO / MRI W ARTH

POSTERIOR SHOULDER DISLOCATION

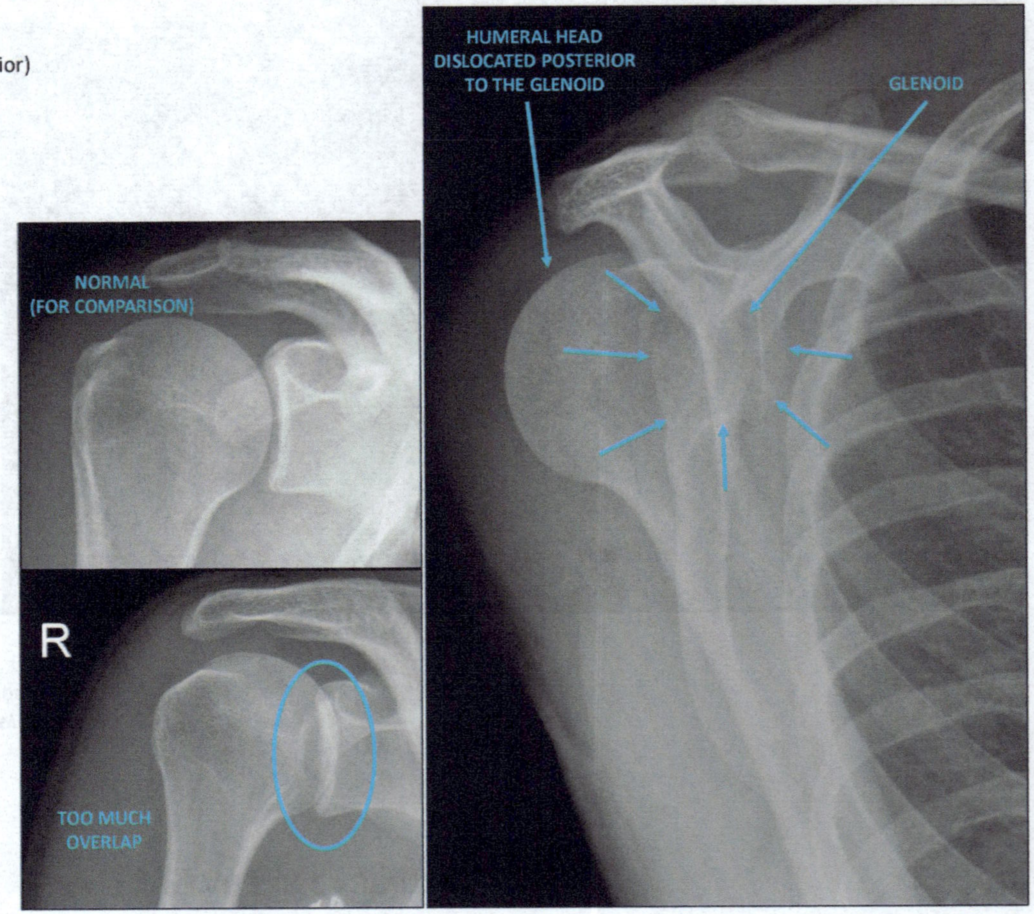

MUSCULOSKELETAL

POSTERIOR HIP DISLOCATION

IMAGING:

Loss of the normal joint congruency between the femoral head and the acetabulum
Radiographic evidence of intra-articular fragments → CT
Femoral head smaller than contralateral side and **superior to acetabulum**
Femur appears adducted

USMLE POINTS:

90% of hip dislocations are posterior
Car accidents → Knee hits dashboard (axial loading on adducted femur)
Injury to the **sciatic nerve and inferior gluteal nerve**
Developmental dysplasia of the hip →Abnormal acetabulum development in newborns

Physical exam: Hip will be **adducted, flexed, and internally rotated**

MODALITIES:

XR → CT WO

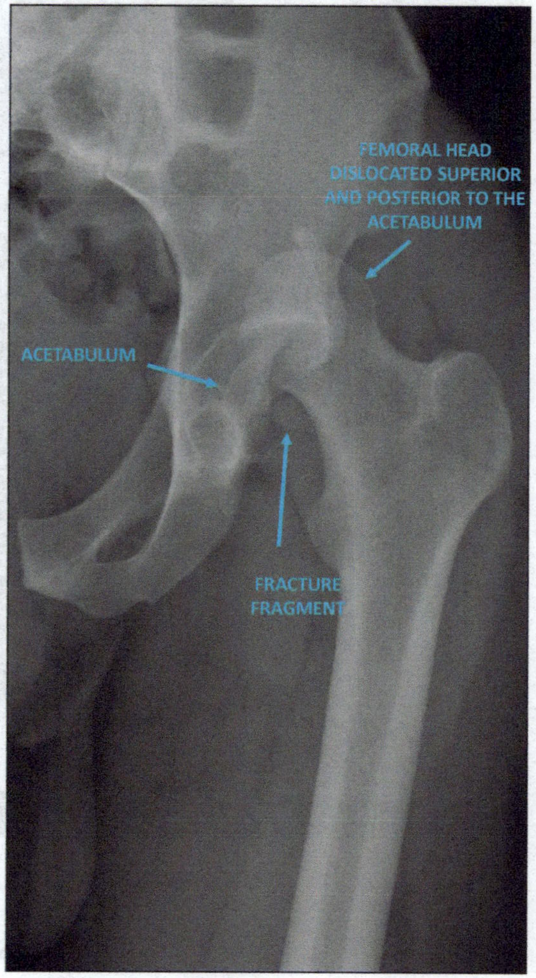

MUSCULOSKELETAL

PREPATELLAR BURSITIS

IMAGING: **Increased fluid/edema and synovitis within the pre-patellar bursa**

USMLE POINTS: Repeated trauma or pressure from excessive kneeling
Anterior knee pain and swelling

Associations: **Repeated trauma/pressure from excessive kneeling**
Manual laborers
'Housemaid's knee"

MODALITIES: US → MRI WO

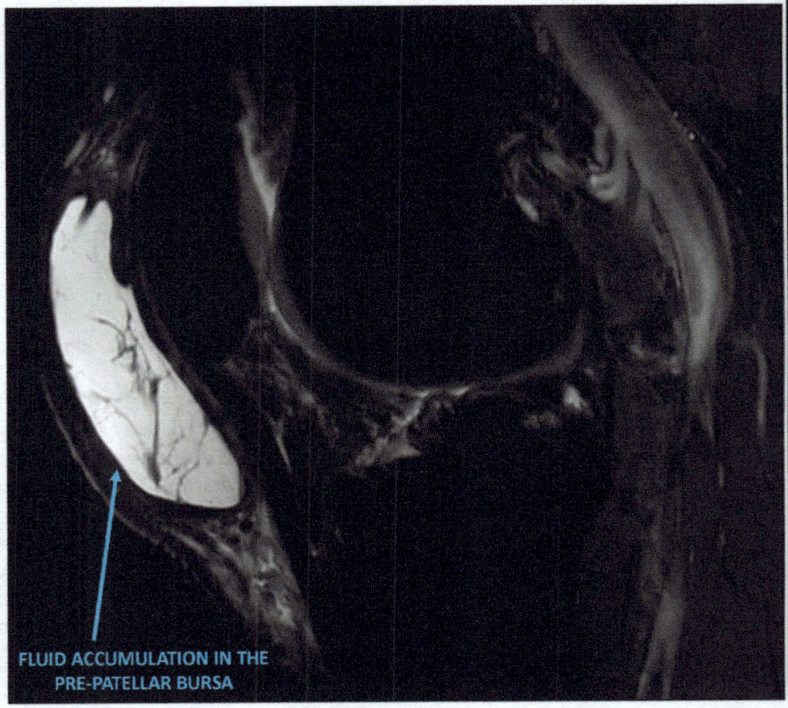

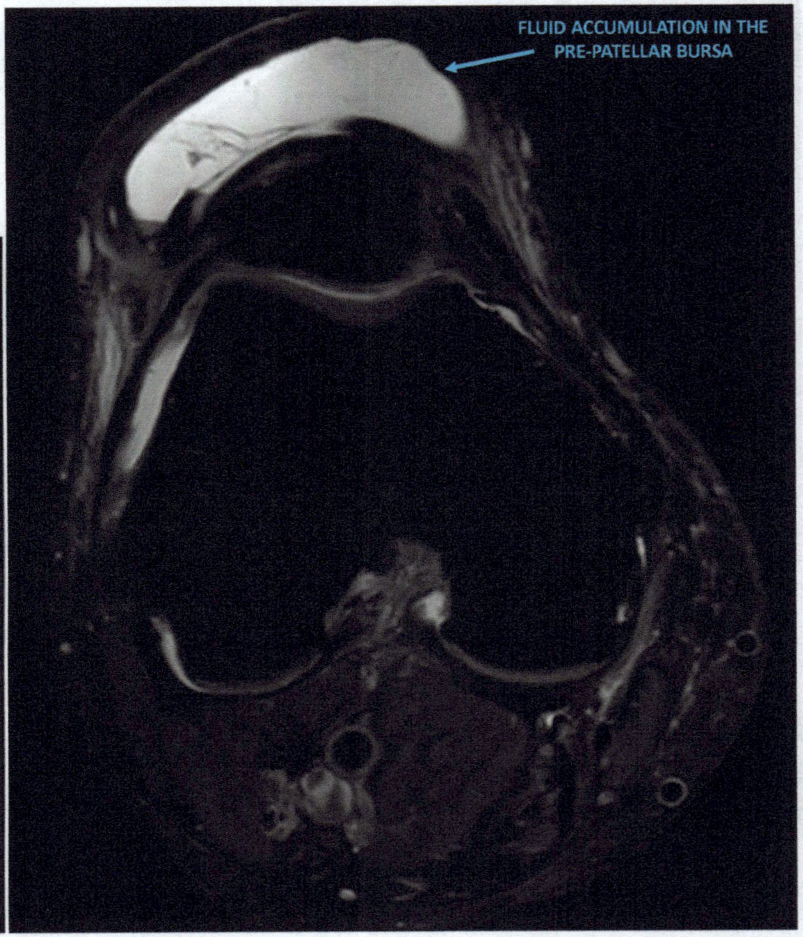

MUSCULOSKELETAL

INTRAMUSCULAR ABSCESS

IMAGING:
Low attenuation organized collections within muscle
May have associated subcutaneous abscess
Overlying skin thickening + subcutaneous induration

USMLE POINTS:
IVDA
Inflammation and collection of pus within muscle
Commonly occurs at site of IM / IV injections
Staph aureus or Streptococcus
Treatment: **Incision & drainage**

MODALITIES: CT W

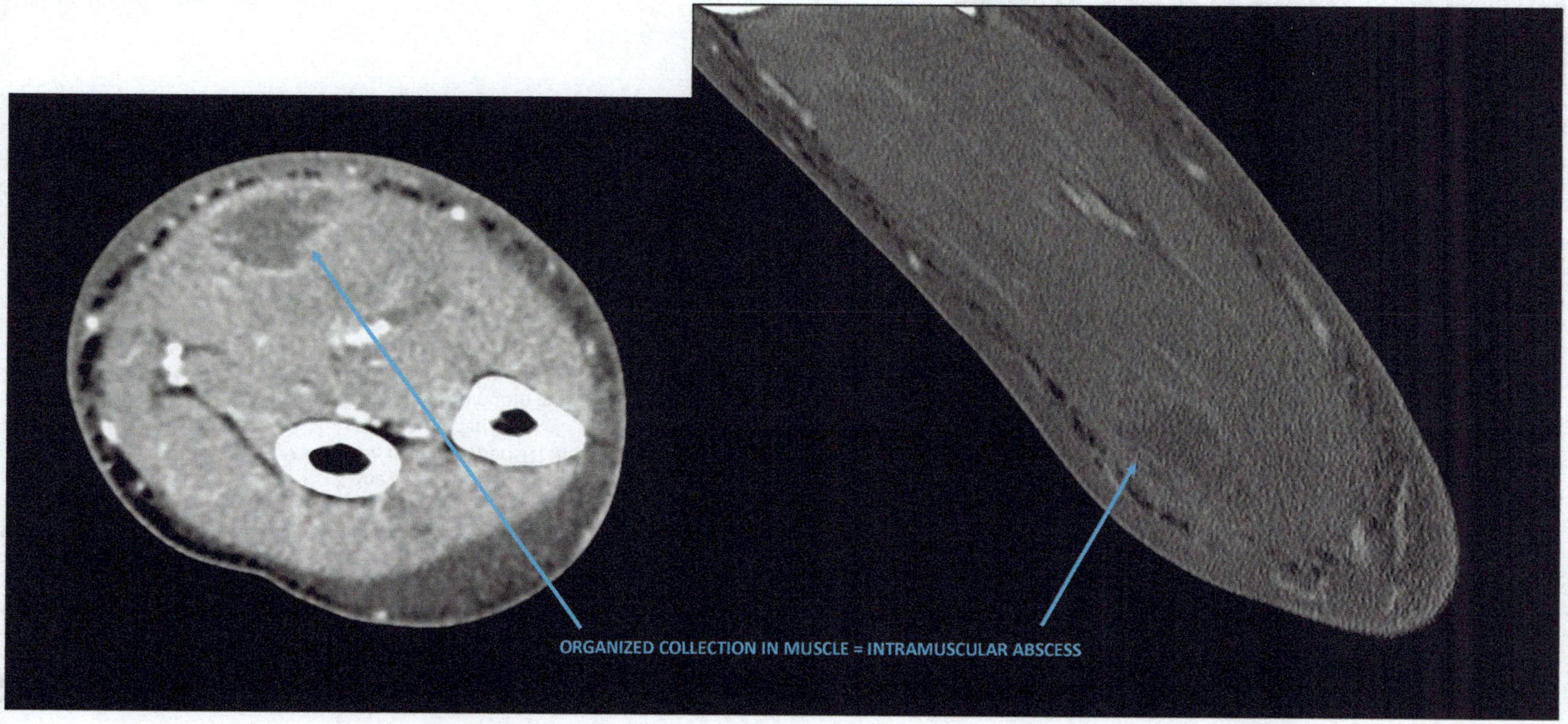

MUSCULOSKELETAL

RENAL OSTEODYSTROPHY

IMAGING: Diffuse osseous sclerosis.
"Rugger-jersey" spine: alternating sclerotic-lucent-sclerotic appearance

USMLE POINTS: **From secondary hyperparathyroidism**
Decreased renal function → Increased phosphate → Decreased calcium → Increased PTH → Bone resorption

Hypercalcemia →	**Stones**	→	Kidney stones
	Bones	→	Bone pain in HyperPTH (bone resorption)
	Groans	→	Lethargy and fatigue
	Moans	→	Constipation (smooth muscle dysfunction)
	Thrones	→	Polyuria and polydipsia
	Psych overtones	→	Confusion, depression, anxiety

MODALITIES: XR / CT WO

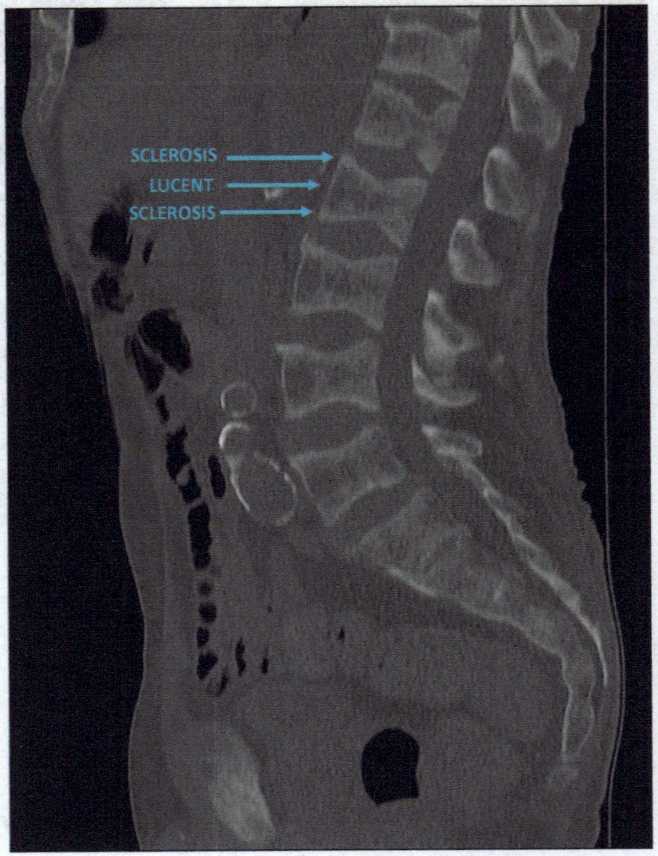

MUSCULOSKELETAL

SICKLE CELL ANEMIA

IMAGING:
Bone infarcts
H-shaped vertebrae
Ground-glass opacities from air-trapping/hypoventilation (Painful inspiration)
Dactylitis

USMLE POINTS:
HbS: Point mutation of ß-globin gene → substitutes valine for glutamic acid (normal Hb has 2 α-globins and 2 ß-globins)
Autosomal recessive

Sickle cell trait:
Resistance to malaria
Papillary necrosis (painless hematuria)

Vaso-occlusive crises:
Obstruction of microcirculation by sickled red blood cells
Bone infarcts (medullary cavities and epiphyses) and subperiosteal hemorrhages
skeletal pain and growth disturbances

MI, CVA, Priapism, Splenic infarct (auto splenectomy)

Infections:
Encapsulated organisms: Strep pneumonia (sepsis / meningitis)
Neisseria meningitidis
Haemophilus type-b
Salmonella (osteomyelitis)

Moya-Moya:
Non-inflammatory, non-atherosclerotic progressive vasculo-occlusive
Involves the terminal supraclinoid internal carotid arteries and circle of Willis
"Puff of Smoke" on Angiogram
Internal carotid artery narrowing which can lead to stroke and development of collateral vessels

Treatment:
Folate, Pneumococcal vaccine, penicillin until 5 years old, transfusion
Hydroxyurea (increases fetal Hb)

MODALITIES:
XR → CT WO
Moyamoya (angiogram)

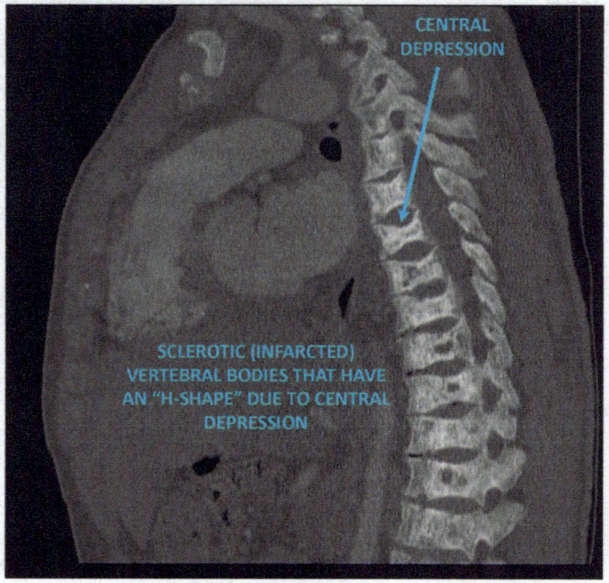

MUSCULOSKELETAL

SICKLE CELL ANEMIA

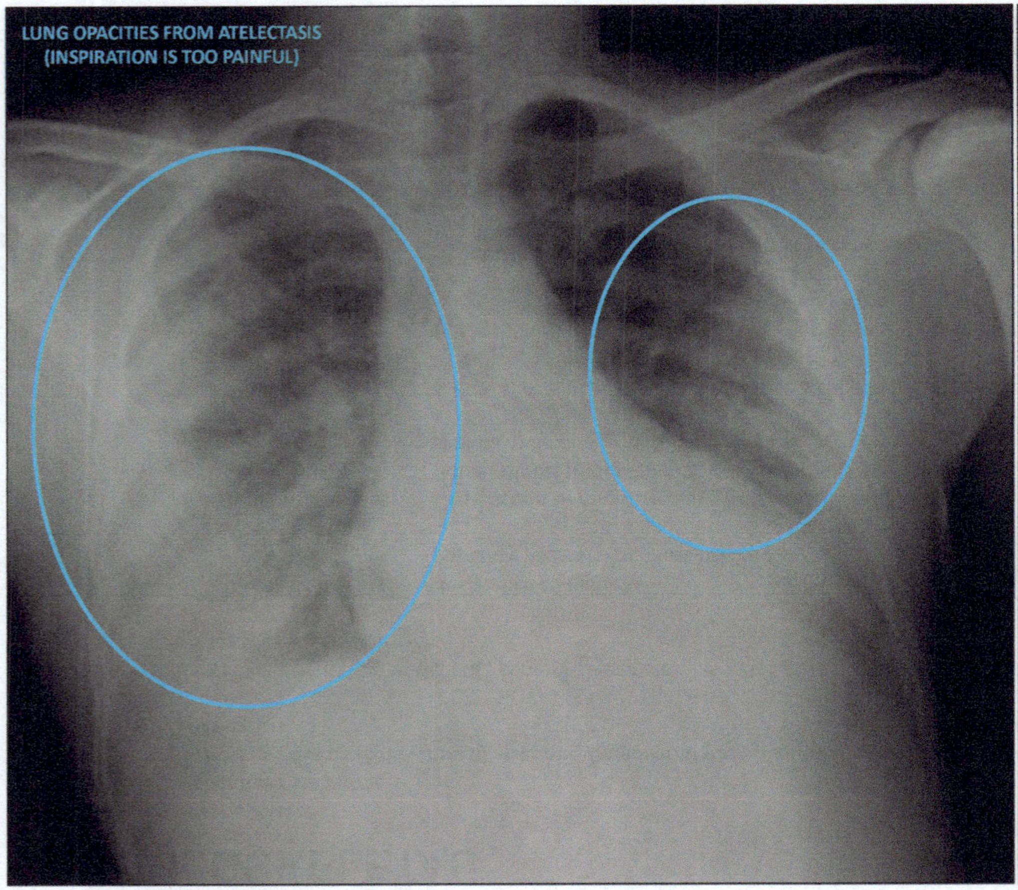

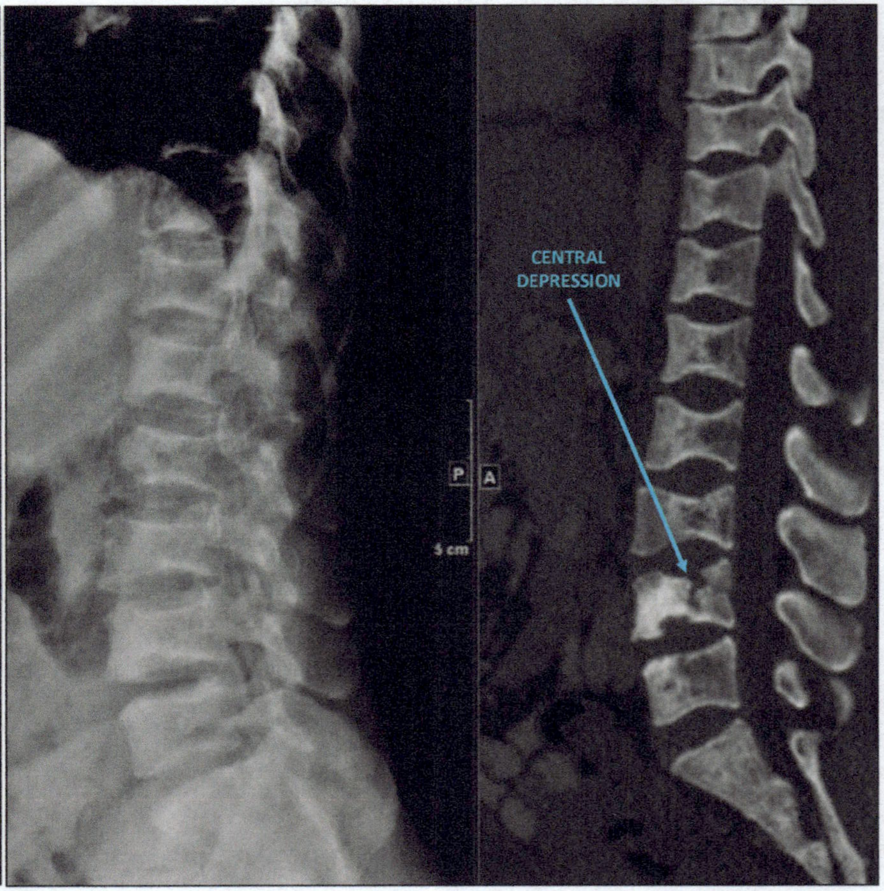

MUSCULOSKELETAL

IMAGING:

Occurs only with **a closed growth plate**
Abuts articular surface
Well-defined with **non-sclerotic margin**
"Soap bubble" appearance

USMLE POINTS:

AKA Osteoclastoma
Multinucleated giant cells and stromal cells that express RANKL
Affects young adults
Epiphysis of long bones (Distal radius, distal femur, or proximal tibia)
Locally aggressive benign tumor

Treatment: Curettage
Marginal excision + bone grafting

MODALITIES:

XR → MRI WO

GIANT CELL TUMOR

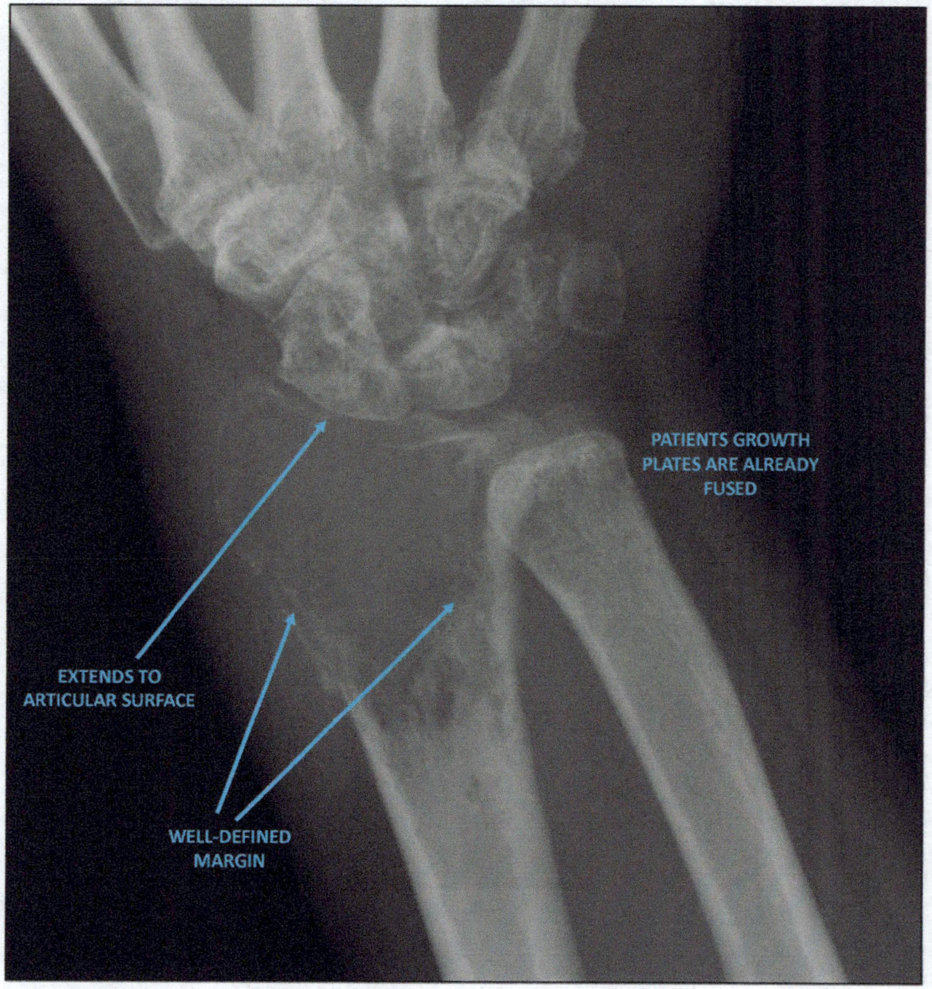

MUSCULOSKELETAL

ACROMEGALY

IMAGING: **Calvarial thickening (inner table), frontal bossing, enlarged paranasal sinuses (especially frontal sinuses)**
"Spade" appearance of distal phalanx tufts

USMLE POINTS: Results from growth hormone excess in adults
Pituitary adenoma (95%)
Increased insulin-like growth factor (IGF-1) mediates effects of GH

Associations: **McCune-Albright syndrome**
MEN
NF
TS

Presentation: Large tongue, hands, feet
Coarsening of facial features
Insulin resistance
Hypertension

Diagnosis: **Increased serum insulin-like growth factor 1**
No decrease in serum GH after oral glucose tolerance test (GH > 1 µg/L)
Pituitary mass on brain MRI

Treatment: Pituitary adenoma resection
Octreotide (somatostatin analog)
Dopamine agonists

MODALITIES: XR

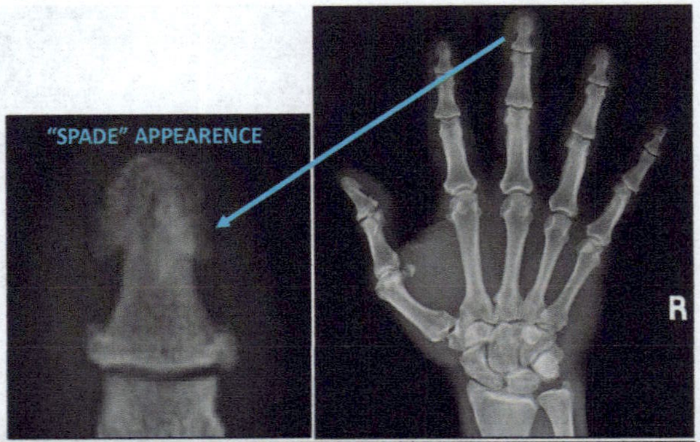

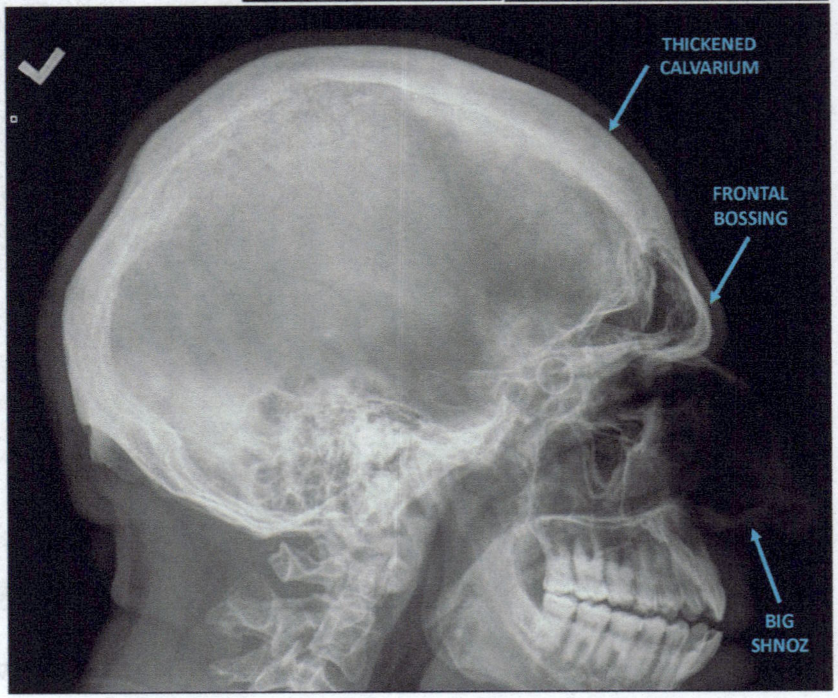

MUSCULOSKELETAL

BONE METASTASIS

IMAGING:

XR:	**Focal lucent/lytic lesion in patient with cancer**
CT:	**Diffuse lytic or blastic lesions**
MRI:	**Marrow replacement – Breach of cortex**

USMLE POINTS:

Metastasis to bone may be bone forming blastic, bone destructive lytic, or mixed
Pathologic fractures

Labs:	CBC, ESR, LFTs, Ca2+, ALP, SPEP, UPEP
Most common:	Breast, Lung, Thyroid, Renal, Prostate
Prostate:	**Often blastic**
Breast:	**Often blastic and/or lytic**
Renal/Thyroid:	**Often lytic**

MODALITIES: XR → MRI WWO

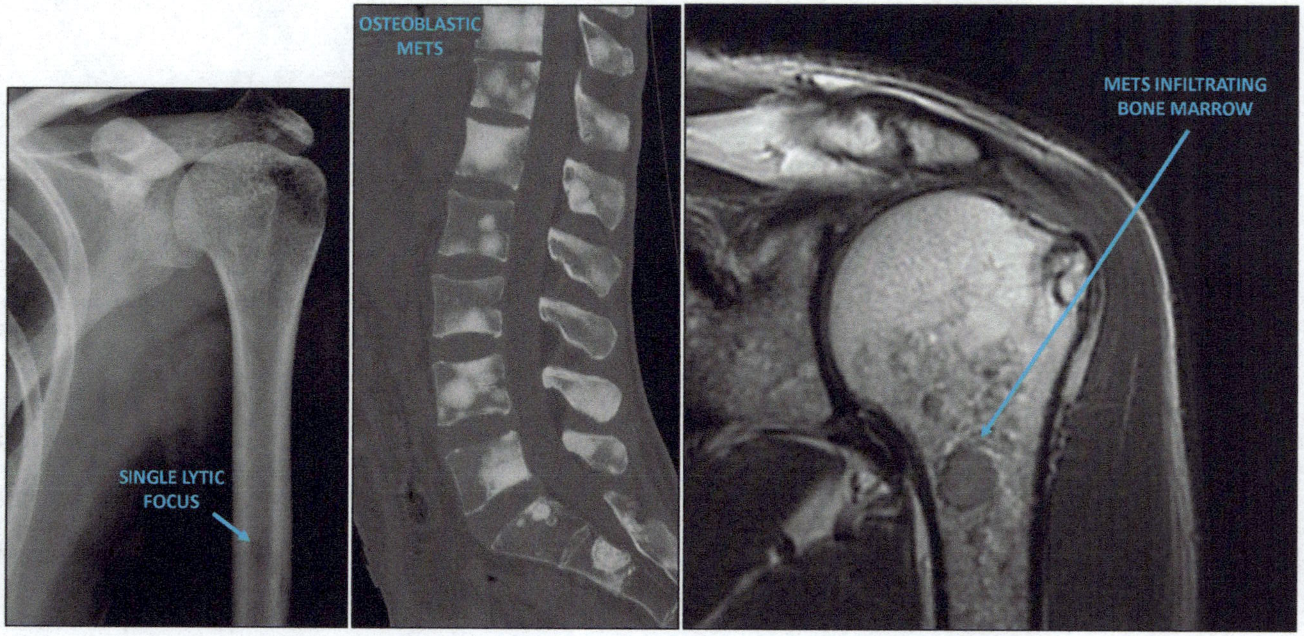

MUSCULOSKELETAL

CRPS / RSD

IMAGING:

XR: **Severe patchy osteopenia, particularly in the periarticular region**
NUC: **Increased tracer uptake in the affected limb**
Diffusely increased juxta-articular activity around all joints of the affected hand or foot on delayed images

USMLE POINTS:

Excess, chronic pain in extremities following surgery, fracture, soft tissue injury
Autonomic dysfunction: Changes in skin temperature
Sweat, edema

Presentation: More than 6 months since trauma
Edema, changes in blood flow, abnormal motor activity, exaggerated pain

Females, 50-70 years old

Treatment: Physical therapy
Medications
Spinal cord stimulation
Peripheral nerve block

MODALITIES:

XR → NUC

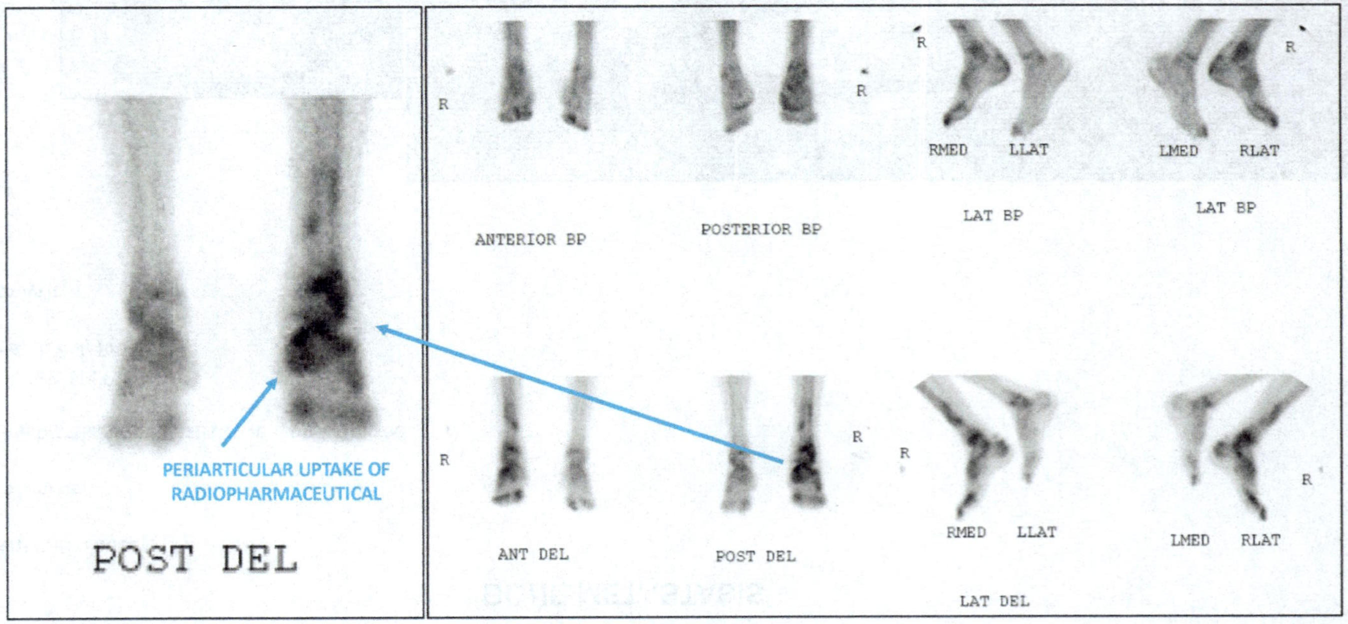

MUSCULOSKELETAL

GAMEKEEPER / SKIER THUMB

IMAGING: Edema / discontinuity of the ulnar collateral ligament of the first MCP

USMLE POINTS:

"Skier thumb" → Acute fall on ski-pole
"Gamekeeper's thumb" (breaking rabbit neck) → Chronic, non-traumatic overuse

Radially-directed force → hyper-abduction of the 1st MCP
May require surgery if **Stener** (interposition of adductor aponeurosis) lesion is present.

MODALITIES: MRI WO

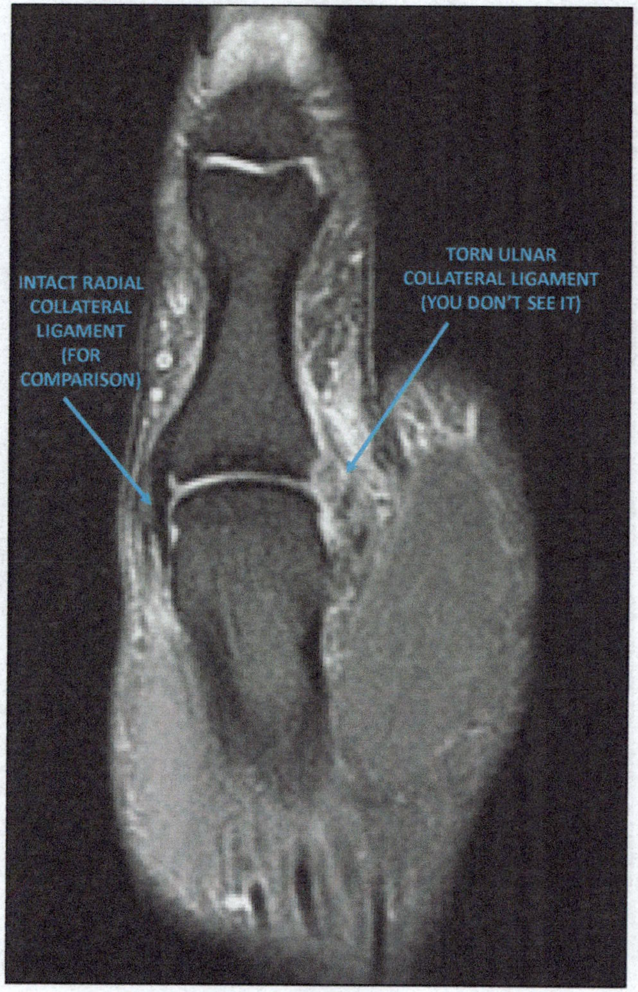

MUSCULOSKELETAL

ILIOPSOAS BURSITIS

IMAGING: **Edema within distal myotendinous junction**
Attaches to **lesser trochanter**

USMLE POINTS: **Psoas sign → pain on passive extension of the right hip**
Anterior hip pain, due to inflammation/irritation of bursa
Often a result of overuse (especially seen in athletes)
Snapping sensation at the front of the hip

Treatment: NSAIDs
Corticosteroid injections
Physical therapy

MODALITIES: MRI WO

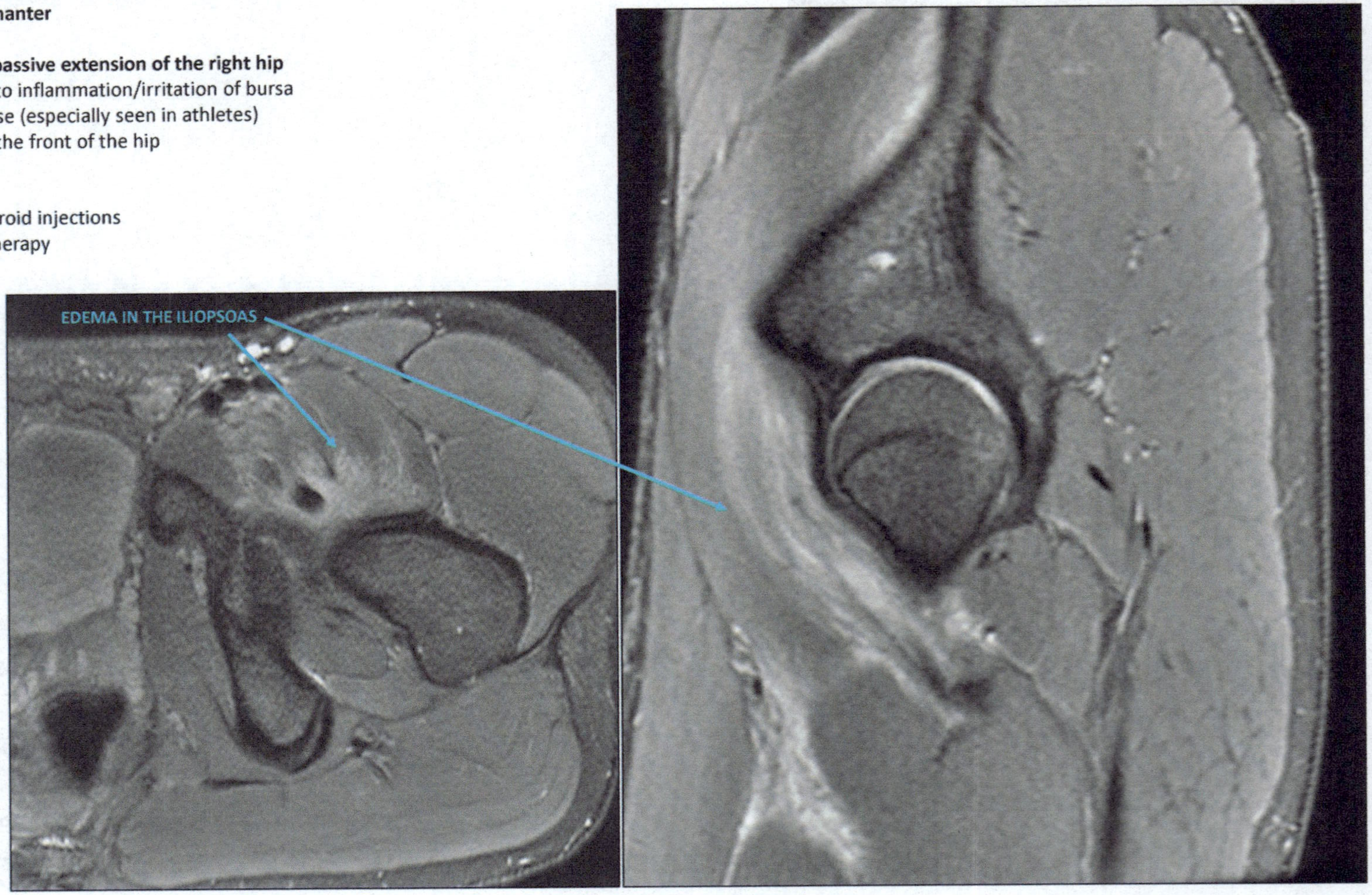

MUSCULOSKELETAL

MAISONNEUVE AND TRIMALLEOLAR FRACTURES

IMAGING:	Maisonneauve:	**Widening of the distal tibiofibular syndesmosis** **Widened medial ankle mortise** **Fracture of the proximal fibula**
	Trimalleolar Fracture:	Ring is completed **Fracture of medial malleolus, lateral malleolus, and posterior-distal tibia**
USMLE POINTS:	Maisonneauve:	**Unstable injury** **Pronation-external rotation**
	Trimalleolar Fracture:	**Unstable injury** **Require ORIF**
MODALITIES:	XR	

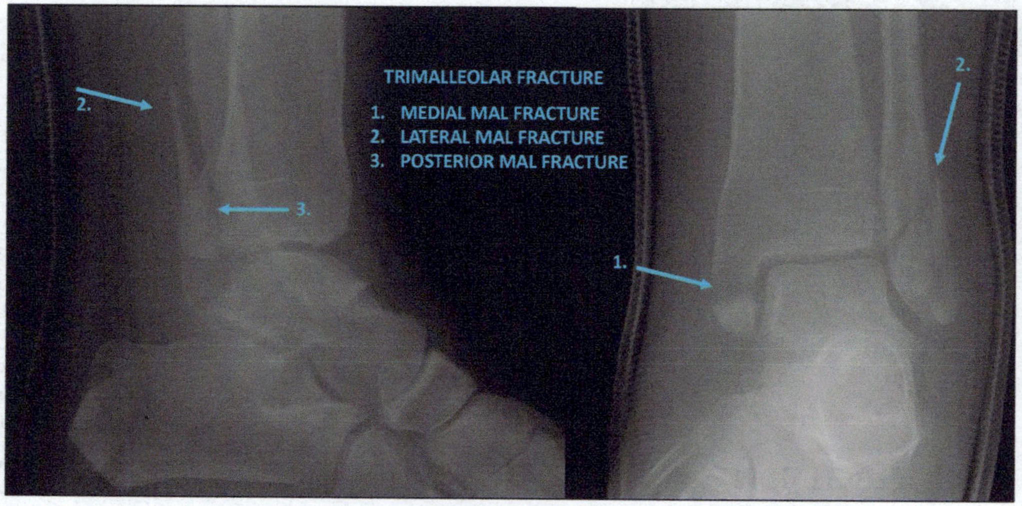

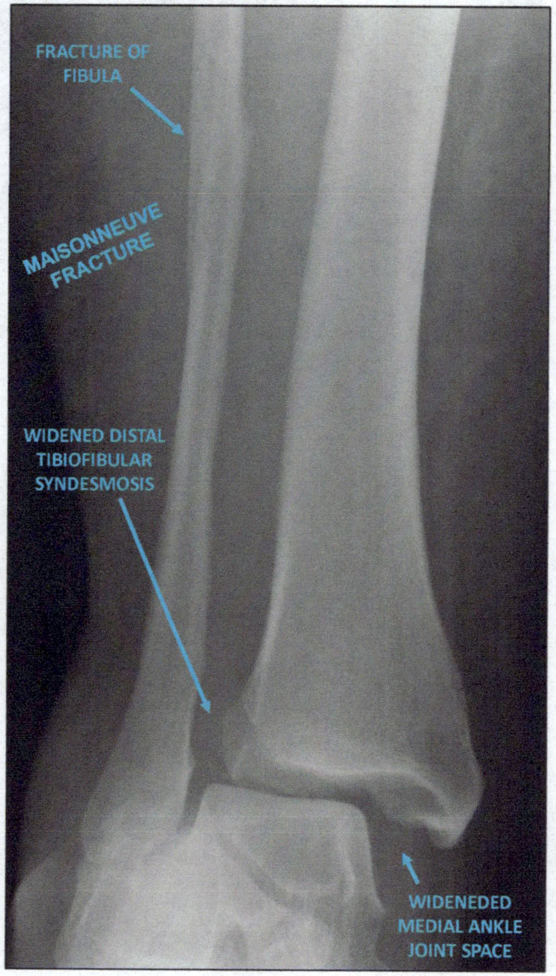

MUSCULOSKELETAL

MCL TEAR

IMAGING:

Grade 1: **Increased signal**
Grade 2: **Partial tear**
Grade 3: **Complete disruption**

USMLE POINTS:

Excessive valgus force tears the MCL
Often associated with tears of the medial retinaculum and MPFL
Valgus test → Increased medial space widening
Unhappy triad:
- ACL
- MCL
- Meniscal tear

MODALITIES: MRI WO

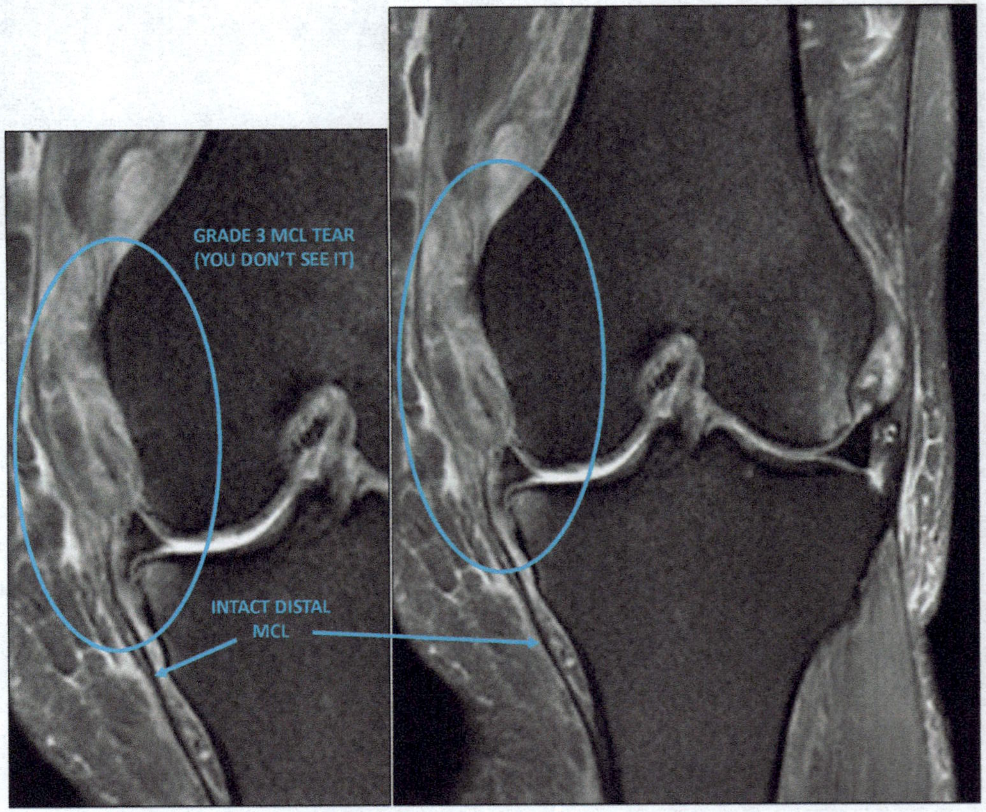

MUSCULOSKELETAL

MORTON'S NEUROMA

IMAGING: **Convex effacement of fat within the plantar intermetatarsal space**

USMLE POINTS: "Interdigital neuritis"
Pain in ball and arch of the foot associated with excessive pronation of the foot
Nerve compression at transverse intermetatarsal ligament
Burning pain between the 3rd & 4th webspace
Treatment: Wide shoes with low heels
Metatarsal padding

MODALITIES: US / MRI WWO

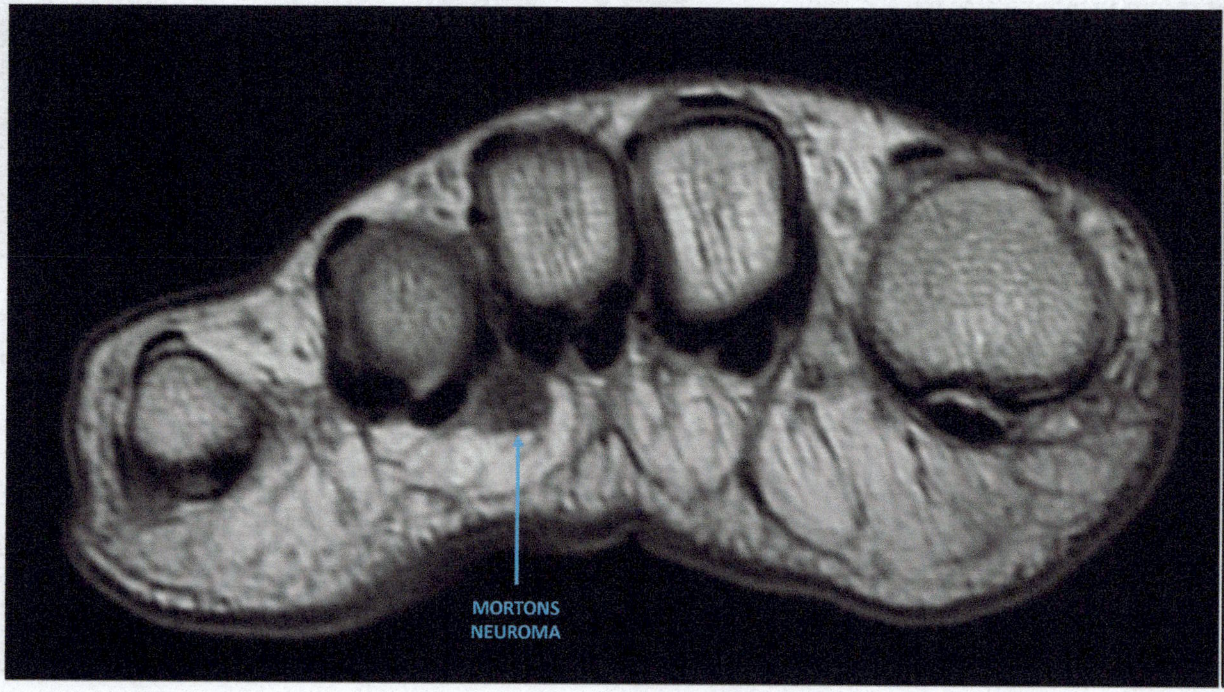

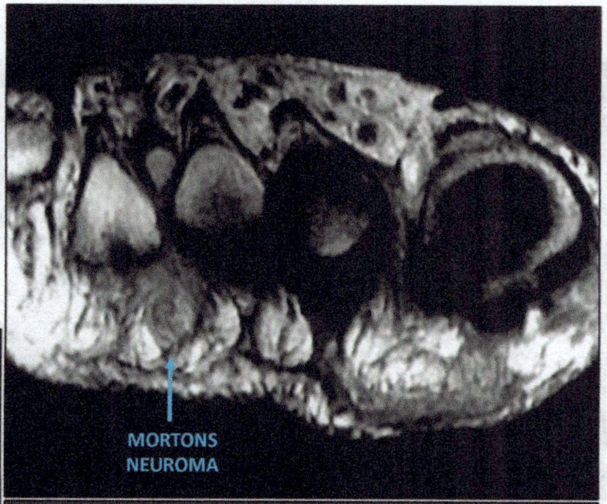

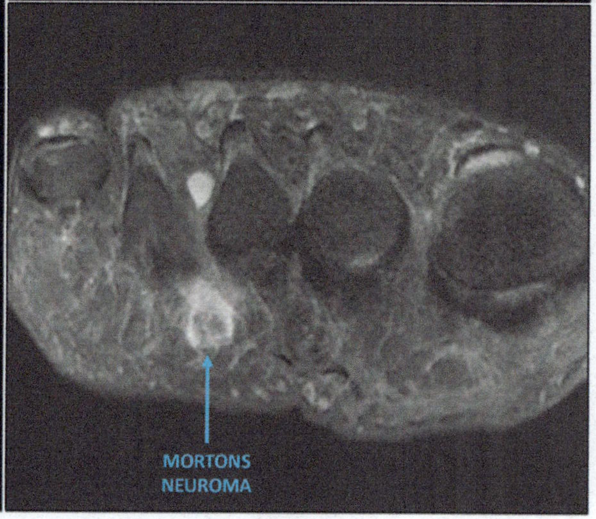

MUSCULOSKELETAL

PSOAS ABSCESS

IMAGING: Look for osteomyelitis-discitis (TB)

USMLE POINTS:
- **Psoas sign → pain on passive extension of the right hip**
- Located in the retrofascial space (retroperitoneal space)
- Result of **hematogenous spread of** an infectious process from an occult source in the body
- Fever, back/flank pain, inguinal mass, and difficulty walking
- May spread to hip joint causing septic arthritis
- **S. aureus**

MODALITIES: CT W

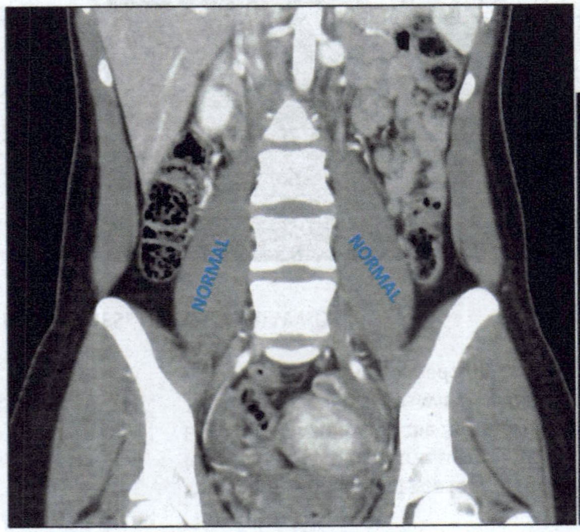

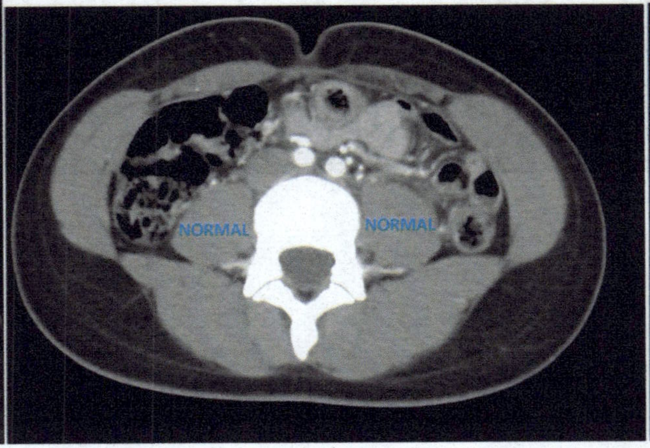

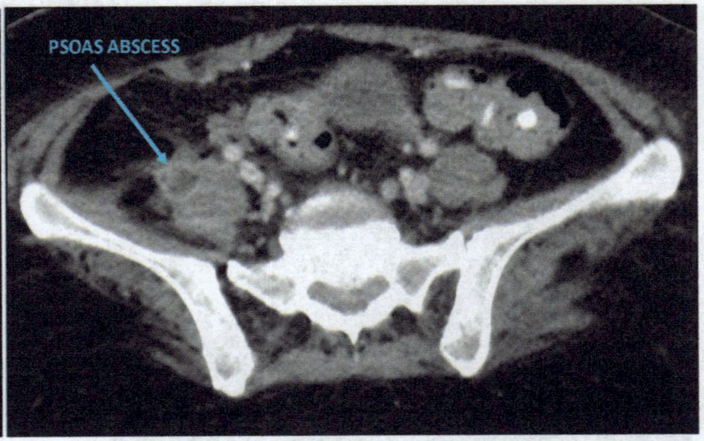

MUSCULOSKELETAL

SACROILIITIS

IMAGING: Asymmetric edema / erosions of the sacroiliac joint

USMLE POINTS: **Pain in buttocks or lower back**
Commonly associated with Ankylosing spondylitis

Psoriatic arthritis	Asymmetric	RF negative / pencil-in-cup deformity / Dactylitis
Ankylosing spondylitis	Symmetric	HLA-B27
Inflammatory bowel disease	Symmetric	UC / Chron's
Reactive (Reiter) arthritis	Asymmetric	Chlamydia trachomatis

Treatment: NSAIDs
PT

MODALITIES: MRI WO

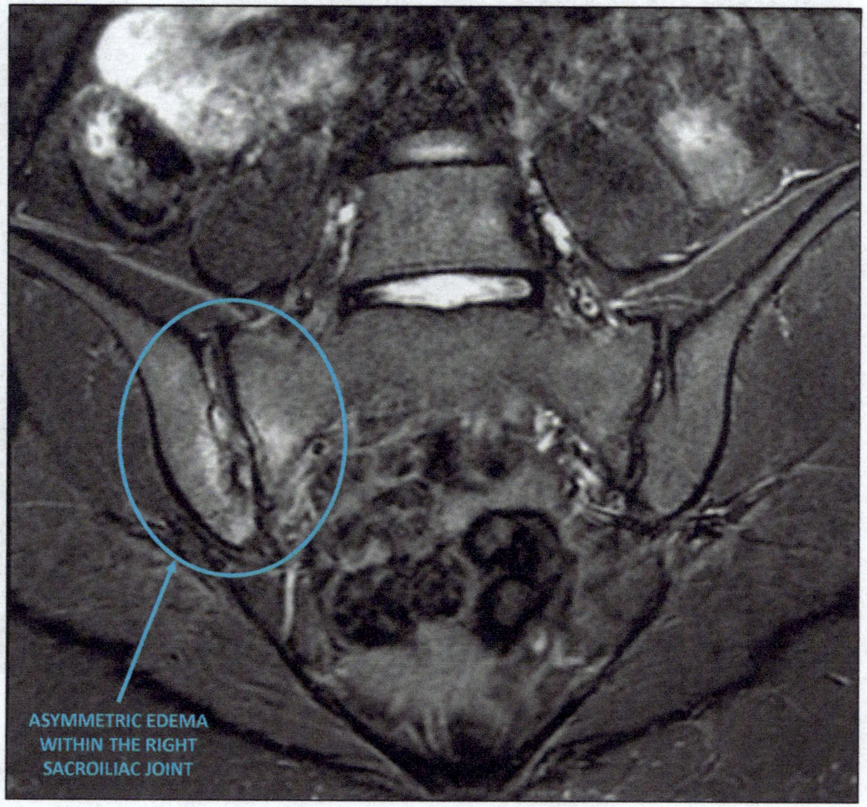

MUSCULOSKELETAL

IMAGING: **Hyperintense signal within the distal supraspinatus**

USMLE POINTS:
Most commonly injured rotator cuff muscle
Innervated by **suprascapular** nerve (C5-C6) along with the infraspinatus
ABducts the arm from 0 – 15 degrees
Shoulder pain exacerbated by overhead reaching
Tendon weakening due to degenerative changes and chronic impingement
Tenderness at the insertion of supraspinatus (anterolateral shoulder)
Treatment: Conservative / PT
NSAIDs
Corticosteroids
Surgical repair (complete tears)

MODALITIES: MRI WO

SUPRASPINATUS (ROTATOR CUFF) TEAR

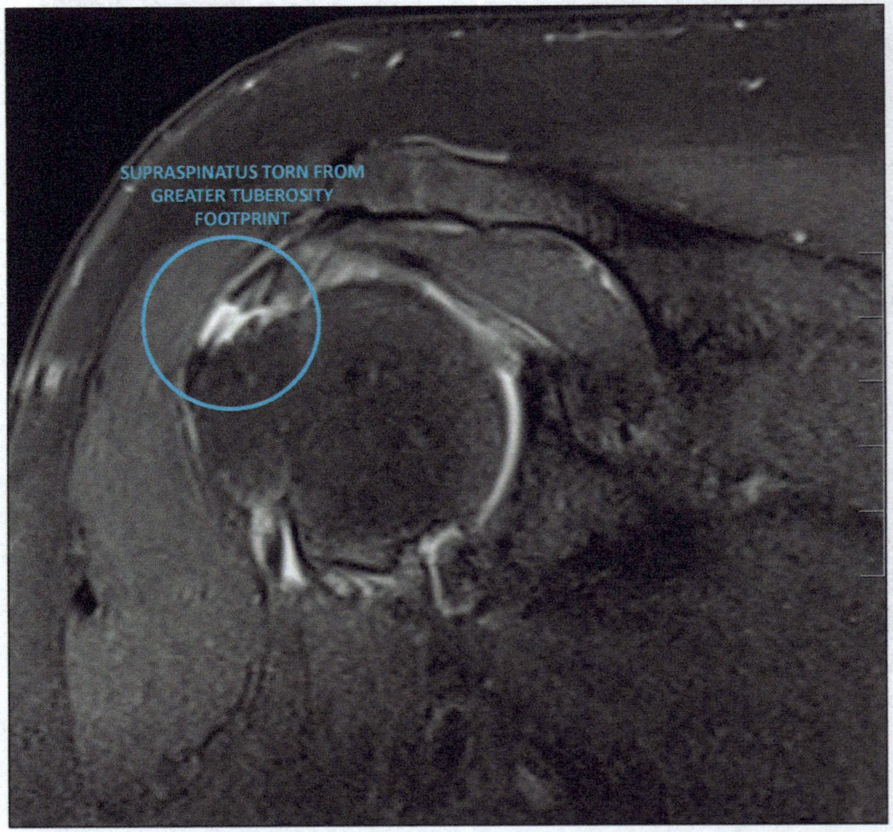

NEURORADIOLOGY

SUBDURAL HEMATOMA

IMAGING: **Crescent shaped** – along cerebral convexity or falx. DDx: Epidural hematoma
Crosses suture lines

USMLE POINTS: **Most common** intracranial hemorrhage **(venous)**
Bleeding at the **bridging veins** caused by head trauma
EtOH + Elderly are more prone due to cerebral atrophy → tension on bridging veins
Common in **anticoagulated** patients

MODALITIES: CT WO

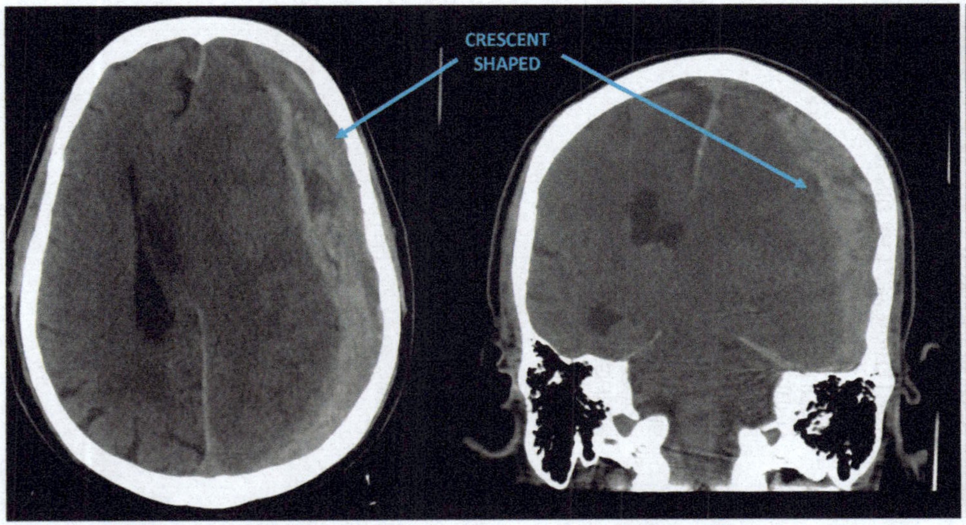

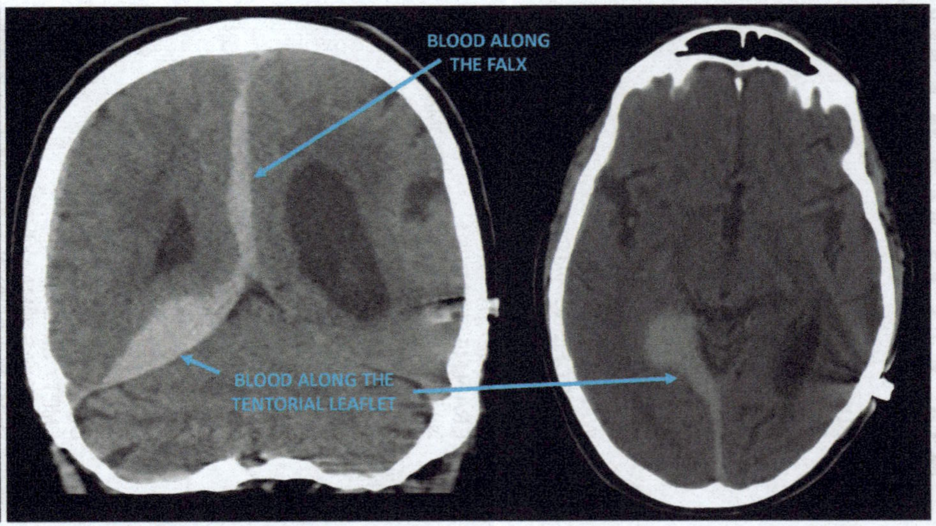

NEURORADIOLOGY

BERRY ANERUSYM

IMAGING: **Saccular** aneurysm – most commonly from **Anterior Communicating Artery**

USMLE POINTS: Junction of two arteries (ACA most common)
Rupture → SAH
Risk factors:
- Ehlers-Danlos Syndrome (vascular type)
- **Aortic coarctation**
- **Autosomal dominant polycystic kidney disease (ADPKD)**
- Advanced age
- **Hypertension**

MODALITIES: CTA OR ANGIO

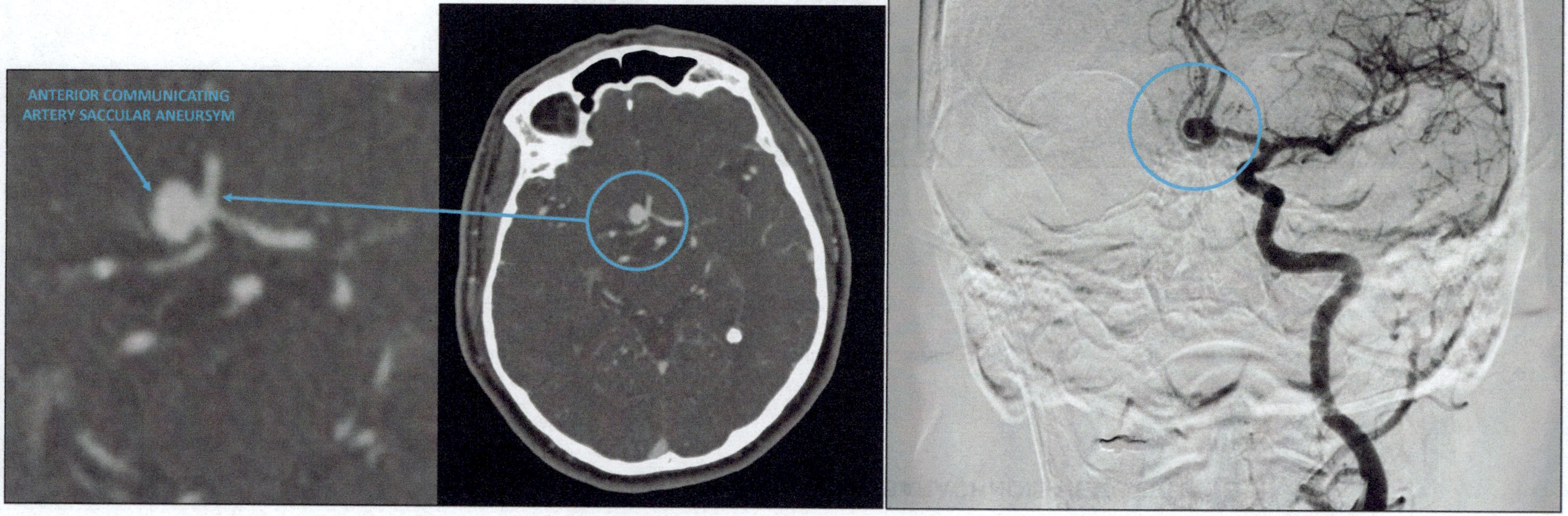

NEUROADIOLOGY

SUBARACHNOID HEMORRHAGE

IMAGING: **Trauma vs. ruptured aneurysm (vs. angio contrast)**
Hemorrhage **within the sulci and perimesencephalic cisterns**

USMLE POINTS: **Trauma (anticoagulated) vs. Ruptured Berry (or saccular) aneurysm**
SAH can cause **vasospasm** → ischemic **stroke in those areas about 3-7 days after initial bleed. Tx: Nimodipine**
Most dangerous/common complication: Rebleeding (1 day after initial bleed)
Risk of developing communicating high pressure and/or **obstructive hydrocephalus** → EVD Shunt catheter
Described as **"worst headache of life"**, can cause photophobia
Xanthochromic (yellow) spinal tap
Polycystic kidney disease (ADPKD) → Berry aneurysm

MODALITIES: CT WO

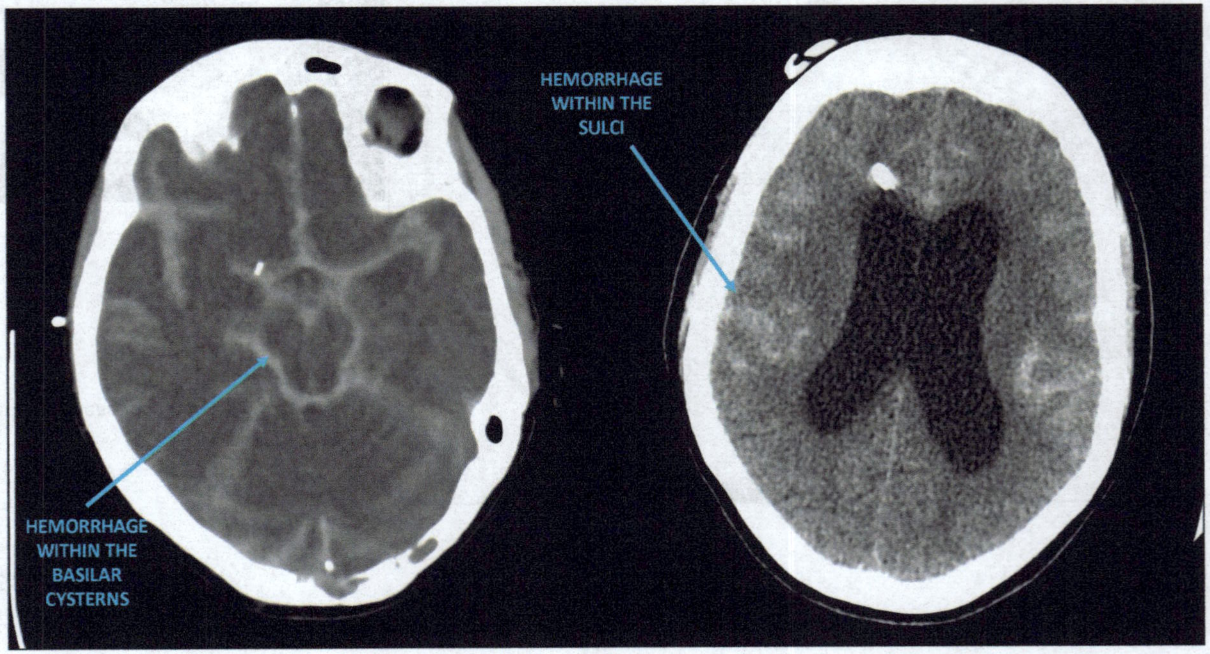

NEURORADIOLOGY

INTRAPARANCHYMAL HEMATOMA

IMAGING: Acute **hyperdense blood within the brain parenchyma (arterial bleed)**
Often surrounding by vasogenic edema
"Swirl-Sign" Low attenuation within acute hyperdense blood indicates active hemorrhage within the CT scan

USMLE POINTS: Most commonly from **hypertension (thalamic) and trauma (frontal lobes)**

Trauma: Hemorrhagic contusions along the inner table of the calvarium → Inferior frontal lobes and temporal lobes

Hypertensive:
- Rupture of small vessels and bleeding
- Charcot-Bouchard microaneurysms (chronic HTN)
- Cerebral amyloid angiopathy (spontaneous intraparenchymal hemorrhage),
- Cavernous hemangiomas
- AV malformation (most common cause of intraparenchymal hemorrhage in children)

MODALITIES: CT WO

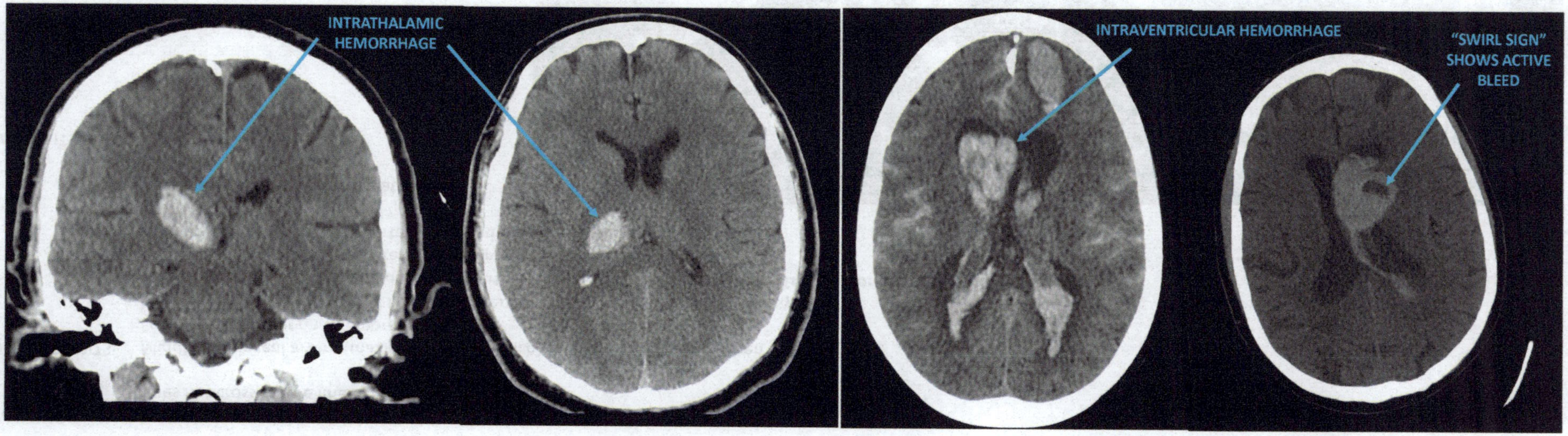

NEURORADIOLOGY

EPIDURAL HEMATOMA

IMAGING: **Hyperdense lens-shaped (biconvex shape) collection** of blood
Does not cross suture lines

USMLE POINTS: **Middle meningeal artery (maxillary artery branch) → Passes through foramen spinosum**
Fracture of the pterion (temporal bone)
Loss of consciousness followed by a **lucid interval up to 48 hours ("talk and die" syndrome)**
Hematoma can rapidly expand due to high arterial pressure → **Brain herniation (Transtentorial / Uncal)**
CN III palsy → Ipsilateral dilated pupil
Cushing reflex → Hypertension, Bradycardia, Respiratory depression

Treatment: Hematoma evacuation

MODALITIES: CT WO

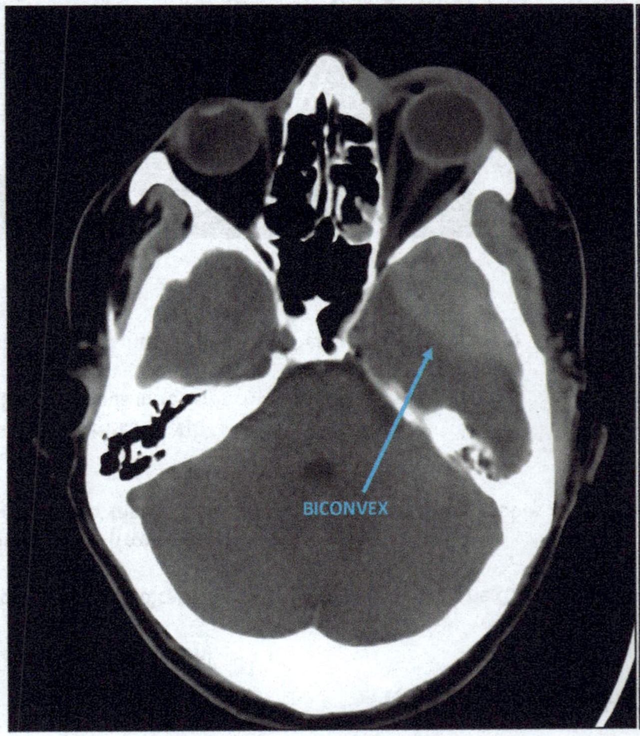

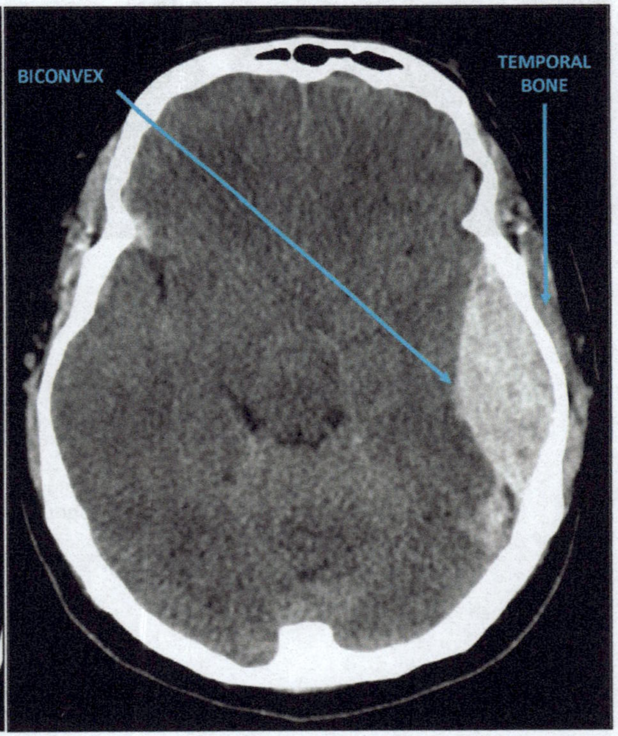

NEURORADIOLOGY

CHIARI MALFORMATIONS 1 & 2

IMAGING:

Chiari 1: **Low-lying tonsils obstructs central canal of spinal cord → Syrinx**

Chiari 2: **Myelomeningocele + Small posterior fossa + Tectal beaking + Tonsillar Herniation + Hydrocephalus**

USMLE POINTS:

Chiari 1:
Downward displacement of the cerebellar tonsils through the foramen magnum
Associated with **syringomyelia** due to obstruction
Often asymptomatic in childhood
Presentation: Paroxysmal occipital headaches and cerebellar symptoms

Chiari 2:
Myelomeningocele → Small posterior fossa → The rest of the manifestations
Downward displacement of the cerebellar vermis and tonsils and the medulla
Aqueduct stenosis → Causing hydrocephalus
Can compress corticospinal tracts leading to upper motor neuron dysfunction

MODALITIES: MRI WO

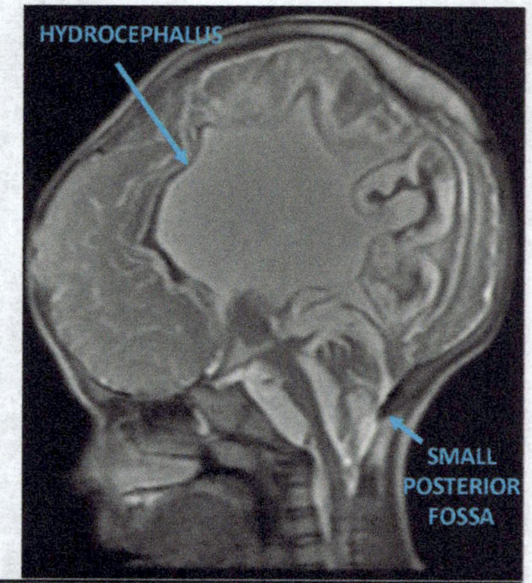

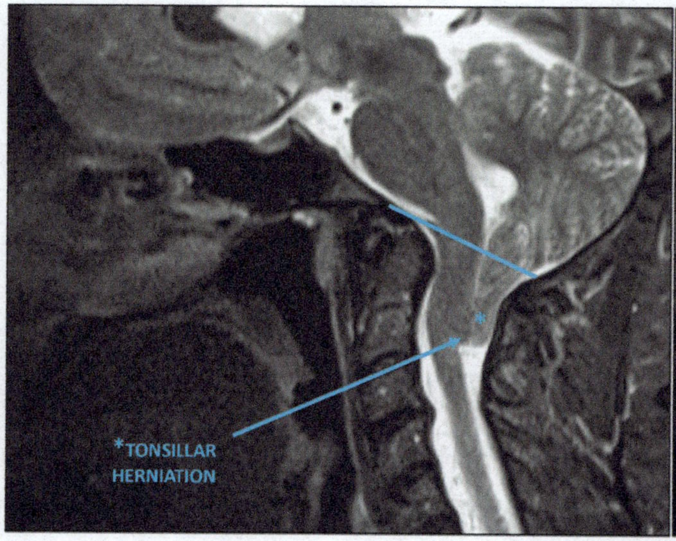

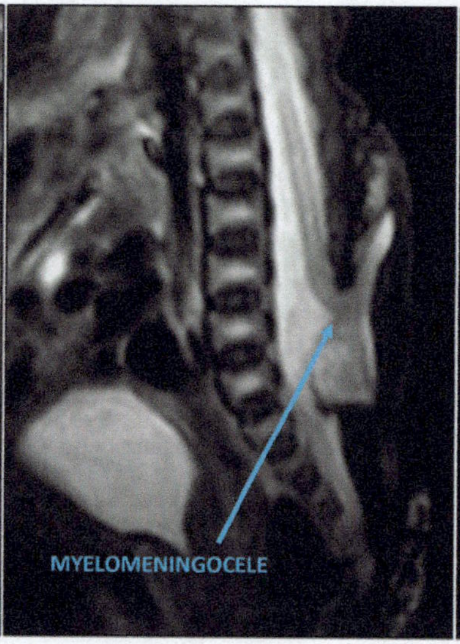

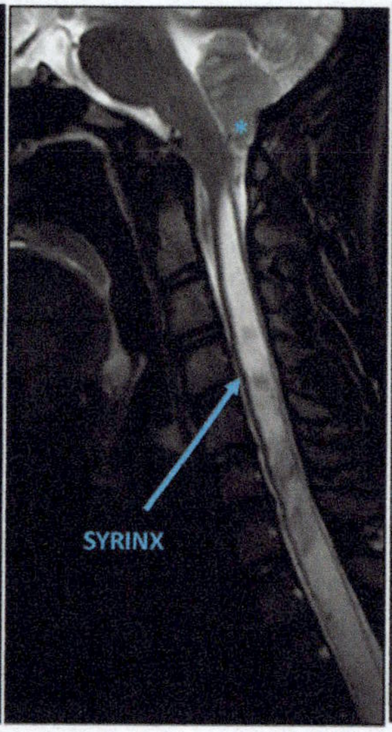

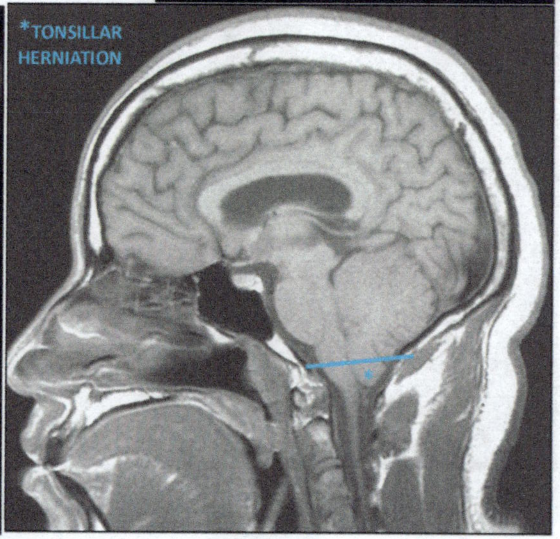

NEURORADIOLOGY

HYDROCEPHALUS & NPH

IMAGING: **Dilation of ventricles with sulcal effacement**

USMLE POINTS: **Communicating vs. Noncommunicating (SAH / Mass)**
Increase in CSF volume that causes ventricular dilation with increased ICP
Newborns: **Cerebral aqueduct stenosis is the most common**

Adults: **SAH** → communicating high pressure and/or obstructive hydrocephalus (EVD shunt catheter)

NPH: **Ventriculomegaly**
Widening of the temporal horns of the lateral ventricles > 6 mm
Dilated Sylvian fissures

Communicating hydrocephalus due to reduced CSF resorption
Elderly, Idiopathic
Normal opening pressure

Presentation:	**Wet**	→	**Urinary incontinence**
	Wacky	→	**Dementia**
	Wobbly	→	**Gait apraxia (wide-based magnetic gait)**

Treatment: Ventriculoperitoneal shunt

MODALITIES: CT WO → MRI WO

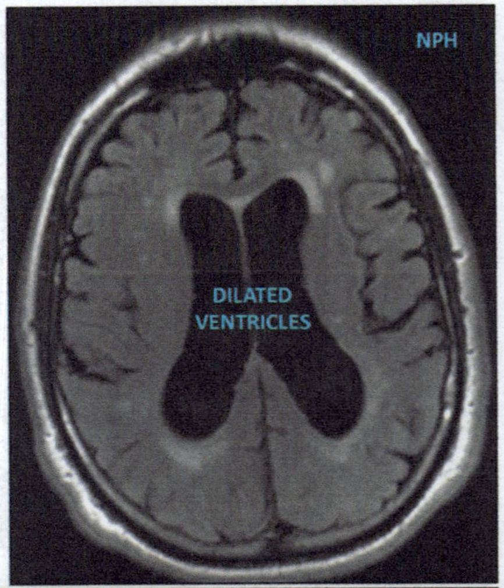

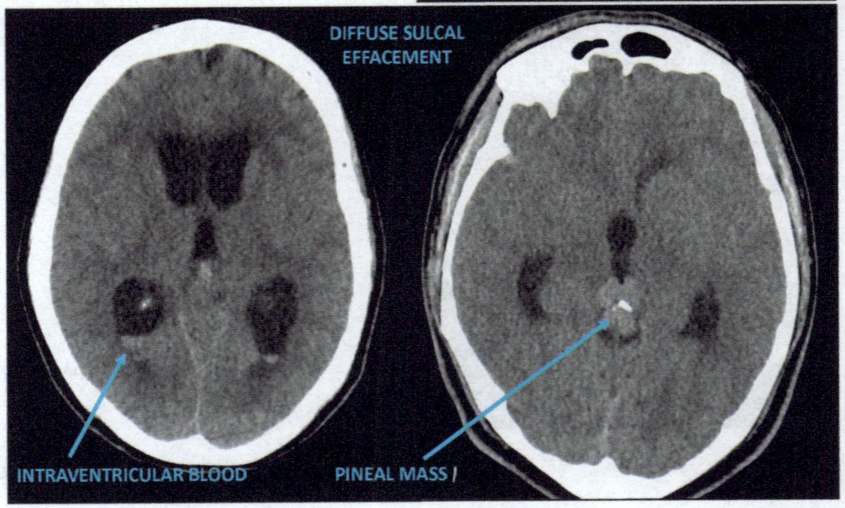

NEURORADIOLOGY

STROKE

IMAGING:

CT: **Loss of gray-white differentiation**
MRI: **Increased signal on DWI**

USMLE POINTS:

Neurological deficits depend on area of brain involved
Risk factors: **Hypertension, DM, Smoking**, Afib, PFO, Hypercoagulable state
Large vessel infarcts are commonly secondary to embolism

MCA Infarct:
- **Contralateral weakness and sensory loss in face & upper limb**
- **Broca's aphasia (superior division MCA)**
- **Wernicke's aphasia (inferior division MCA)**

Lenticulostriate artery infarct:
- **Pure, unilateral motor weakness**
- **Pure, unilateral sensory weakness**
- **Dysarthria-clumsy hand syndrome**

tPA contraindications:

Intracranial hemorrhage

Stroke or head trauma	**in the past 3 months**
Major surgery	**in the past 2 weeks**
GI or urinary tract bleeding	**in the past 3 weeks**
Myocardial infarction	**in the past 3 months**

Persistent hypertension SBP > 185 mmHg or DBP > 110 mmHg

Direct thrombin inhibitors (such as dabigatran or argatroban)
Platelets < 100,000
INR > 1.7 or PT > 15 seconds if on warfarin

Intracranial neoplasm, arteriovenous malformation, or aneurysm

MODALITIES: CT WO + CTA / MRI WO (DWI)

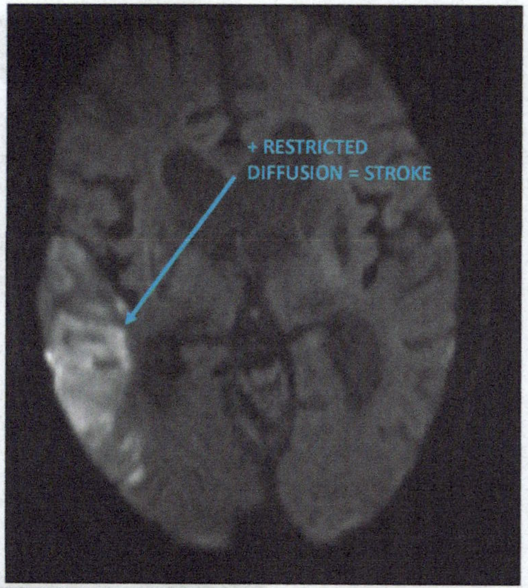

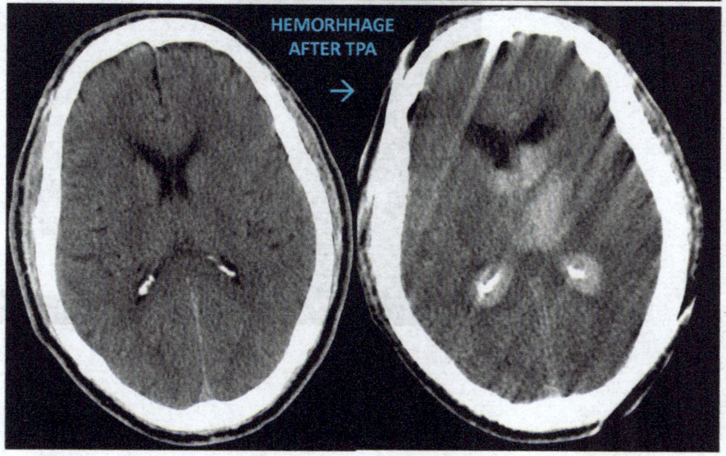

STROKE

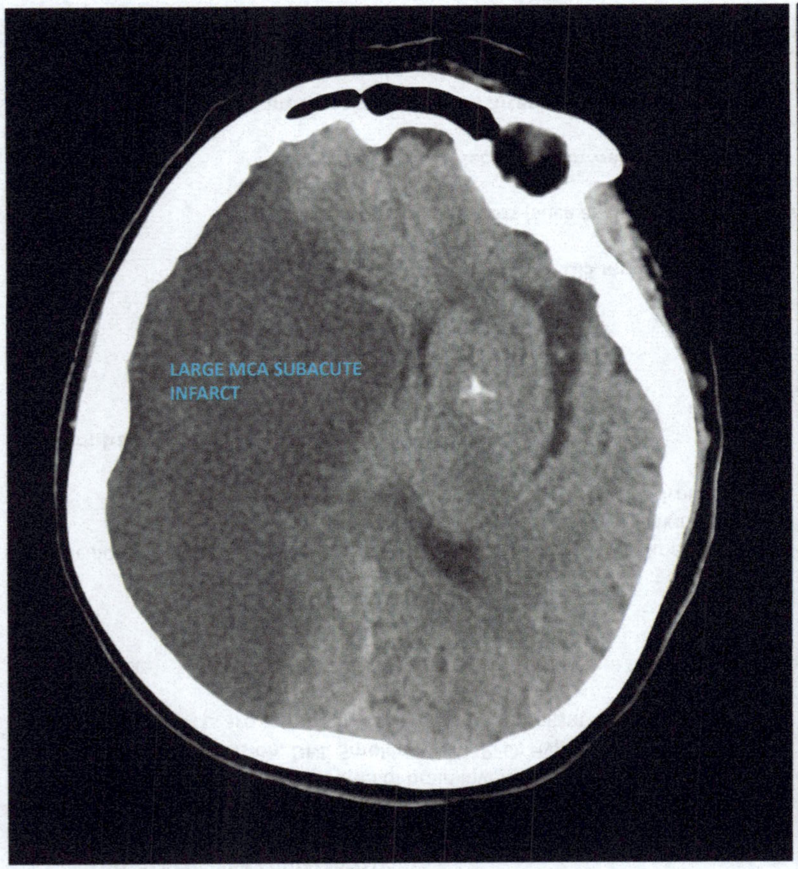

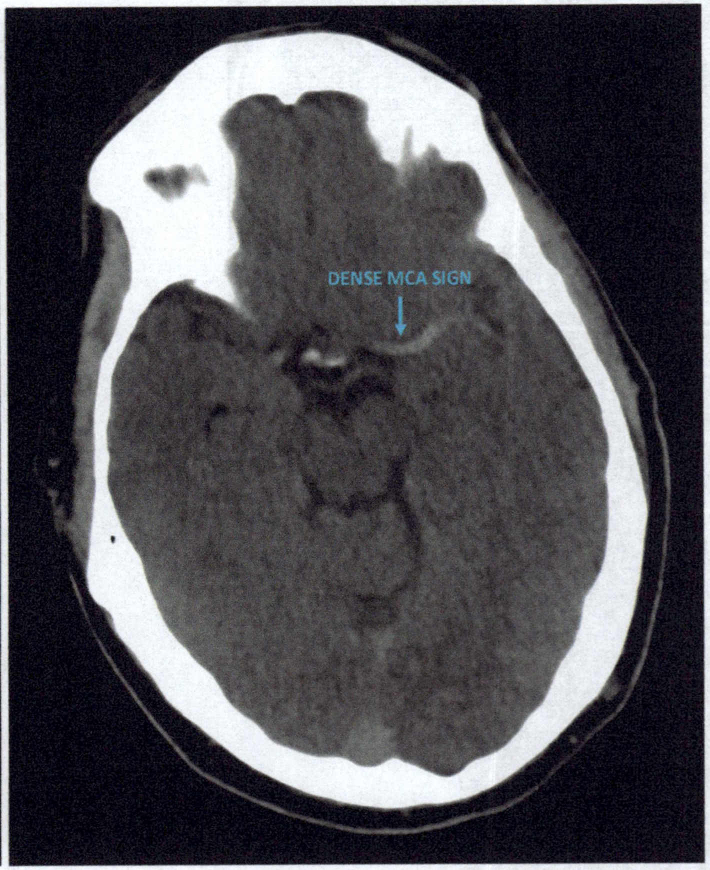

MULTIPLE SCLEROSIS

IMAGING:
T2/FLAIR signal changes
"Dawson Fingers" – Perpendicular to long-axis of the CC

USMLE POINTS:
Women & young adults
Axonal destruction by CD8+ lymphocytes and macrophages
MRI is gold standard for MS diagnosis
LP → Oligoclonal bands + Elevated IgG index
Periventricular plaques can be seen extending from corpus callosum (also known as Dawson's fingers)
Areas of oligodendrocyte loss and reactive gliosis with preservation of axons

McDonald 2017 Criteria: Symptoms differing in space and time

Presentation:
Unilateral motor / sensory deficits
Intranuclear ophthalmoplegia
Nystagmus, vertigo
Optic neuritis

Treatment:
IV Methylprednisolone
Natalizumab (PML) → Need to test for JC virus
Baclofen & Tizanidine for spasticity

MODALITIES: MRI WWO

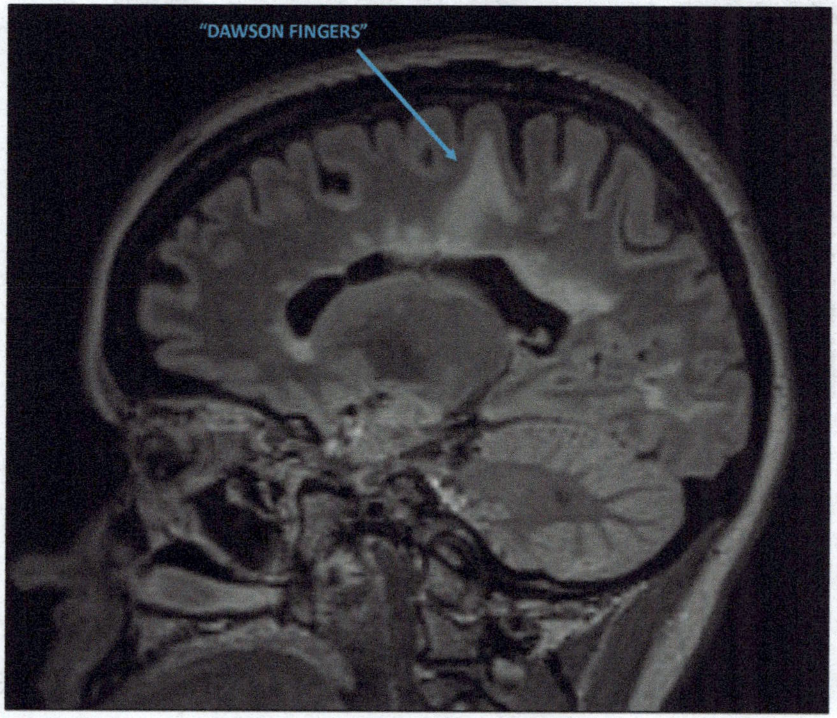

NEURORADIOLOGY

OSMOTIC DEMYELINATION

IMAGING: **Increased DWI signal within the pons**
Basal ganglia, midbrain and subcortical white matter

USMLE POINTS: "Locked-in" syndrome
Massive **axonal demyelination** of the pons
Rapid sodium correction **(> 8-10 mEq/day)**
Serious complication of **correcting SIADH-induced hyponatremia too** quickly (with **–vaptans**)

DDX: **Wernicke's encephalopathy** → **Gait ataxia + oculomotor dysfunction + encephalopathy**

MODALITIES: MRI WO

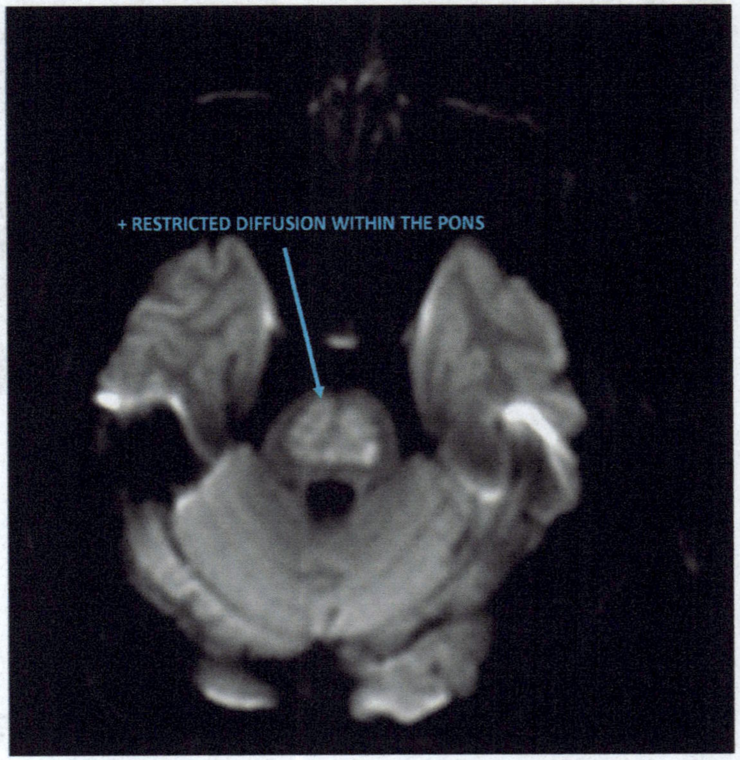

NEURORADIOLOGY

WALLENBURG SYNDROME

IMAGING: Signal change (DWI) within the **lateral medulla**

USMLE POINTS: **"PICA" or Lateral Medullary Syndrome**

Presentations:

Contralateral	**Sensory deficits that affect the trunk and extremities**
Ipsilateral	**Sensory deficits of the face and cranial nerves**

Caused by occlusion of the **posterior inferior cerebellar artery (PICA)**

Traumatic vascular dissection / occlusion of the distal vertebral artery

MODALITIES: MRI WO

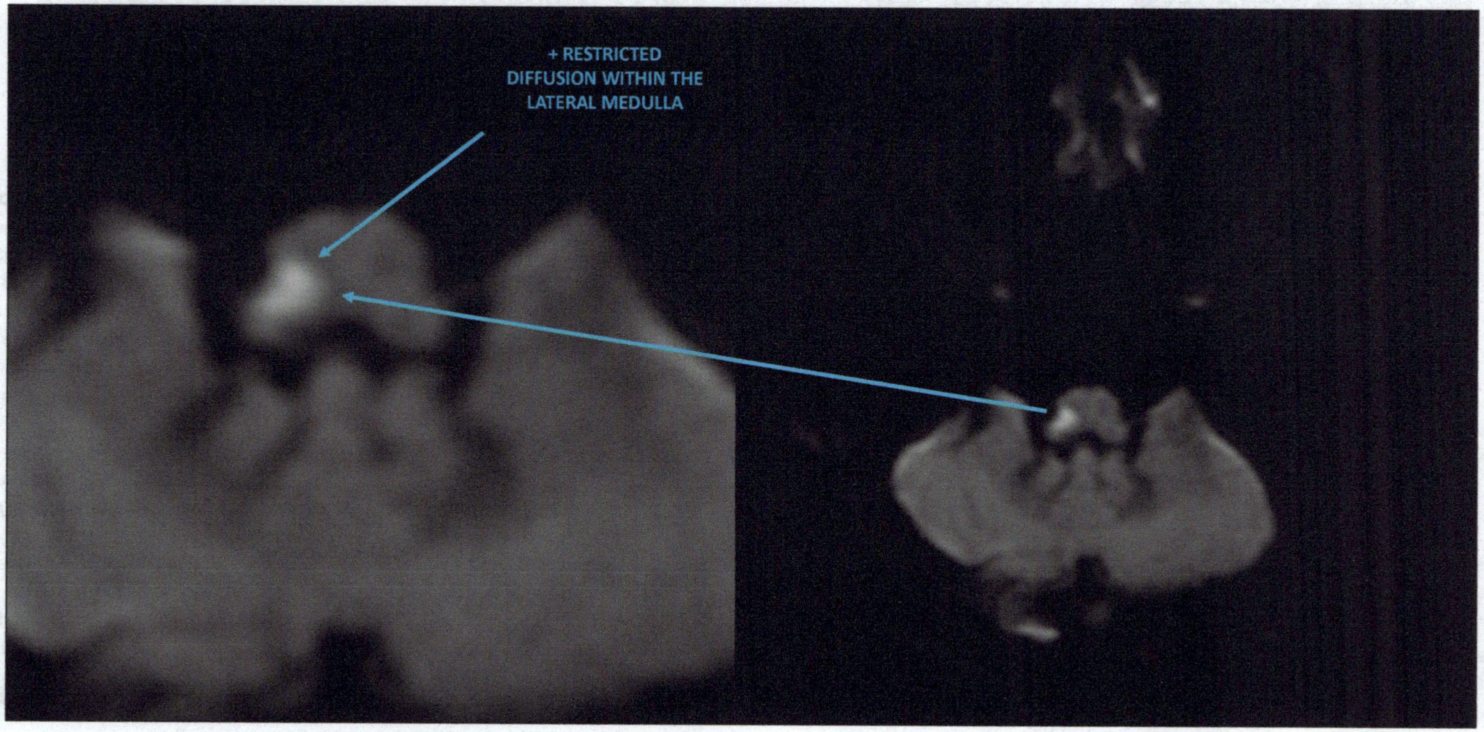

NEURORADIOLOGY

NEUROFIBROMATOSIS TYPE 1

IMAGING: **Vestibular Schwannoma (CP angle)**
Plexiform neurofibromas

USMLE POINTS: von-Recklinghausen disease
Vestibular schwannoma (acoustic neuroma) → Schwann cells in the vestibular nerve
Typically located on CN VIII in the internal acoustic meatus → May extend to CP angle
Deficits in CNVIII, CNVII, and CNV
Stain S100+

Autosomal dominant disease associated with NF1 tumor suppressor gene on chromosome 17
Associations:
- **Cafe-au-lait spots**
- **Cutaneous neurofibromas**
- **Lisch nodules**
- **Optic gliomas**
- **Pheochromocytomas**
- **Sphenoid dysplasia, scoliosis, and congenital pseudoarthrosis**
- **Plexiform neurofibromas are associated with NF1**

MODALITIES: MRI WWO

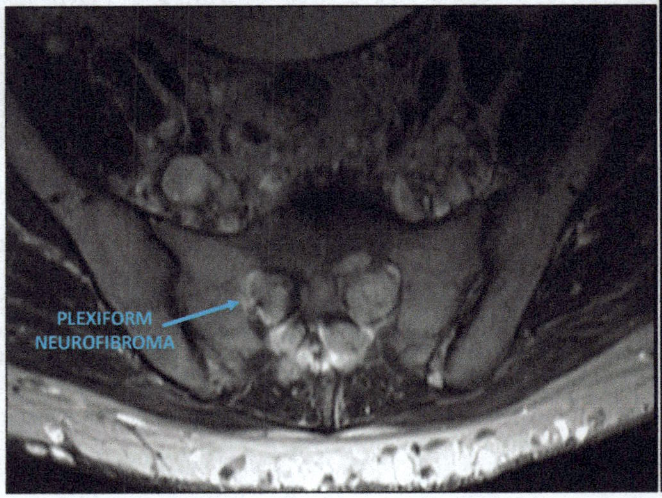

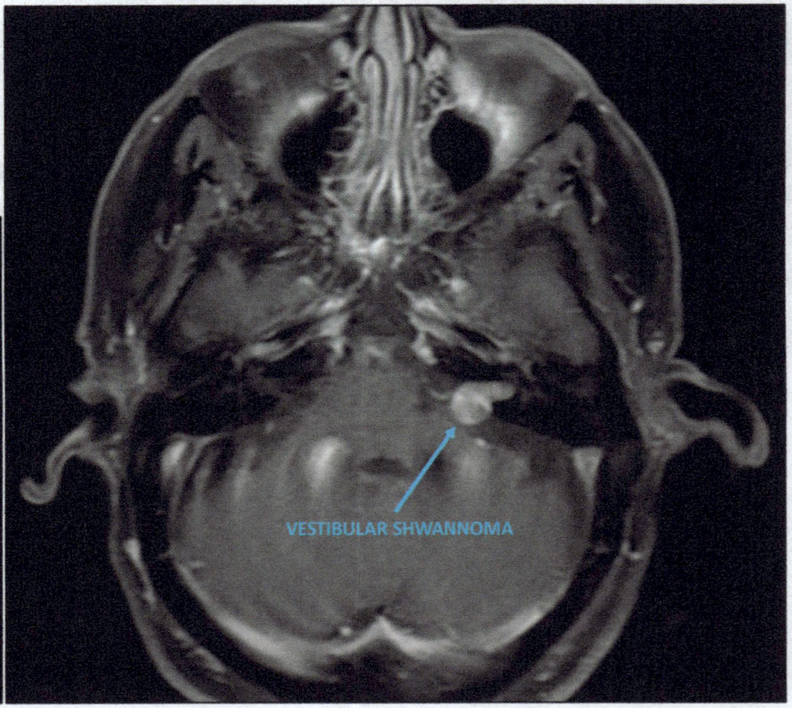

NEURORADIOLOGY

IMAGING:

MISME
Bilateral vestibular schwannomas are diagnostic
Intracranial and spinal meningioma
Intraspinal-intramedullary ependymoma

USMLE POINTS:

NF2 gene encodes a TSG → merlin (schwannomin)
Autosomal dominant. Chromosome 22

Presentation:
- Hearing loss
- Tinnitus
- Vertigo
- Sensorineural hearing loss

DDx NF1:
- **Café-au-lait macules**
- **Irish hamartomas (Lisch nodules)**
- **Neurofibromas**

MODALITIES: MRI WWO

NEUROFIBROMATOSIS TYPE 2

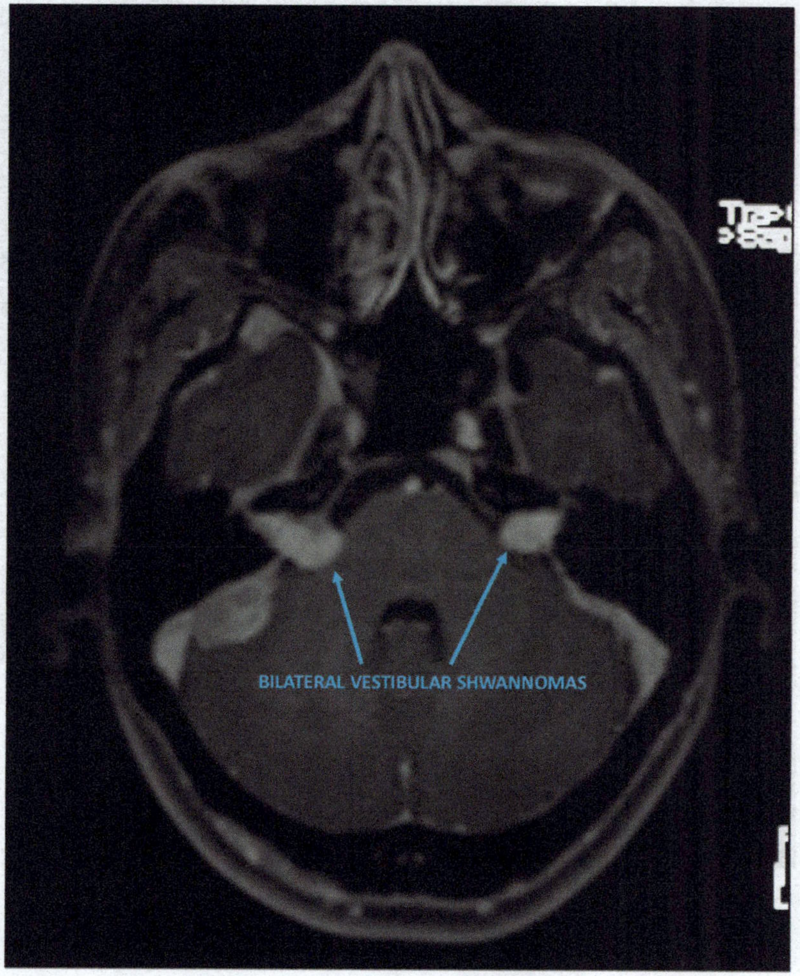

NEURORADIOLOGY

AVM

IMAGING:	**Tangle of vessels with flow voids** **Subarachnoid hemorrhage**
USMLE POINTS:	Most common cause of intraparenchymal hemorrhage in children Presentation: Intracranial hemorrhage, seizure, headache, or focal neurologic deficits Associations: **Hereditary Hemorrhagic Telangiectasia**
MODALITIES:	CTA / MRA / ANGIO

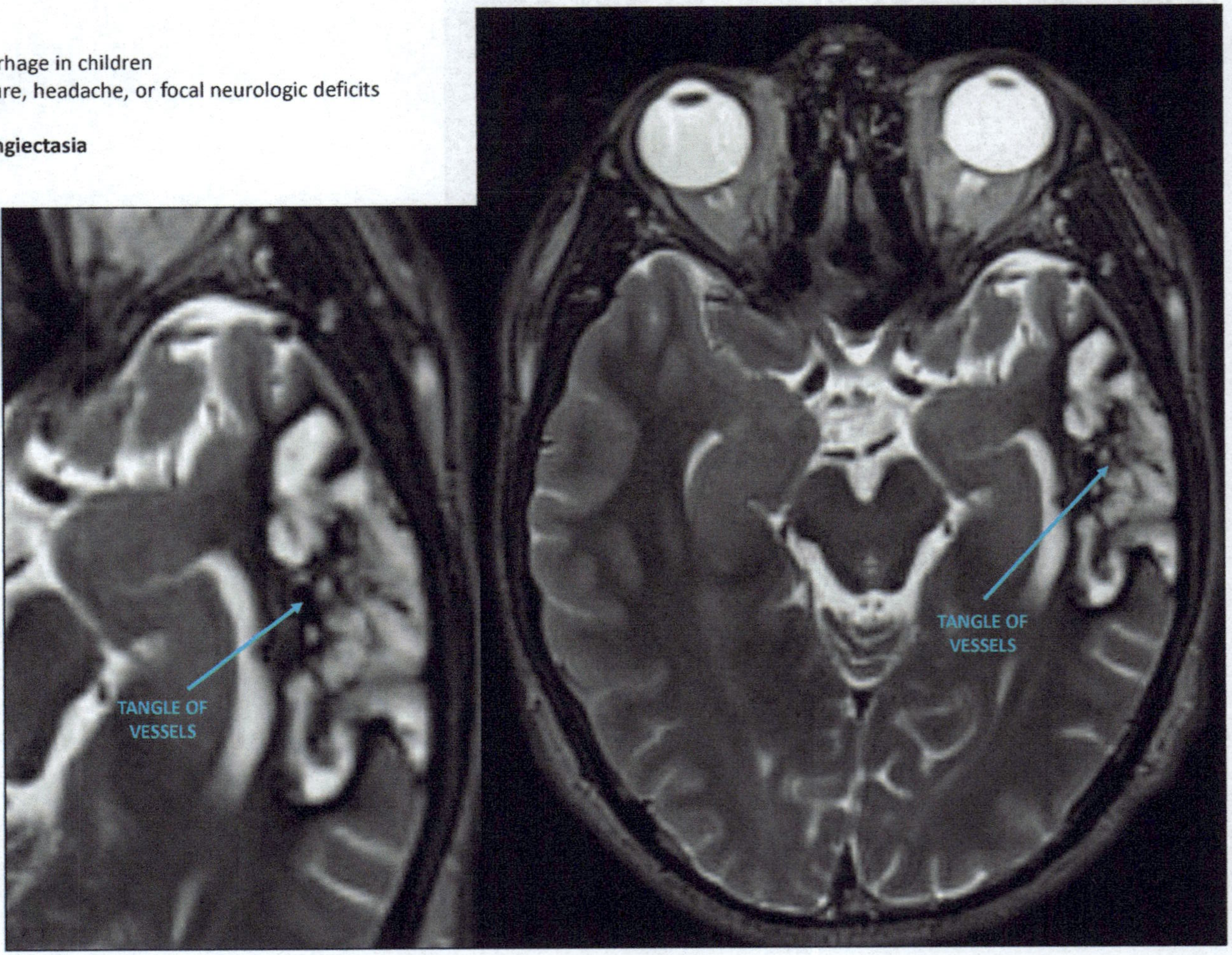

NEURORADIOLOGY

BRAIN DEATH

IMAGING:

CT: **Diffuse sulcal effacement**
Loss of gray-white differentiation

NUC: **Lack of radiotracer in the brain + ICA**
Hot-Nose sign

USMLE POINTS:

Hippocampus (CA1 pyramidal neurons) are affected first due to high metabolic demand
Loss of brain-stem reflexes: Corneal, pupillary, jaw-jerk, oculovestibular, gag reflex
No respiratory response with a PaCO2 > 60 mmHg

MODALITIES:

CT WO / NUC
Cerebral angiography "gold standard"

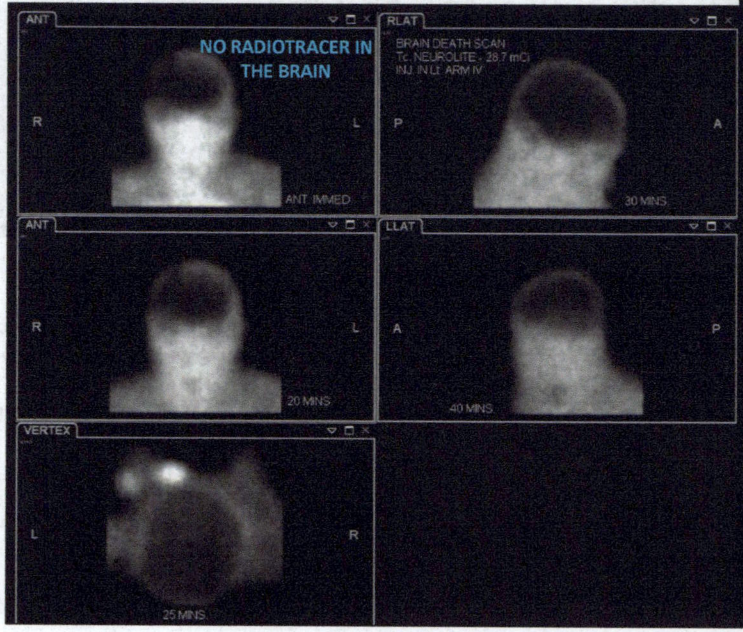

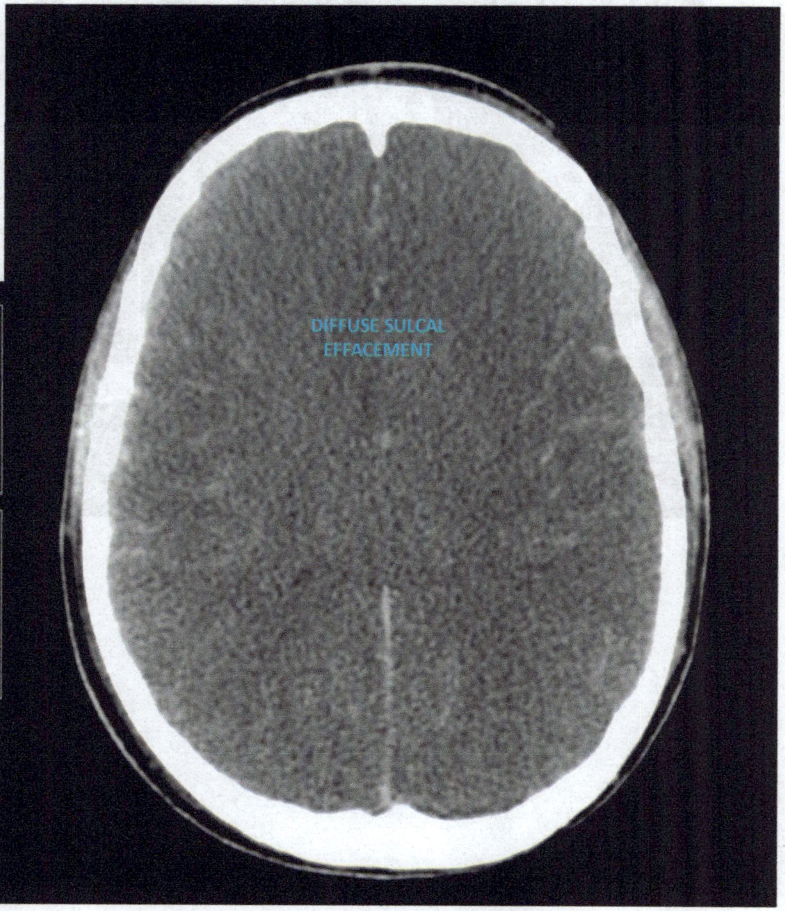

NEURORADIOLOGY

BRAIN METASTASES

IMAGING:
Multiple lesions
Gray-white junction
Vasogenic edema
DDX: Septic emboli (based off clinical history / emboli more likely to cavitate)

USMLE POINTS:
Lung > Breast > Melanoma, Colon, Kidney

Treatment: Dexamethasone for increased ICP
Phenytoin for seizures

MODALITIES:
MRI **WWO**

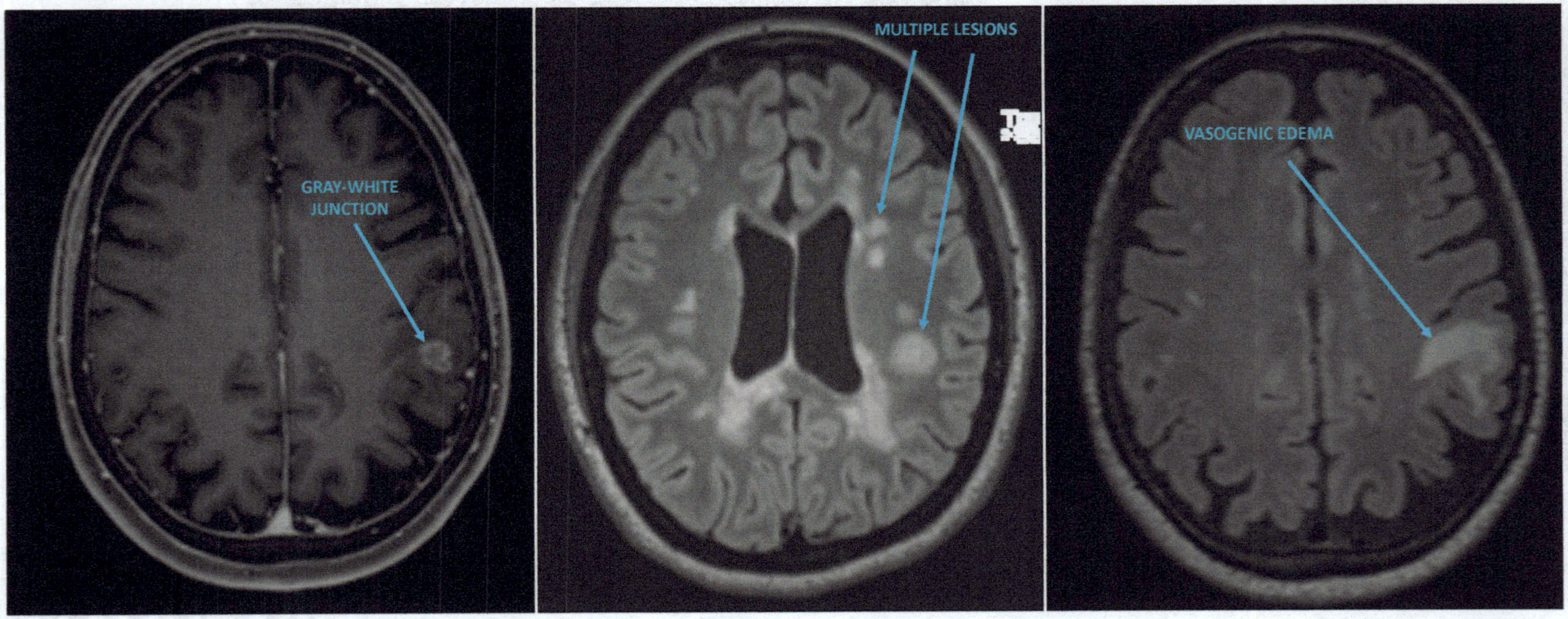

NEURORADIOLOGY

NASOPHARYNGEAL CARCINOMA

IMAGING: **Soft-tissue mass within the nasopharynx**

USMLE POINTS:
Epstein-Barr virus
Asian adults or African children
Associated with **smoking / tobacco, HPV-16, Betel nut, Radiation**

Presentation: Nasal congestion with epistaxis, headaches, and spread to the cervical lymph nodes.
Histology: **90-95% Squamous cell carcinoma →** Pleomorphic keratin-positive epithelial cells in a background of lymphocytes

MODALITIES: CT W

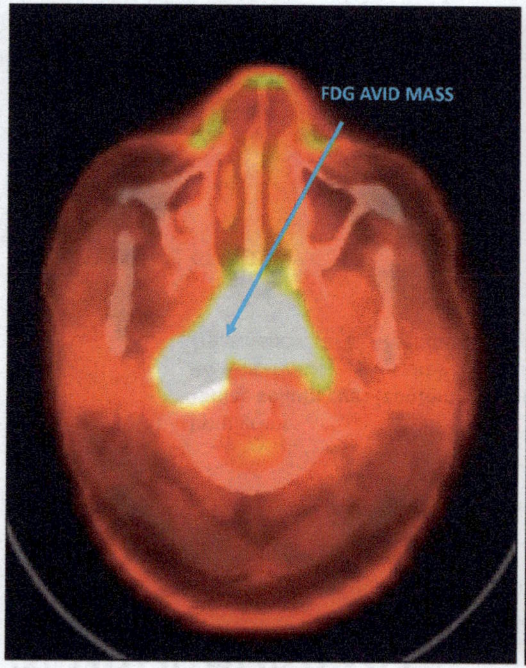

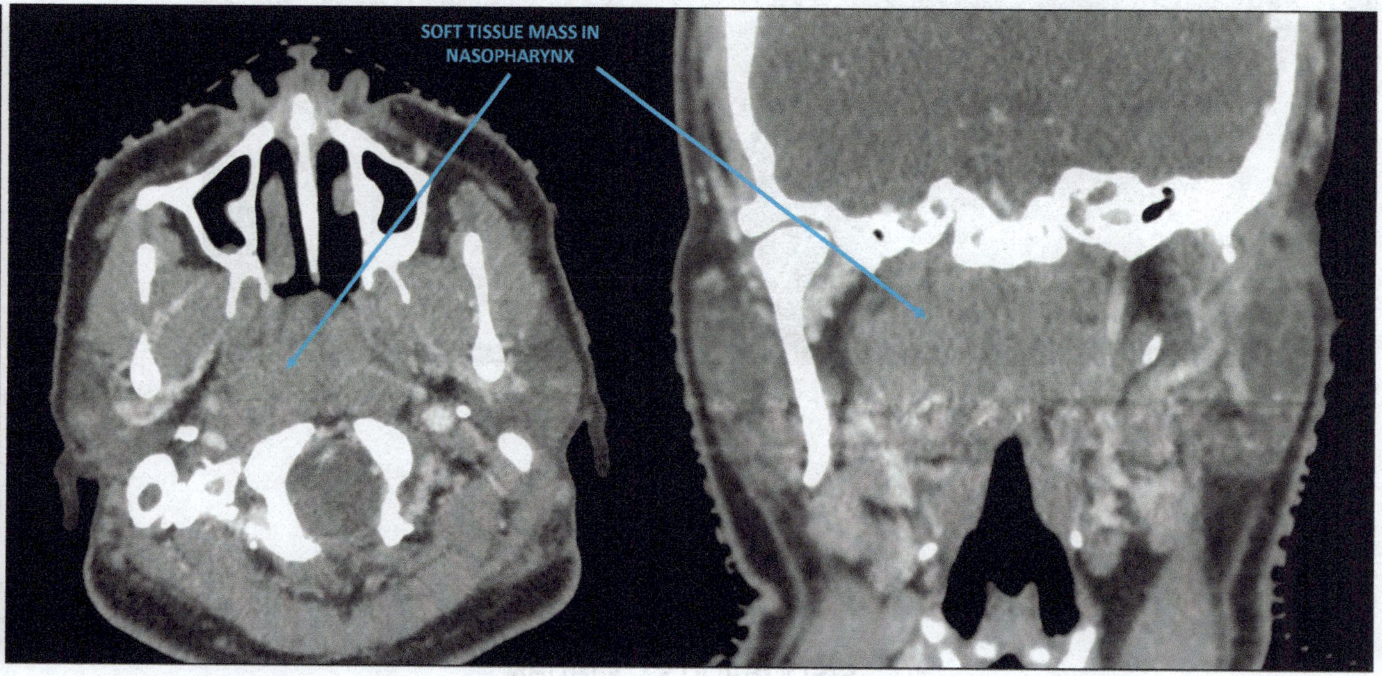

NEURORADIOLOGY

NEUROCYSTICERCOSIS

IMAGING: **Multiple scattered calcified densities**

Several cystic lesions surrounded by edema ("swiss-cheese" appearance on scan)

4 Stages:
- **Vesicular**
- **Colloidal vesicular**
- **Granular nodular**
- **Nodular calcified**

USMLE POINTS: **Immigrant**

Taniae solium eggs (contaminated pork)

Presentation: Seizures & hydrocephalus

Treatment: **Albendazole + corticosteroids**

MODALITIES: CT WO

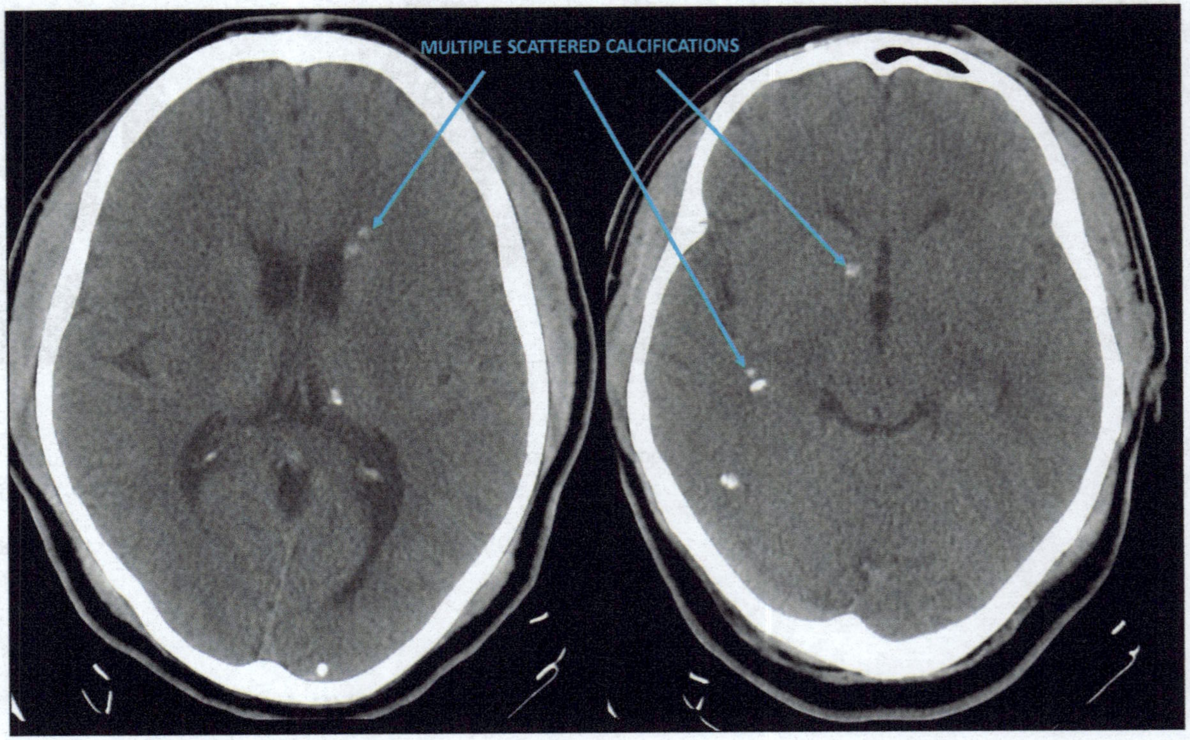

NEURORADIOLOGY

PROGRESSIVE MULTIFOCAL LEUKOENCEPHALOPATHY

IMAGING:

Extensive white matter – Nonenhancing (DDx, other etiologies such as tumor / toxoplasmosis)
Multifocal, asymmetric periventricular and subcortical involvement
Subcortical U-fiber involvement is an important feature of lesions of multiple sclerosis
Parietal and occipital area

USMLE POINTS:

HIV History
Reactivation of **latent JC virus** in the immunocompromised (AIDS, leukemia)
Adverse effect of **Rituximab or Natalizumab (MS treatment)**
Destruction of oligodendrocytes and astrocytes

MODALITIES:

MRI WWO

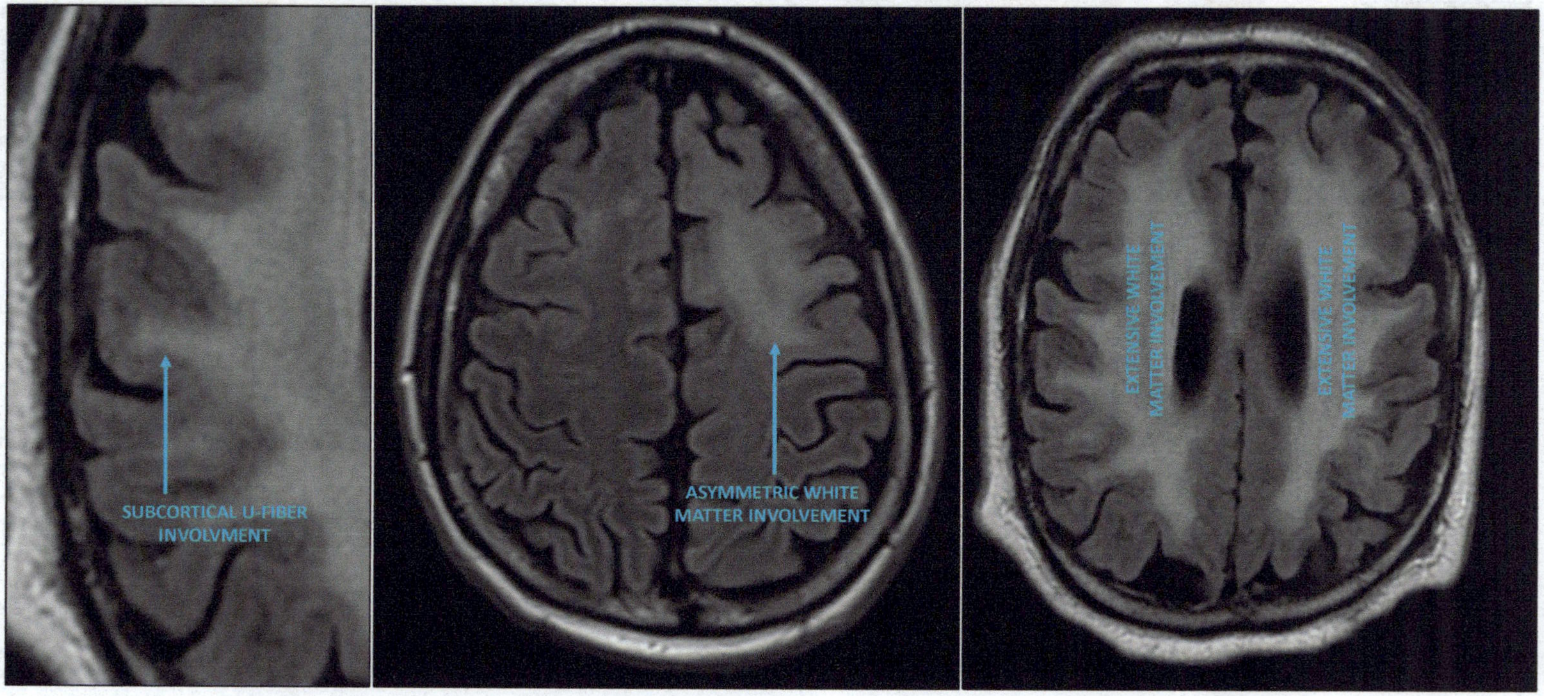

NEURORADIOLOGY

ALZHEIMER DEMENTIA

IMAGING:

Hippocampal or parahippocampal volume loss
SPECT and PET can detect regional **hypoperfusion/hypometabolism in a biparietal and bitemporal** distribution

USMLE POINTS:

Diffuse cortical and subcortical atrophy
Impaired declarative episodic memory
Most common cause of dementia
Hippocampal atrophy (hippocampus is particularly sensitive to damage)
Build up of beta-amyloid plaques and tau tangles
Trisomy 21
APOE4 is associated with an increased risk

MODALITIES:

CT WO / MRI WO / NUC

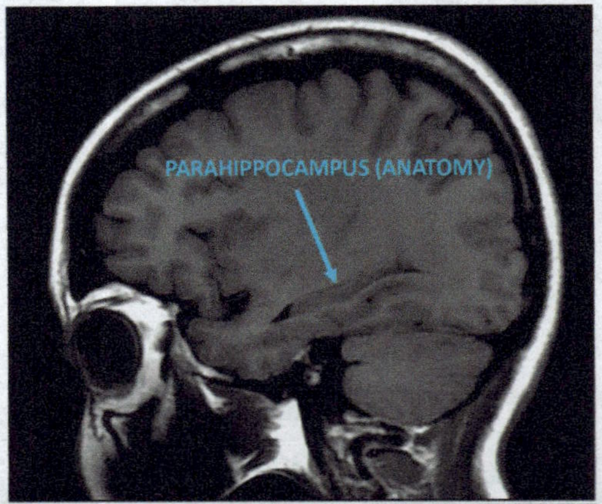

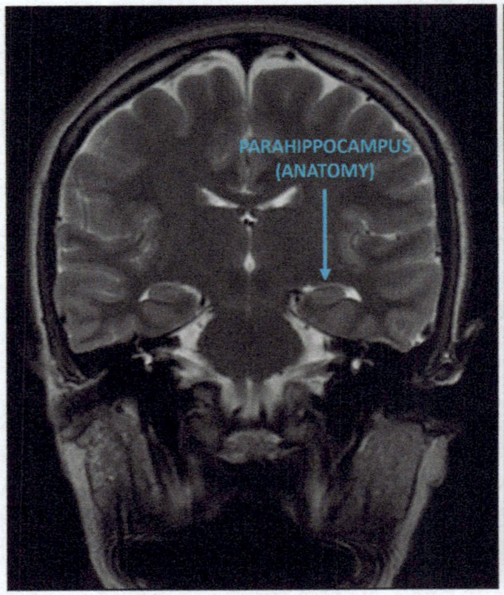

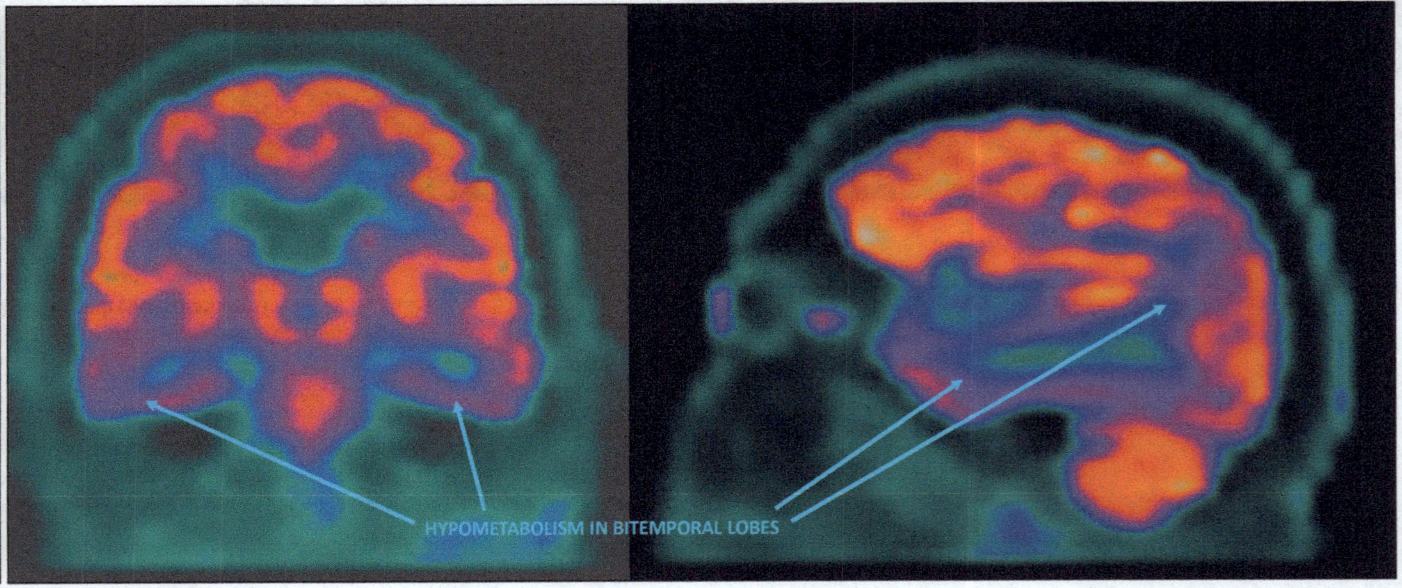

NEURORADIOLOGY

FRONTOTEMPORAL DEMENTIA

IMAGING: Asymmetric **atrophy of the frontotemporal lobes**

USMLE POINTS:
Pick's disease
Degenerative disease of frontal and temporal lobes
Behavioral (disinhibitions) and language problems early in the disease → Dementia
Histology: Pick Bodies → Ubiquinated TDP-43 & round aggregates of hyperphosphorylated tau protein
Silver stain+

MODALITIES: CT WO / MRI WO

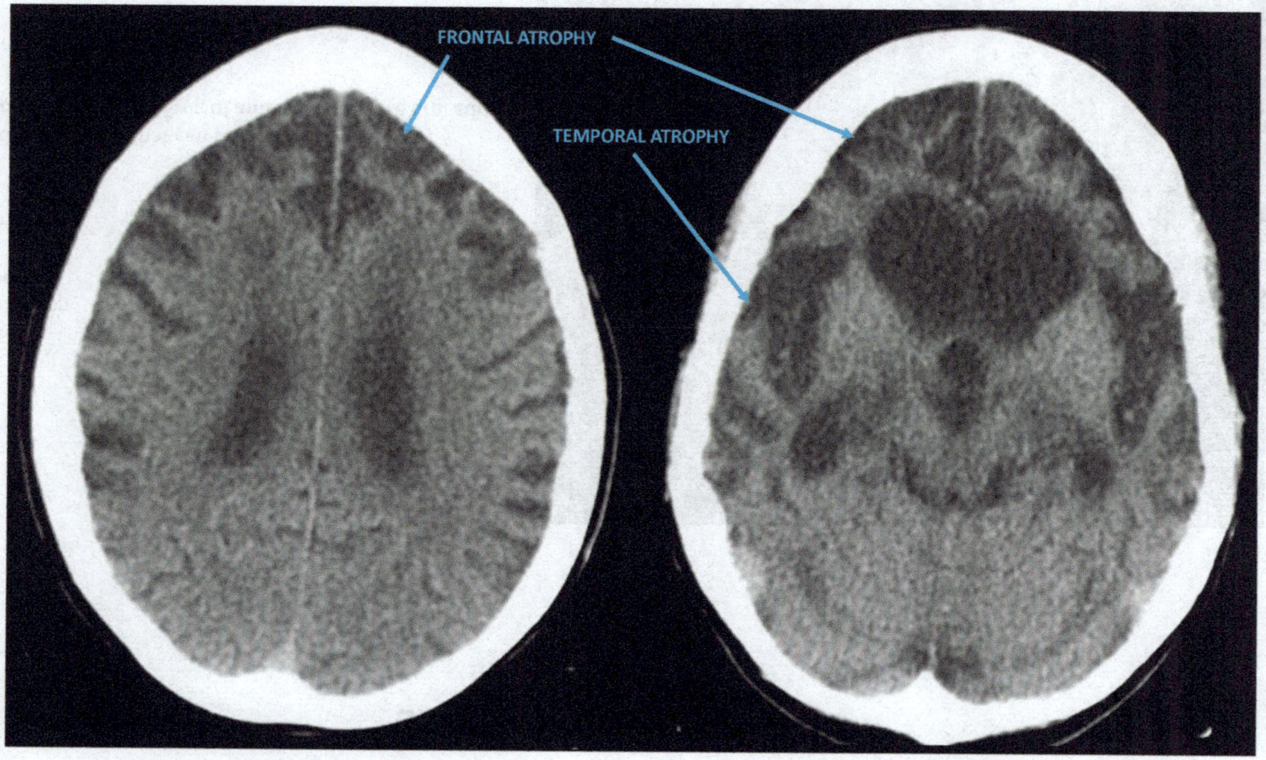

NEURORADIOLOGY

BRAIN ABSCESS

IMAGING: Rim enhancing lesion (MAGIC DR)

Mets
Abscess
Gliomastoma
Infarct
Contusion

Demyelinating (incomplete ring)
Radiation necrosis

USMLE POINTS:

Associated with liquefactive necrosis
Infection is often polymicrobial
Infections of contiguous structures: Otitis media, Dental infection, Mastoiditis

Treatment: Ceftriaxone / Cefotaxime + **Metronidazole**
Vancomycin

Nocardia: Filamentous-branching gram-positive organism that can cause brain abscess
Suspect this is patient had recent **dental work** (2000mg of **amoxicillin** before procedure)

MODALITIES: MRI WWO

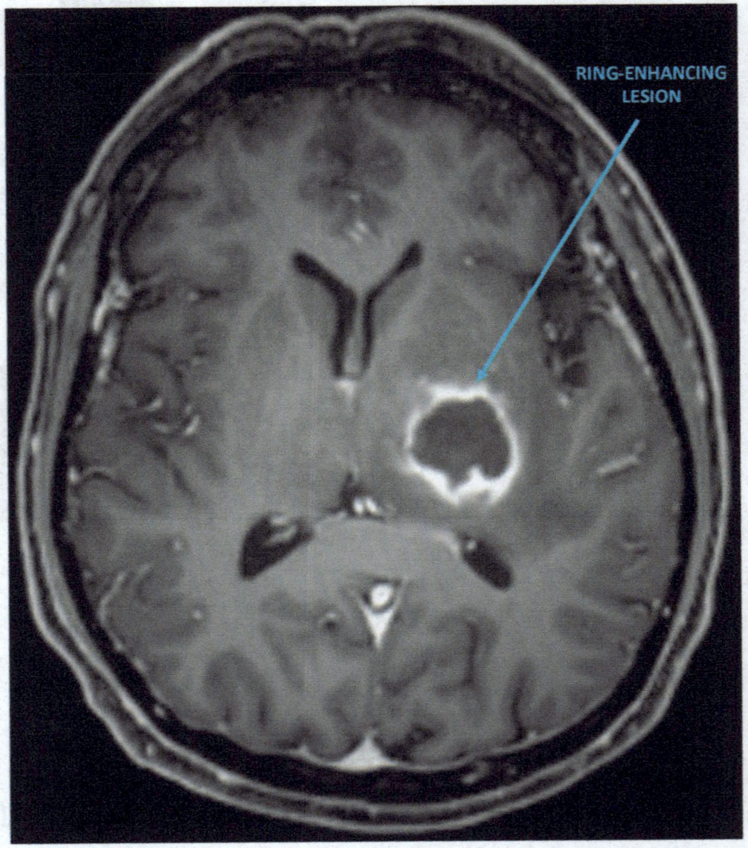

NEURORADIOLOGY

TOXOPLASMOSIS

IMAGING:

CT: Multiple hypodense regions predominantly in the **basal ganglia** and at the corticomedullary junction

MRI: **Ring enhancement or nodular enhancement within the basal ganglia**

USMLE POINTS:

Cat stuff (dirty cat litter)

Protozoa → encephalitis and ring enhancing lesions in HIV patients

May cross placenta → Congenital chorioretinitis, hydrocephalus, intracranial calcifications, and deafness

Treatment: **Pyrimethamine/Sulfadiazine**

TMP-SMX prophylaxis is indicated in AIDS patients with a CD4 count of less than 100

MODALITIES: MRI WWO

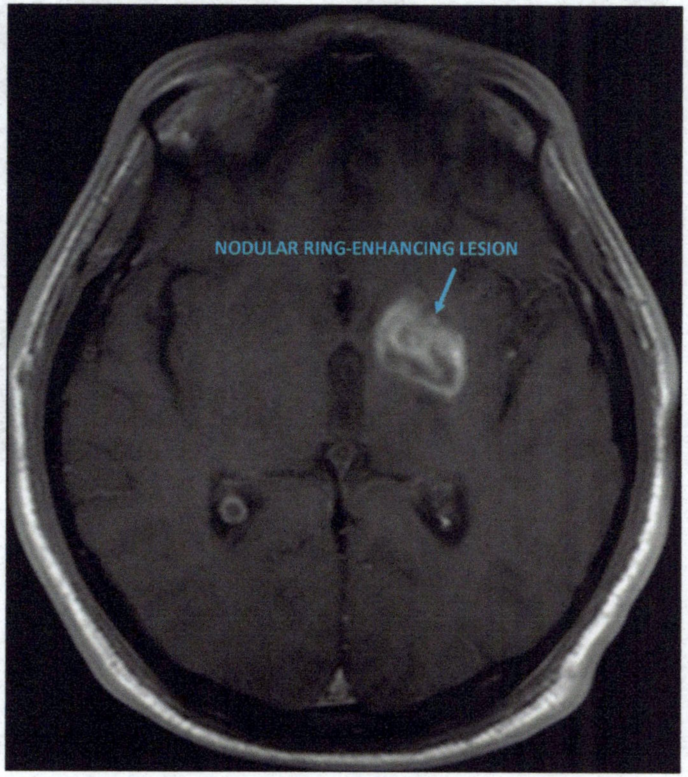

NEURORADIOLOGY

BROWN-SEQUARD SYNDROME

IMAGING: Damage to right or left side of **hemi-cord**

USMLE POINTS: Presentation:

Ipsilateral	**Loss of vibration, proprioception, and touch below the level of the lesion**	→	**Due to dorsal column damage**
Ipsilateral	**Upper motoneuron signs below the level of the lesion**	→	**Due to corticospinal tract damage**
Contralateral	**Loss of pain and temperature below the level of the lesion**	→	**Due to spinothalamic tract damage**
Ipsilateral	Loss of all sensation at the level of the lesion		
Ipsilateral	Lower motoneuron signs at the level of the lesion		

MODALITIES: MR WO

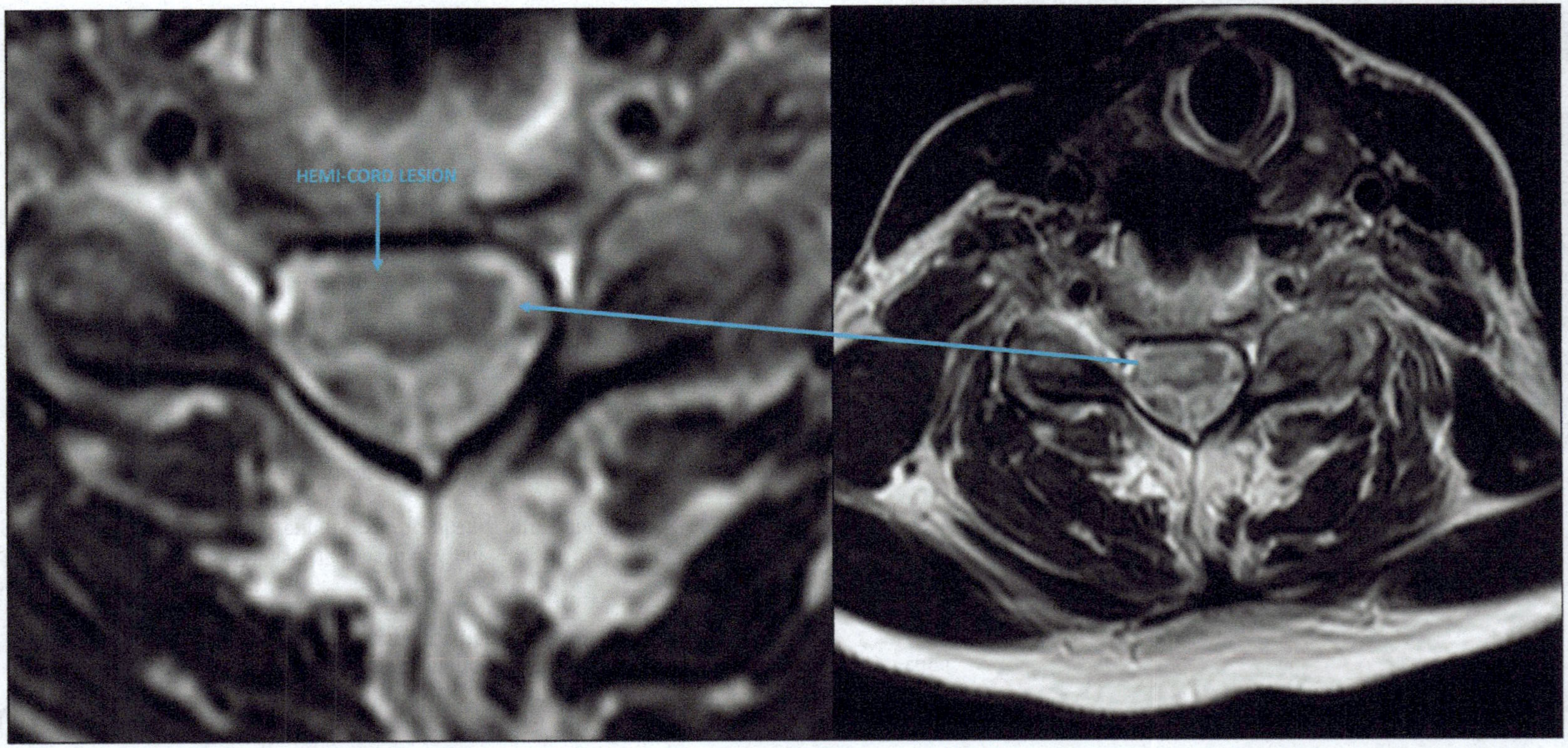

NEURORADIOLOGY

SUBACUTE COMBINED DEGENERATION

IMAGING: **Symmetric, bilateral increased signal within the dorsal columns**

USMLE POINTS: Due to **Vitamin B12 deficiency**
Demyelination of spinocerebellar tracts, lateral corticospinal tracts, and dorsal columns
Loss of vibration and proprioception in the hands and feet
Eventual progression to sensory loss of all modalities, sensory gait ataxia, and distal muscle weakness
Physical exam:
- + Romberg
- + Babinski
- Spastic paresis in legs
- Lower extremity hyperreflexia

MODALITIES: MRI WO

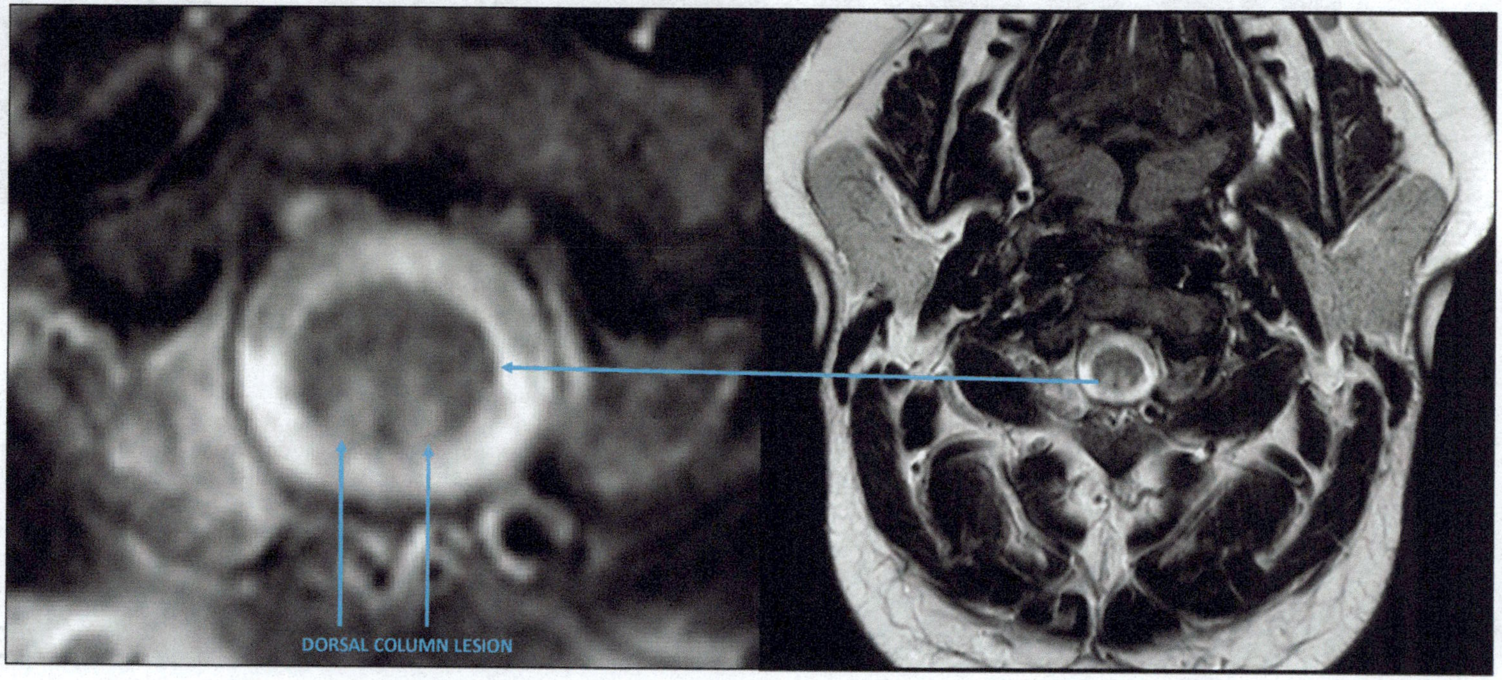

NEURORADIOLOGY

CAUDA-EQUINA SYNDROME

IMAGING:
Compression of the cauda equina nerve **roots (L2 and below)**
Fracture, Infection, Mass/Tumor
Collection of L1-S5 peripheral nerves within the lumbar canal

USMLE POINTS:
Presentation: Gradual, severe radicular pain, asymmetrical weakness, **saddle anesthesia and bowel/bladder dysfunction**
Cauda equina compression interrupts the nerves forming the bladder reflex arc

Bladder innervations:

Parasympathetic	→	Promotes urination
Sympathetic	→	Promotes urinary retention

Spinal cord tumors:

Intramedullary	→	Inside the spinal cord	→	**Ependymoma / Astrocytoma**
Intradural extramedullary	→	Outside the spinal cord but in the spinal sac	→	**Meningioma / Schwannoma / Neurofibroma**
Extradural	→	Outside the spinal canal	→	Degenerative disc disease

MODALITIES: MRI WO

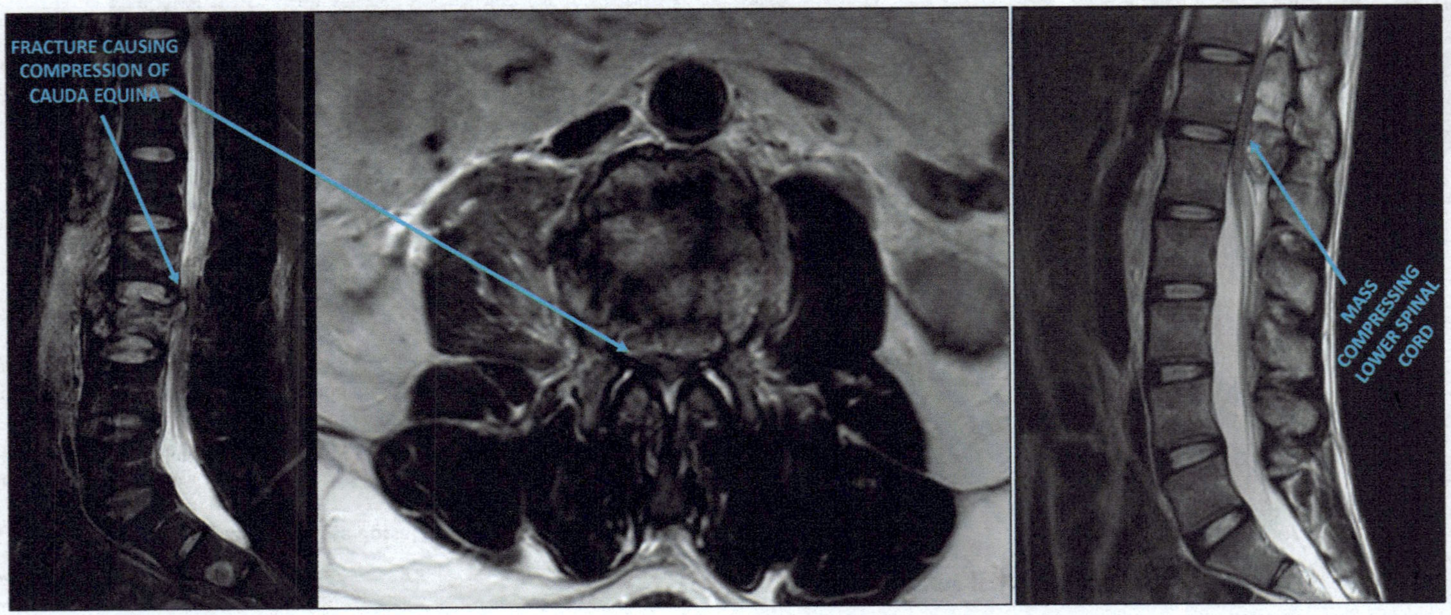

NEURORADIOLOGY

CREUTZFELDT-JACOB DISEASE

IMAGING: **Pulvinar ("hockey-stick") sign**
Cortical Ribbon sign

USMLE POINTS: Abnormal **prion** proteins
Rapidly progressive dementia + ataxia & myoclonus

EEG: **Periodic sharp wave complexes**

Association: Increased **14-3-3** protein in CSF
Neuropathologist / Neurosurgical transmission

Histology: Vacuole formation in grey matter structures that develops into cysts

MODALITIES: MRI WWO

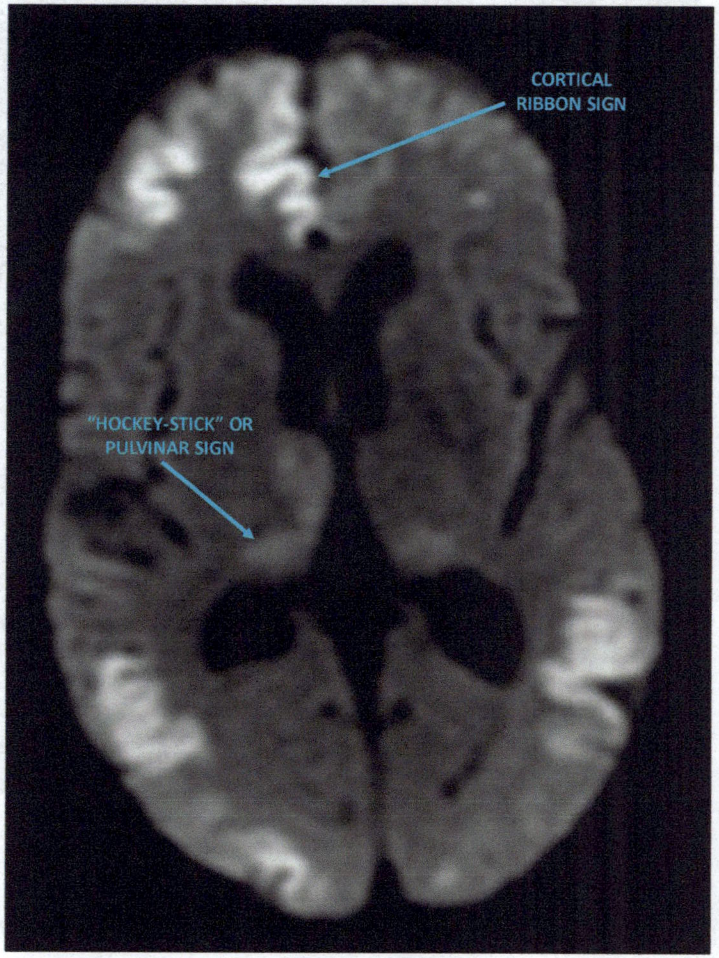

NEURORADIOLOGY

CRANIOPHARYNGIOMA

IMAGING: **Calcified suprasellar mass in a child**

USMLE POINTS: CN 3 Compression → **Bitemporal hemianopsia (loss of peripheral vision)**
Commonly occur in pituitary stalk, causing hypopituitarism
Childhood tumor:
- Benign CNS tumor from epithelial **remnants of Rathke's pouch**
- Filled with cholesterol crystals and calcification
- Tend to recur after resection

Suprasellar Masses:
- S: Sarcoid
- A: Aneurysm, **Adenoma**
- T: Teratoma or tuberculosis (and other granulomatous diseases)
- C: **Craniopharyngioma**, cleft cyst (Rathke's), chordoma
- H: Hypothalamic glioma, hamartoma of tuber cinereum, histiocytosis
- M: Meningioma, metastasis
- O: Optic nerve glioma

MODALITIES: MRI WWO

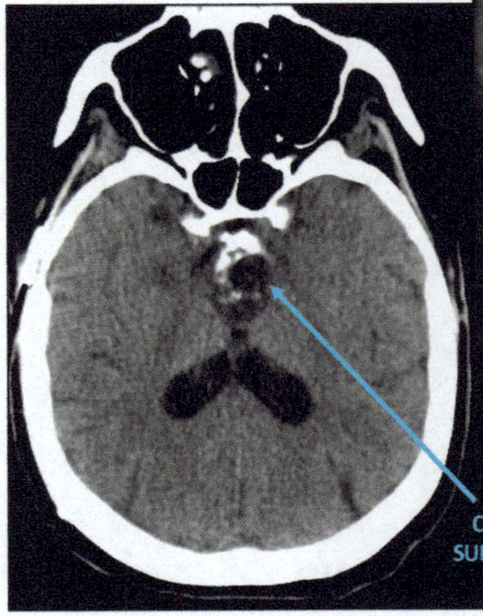

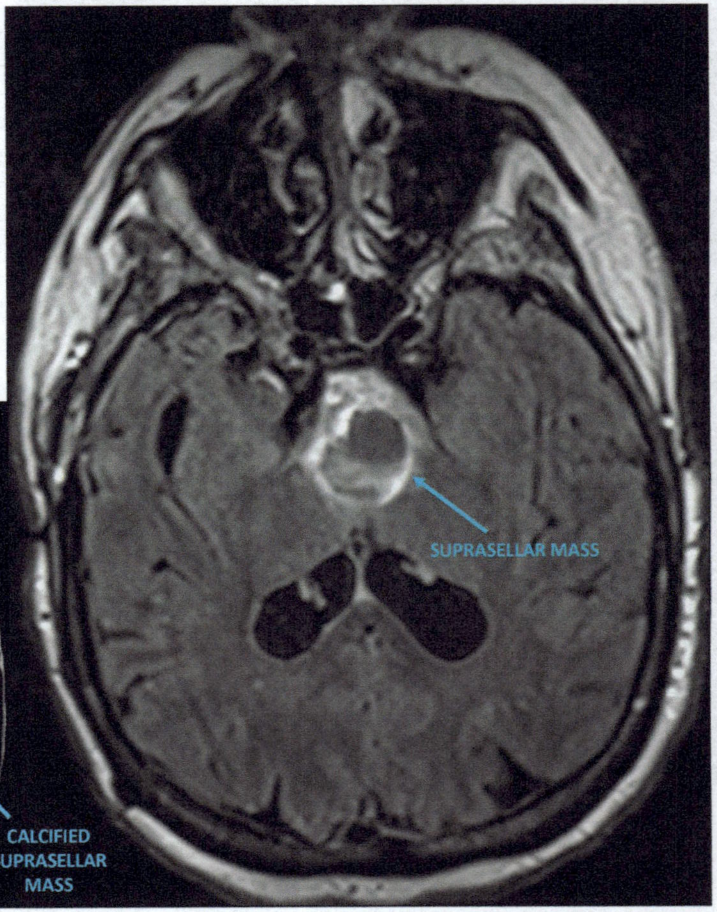

NEURORADIOLOGY

DIFFUSE AXONAL INJURY

IMAGING: **Punctate hemorrhages at the grey-white matter junctions**
Commonly affects the corpus callosum and brain stem

USMLE POINTS: Significant neuronal damage → **Decerebrate or decorticate posturing, coma**
Type of brain injury that typically occurs from traumatic **acceleration/deceleration shearing forces** → Due to different moments of inertia
Often from MVA

MODALITIES: CT WO → MRI WO (SWI)

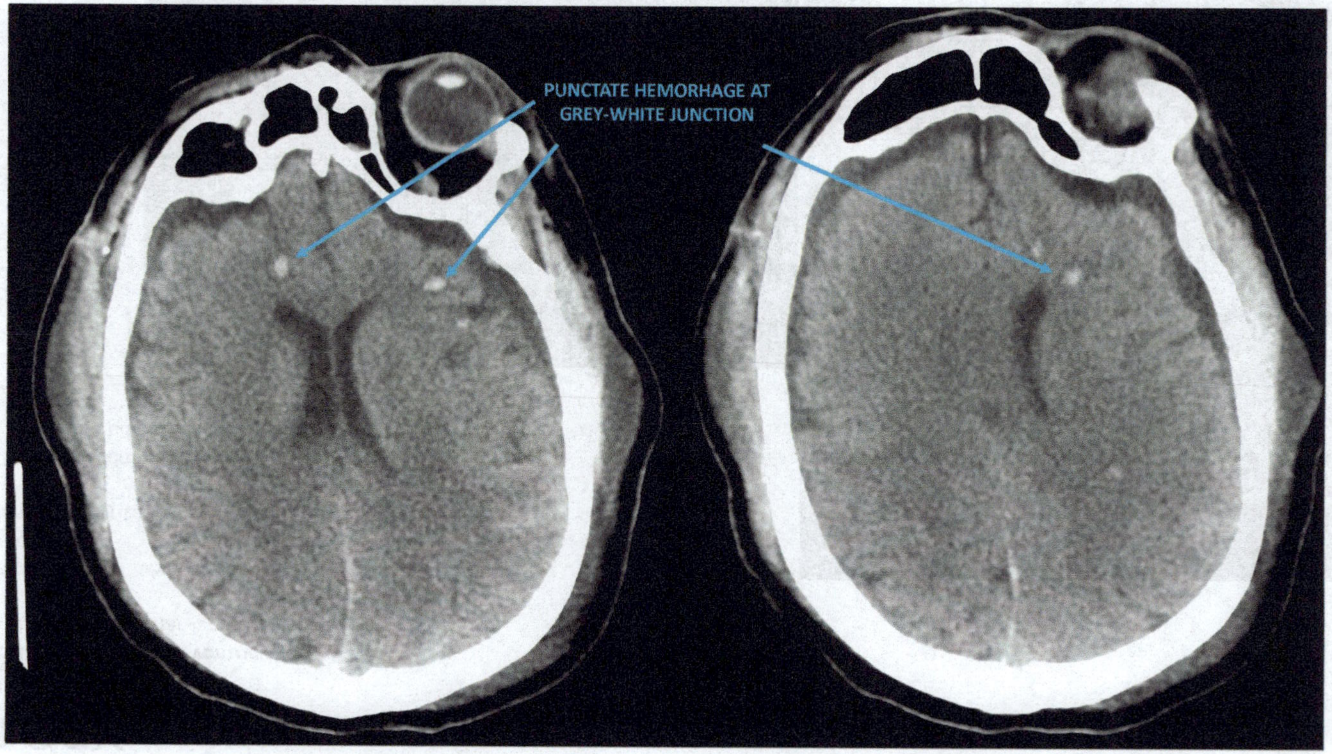

NEURORADIOLOGY

DANDY-WALKER SYNDROME

IMAGING:

Hypoplasia of the vermis
Massive cystic dilation of the 4th ventricle
Enlarged posterior fossa (torcular-lambdoid inversion)

USMLE POINTS:

Due to congenital failure of development of the cerebellar vermis
Cause of macrocephaly
May require ventriculoperitoneal shunt catheter

Associations: Non-communicating hydrocephalus
Spina bifida

MODALITIES: MRI WO

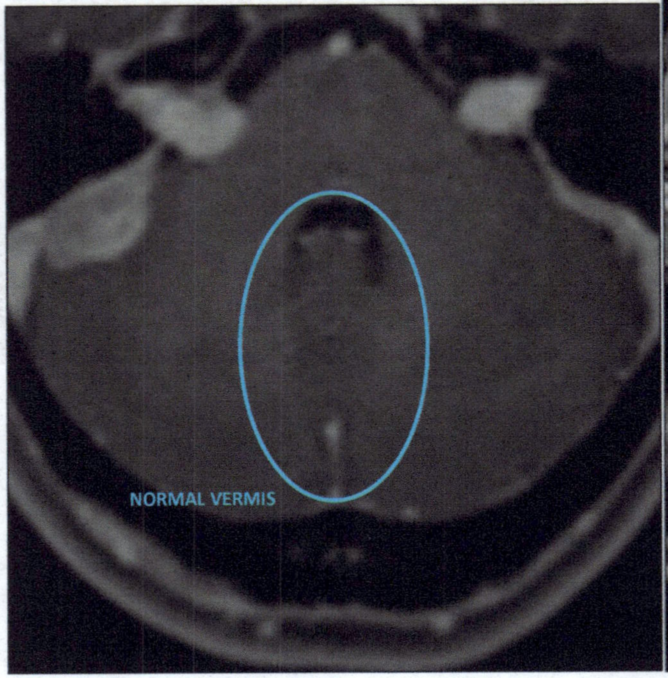

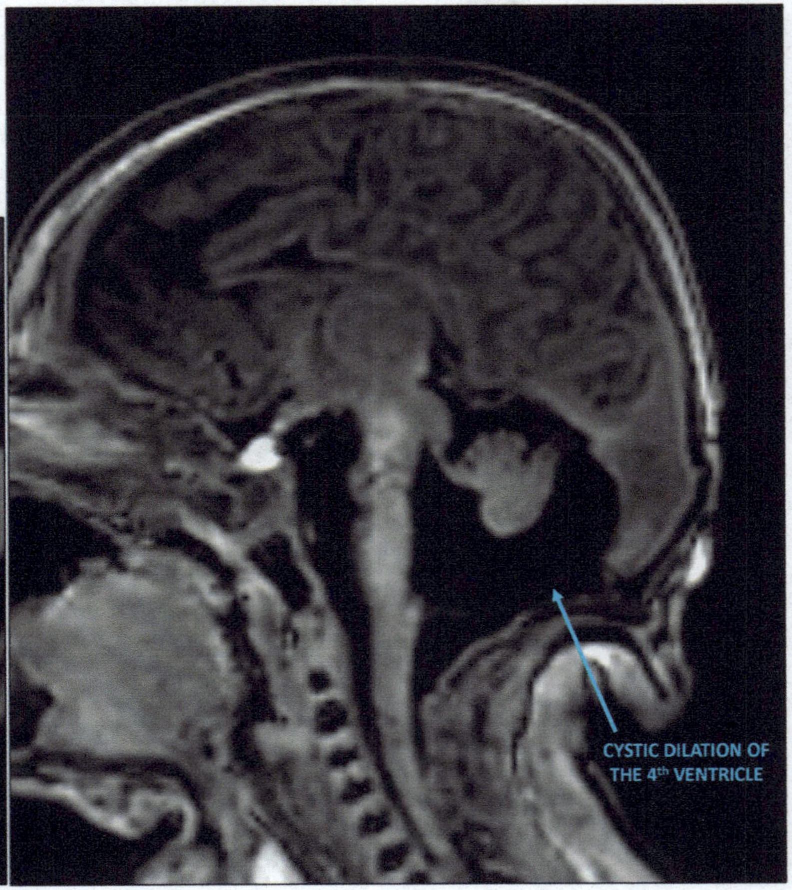

NEURORADIOLOGY

DURAL SINUS THROMBOSIS

IMAGING: **Filling defect within the dural venous sinuses**
Superior sagittal sinus, Transverse sinus, straight sinus, sigmoid sinus

USMLE POINTS: Associated with hypercoagulable states: **Female on OCP**
Factor-V Leiden mutation, Factor-V Leiden mutation, protein C / S deficiency, Antithrombin deficiency
J&J Covid-vaccine

May cause cerebral infarct that doesn't adhere to arterial distribution

MODALITIES: CTV / MRV

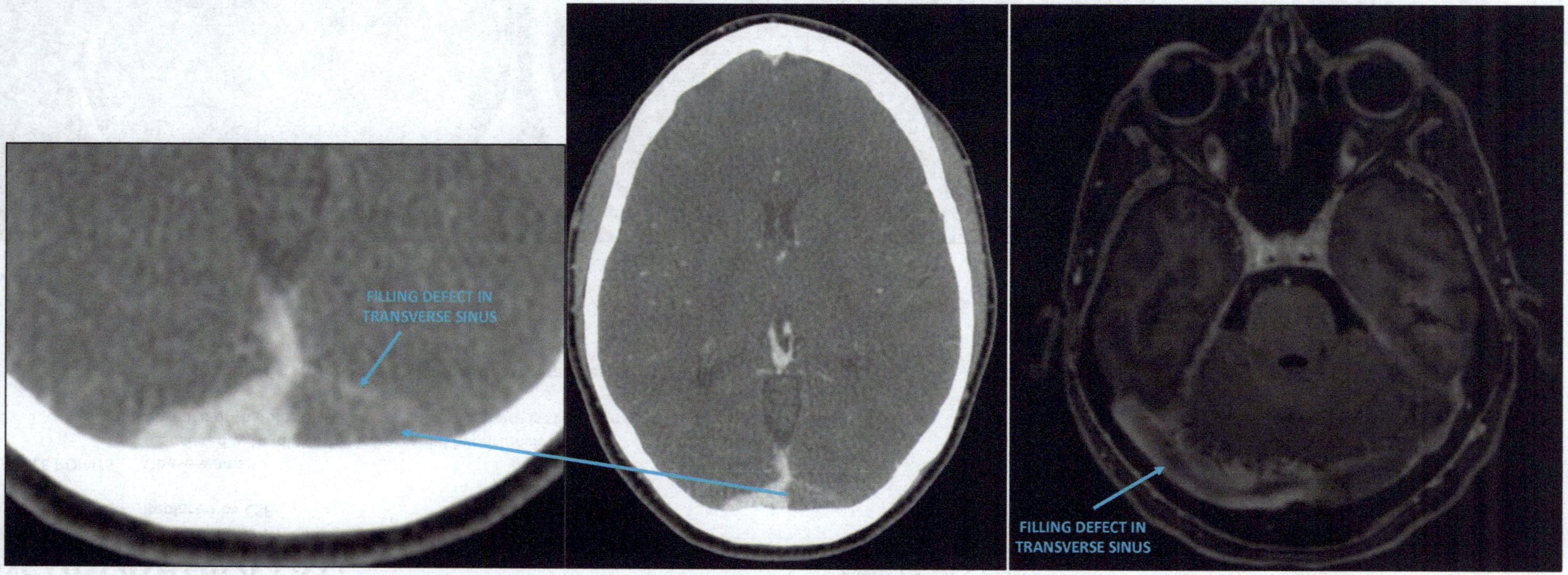

NEURORADIOLOGY

EMPTY SELLA

IMAGING: **Pituitary fossa which is largely empty**
Replaced by CSF

USMLE POINTS: **Obese** woman
Associated with **Idiopathic intracranial hypertension**
Absence of the pituitary gland on imaging (there is still some functional pituitary tissue)

Neurohypophysis: Hyperintense (neurosecretory granules)
Vasopressin (ADH) & Oxytocin
Arises from neuroectoderm

MODALITIES: MRI WO

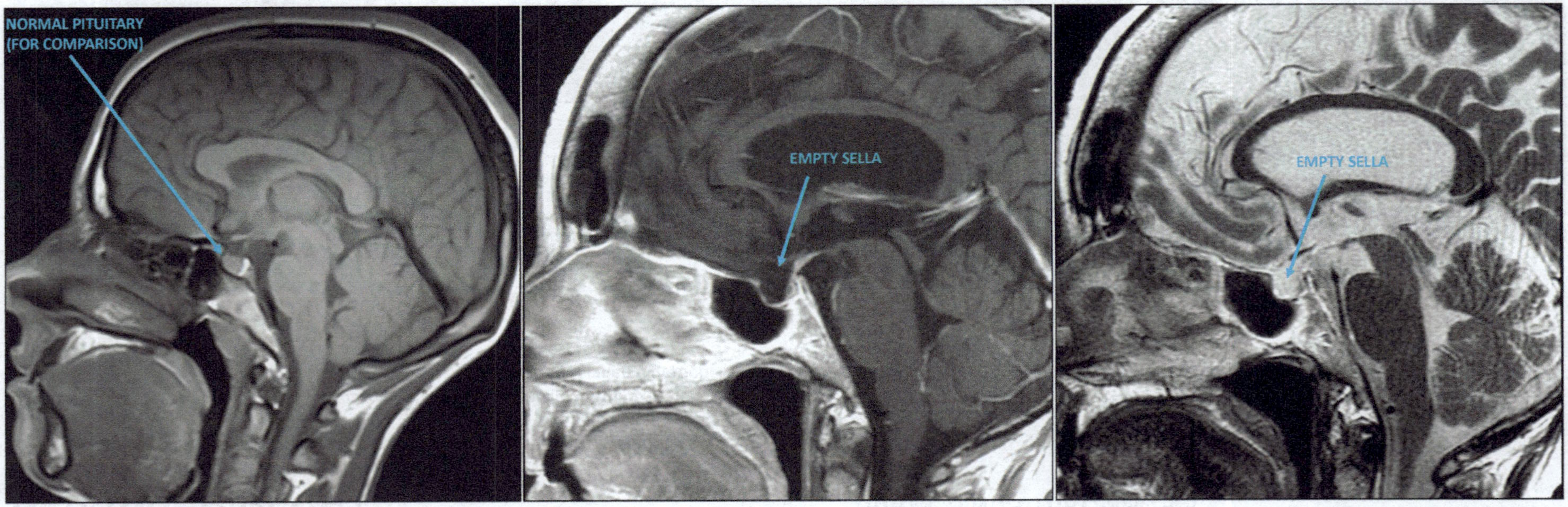

NEURORADIOLOGY

GLIOBLASTOMA MULTIFORME

IMAGING:

Large, aggressive brain neoplasm
Thick, irregular-enhancing margins
Central necrotic core (hemorrhage)
Crosses corpus callosum → **"Butterfly" glioma**
Midline crossing lesions → MS, Lymphoma, GBM

USMLE POINTS:

Most common primary malignant CNS tumor in adults
High-grade tumor of astrocytes **(High grade astrocytoma)**
Characterized by endothelial cell proliferation
Poor prognosis, **1-year median survival**
GFAP+

Histology: **Pseudo-palisading tumor cells (tumor** cells surrounding regions of necrosis)

Associations:
Turcot syndrome
Li-Fraumeni syndrome
Lynch syndrome
Cowden syndrome

MODALITIES: MRI WWO

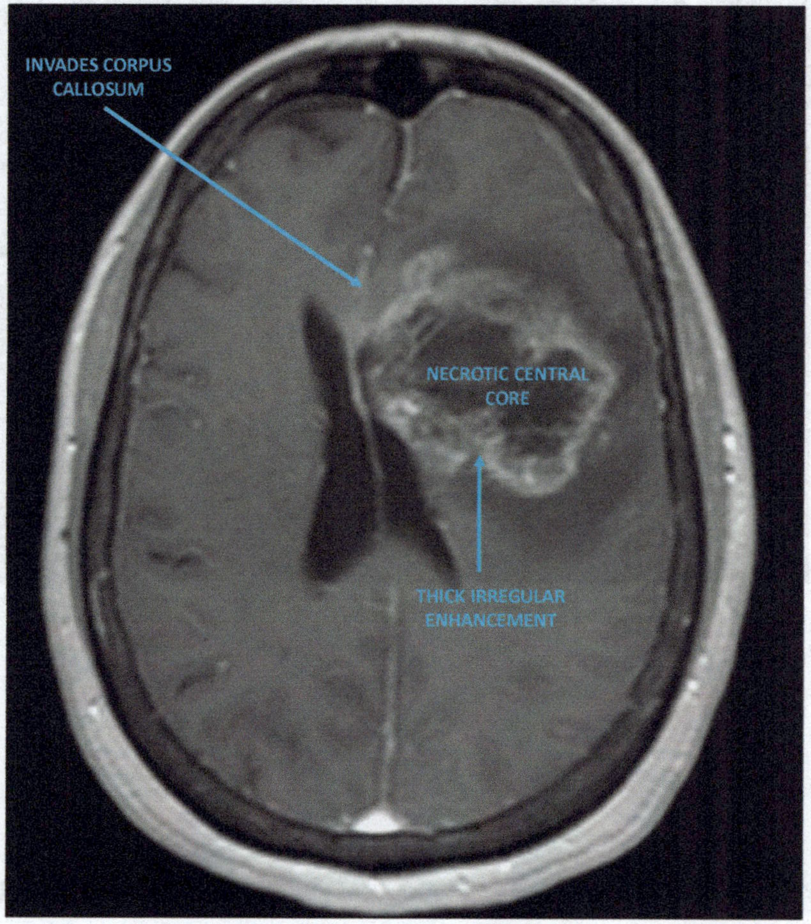

NEURORADIOLOGY

HEMANGIOBLASTOMA

IMAGING: Posterior fossa tumor with **cyst + enhancing mural nodule**
- Adult: **Hemangioblastoma**
- Kid: Astrocytoma (GAME)

USMLE POINTS:
- Associated with **VHL (Chromosome 3)**
- Occur in the **cerebellum and retina**
- PAS+ and are prone to rupture & subsequent hemorrhage
- Tumor may produce **erythropoietin**

VHL:
- **Hemangioblastoma**
- **RCC (clear-cell)**
- Retinal capillary hemangioblastoma
- **Pheochromocytoma**
- Endolymphatic sack tumor
- Pancreatic tumors

MODALITIES: MRI WWO

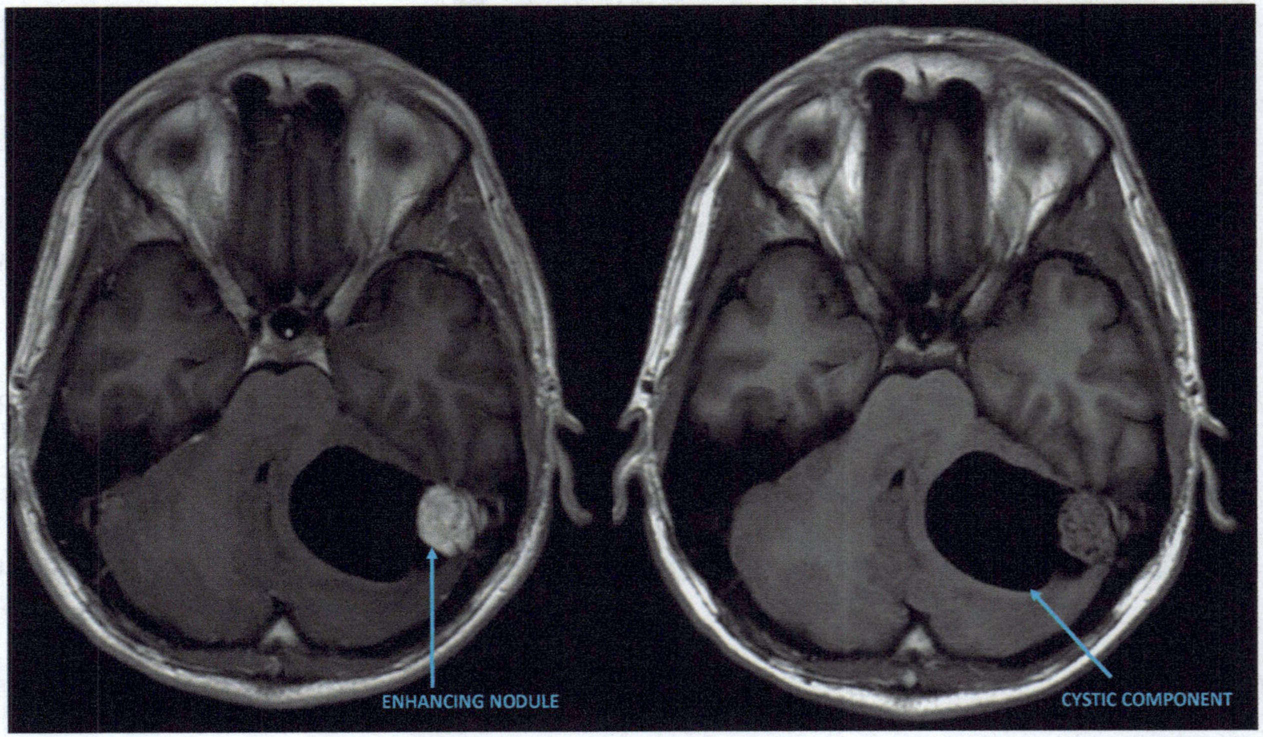

NEURORADIOLOGY

HERPES ENCEPHALITIS

IMAGING: **Asymmetric signal changes in a temporal lobe**
Basal ganglia are typically spared, helping distinguish it from an MCA infarct

USMLE POINTS: **HSV-1**
Edema and hemorrhagic necrosis of the temporal lobe (basal ganglia spared)

Presentation: Seizures, Fever, Headache, N/V

Diagnosis: **PCR** – gold standard

Treatment: **Acyclovir ASAP (IV** fluids to prevent crystalline nephropathy)
Foscarnet for acyclovir-resistant herpes

LP:

Bacterial:	Increased opening pressure	Increased PMN	Decrease glucose
Viral:	**Normal opening pressure**	**Increased lymphocytes**	**Normal glucose**
Fungal:	Increased opening pressure	Increased lymphocytes	Decreased glucose

MODALITIES: MRI WO

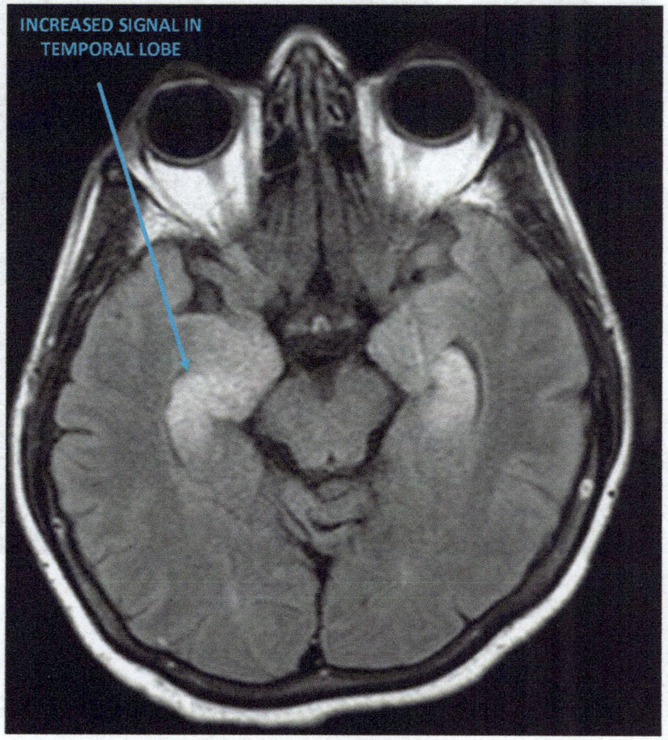

NEURORADIOLOGY

CAROTID ARTERY DISSECTION

IMAGING: **Blood entering the media through a tear in the intima – Can often see dissection flap**
Hyperintense crescent-shaped rim and decreased lumen

USMLE POINTS: Stroke in young patient
Most commonly caused by neck trauma (strangulation / MVA)

Triad: Ipsilateral neck pain
Horner syndrome
Cerebral or retinal ischemia

Treatment: tPA
Antithrombotic or antiplatelet therapy
Endovascular / Surgical repair

MODALITIES: CTA / MRA

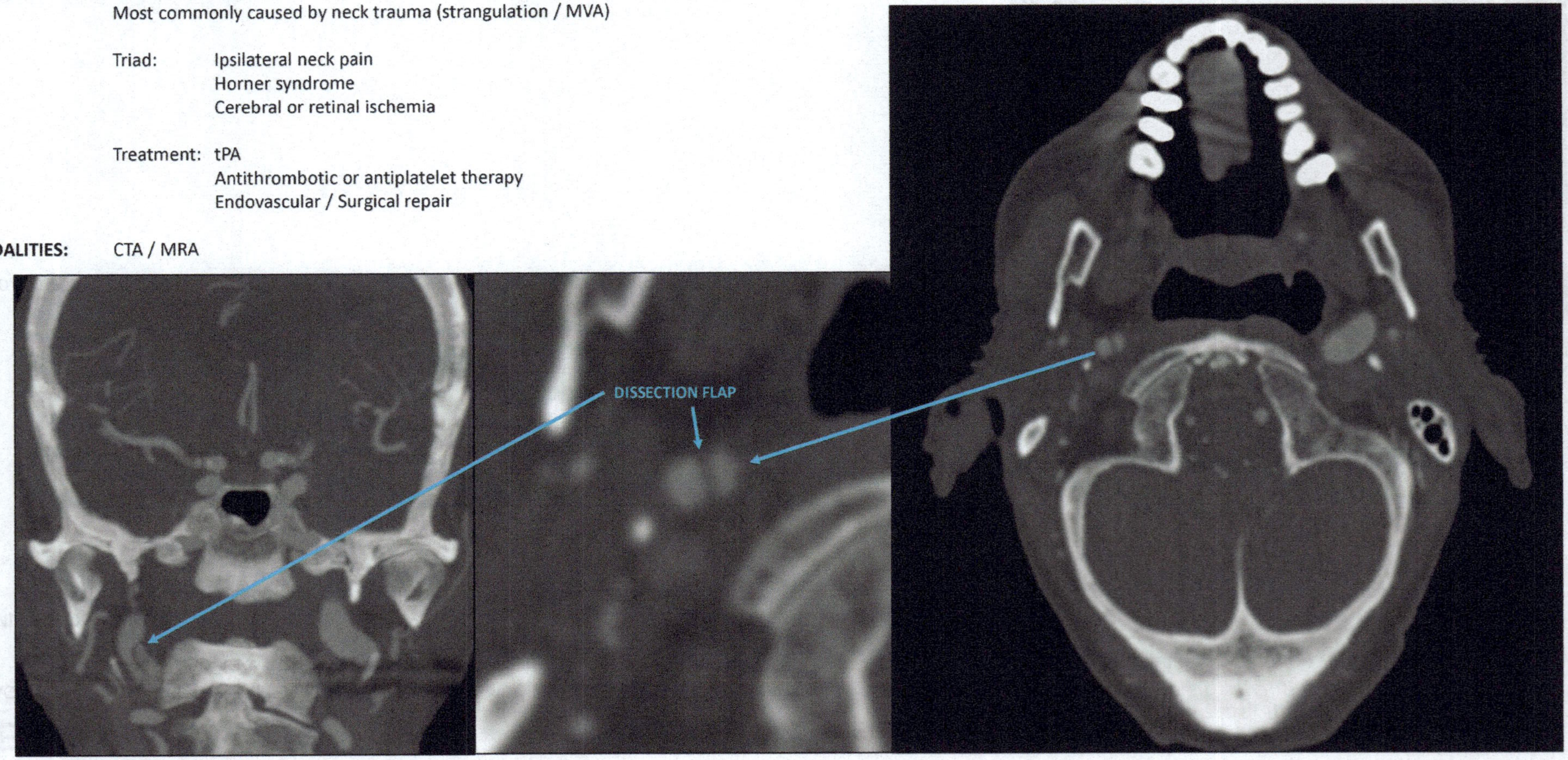

NEURORADIOLOGY

VERTEBRAL ARTERY DISSECTION

IMAGING: **Blood entering the media through a tear in the intima**

USMLE POINTS:
Chiropractic manipulation
Most common cause of **Wallenberg Syndrome (lateral medullary syndrome)**
Course through the transverse foramina in the neck and thus can easily be injured by cervical spinal trauma

MODALITIES: CTA / MRA

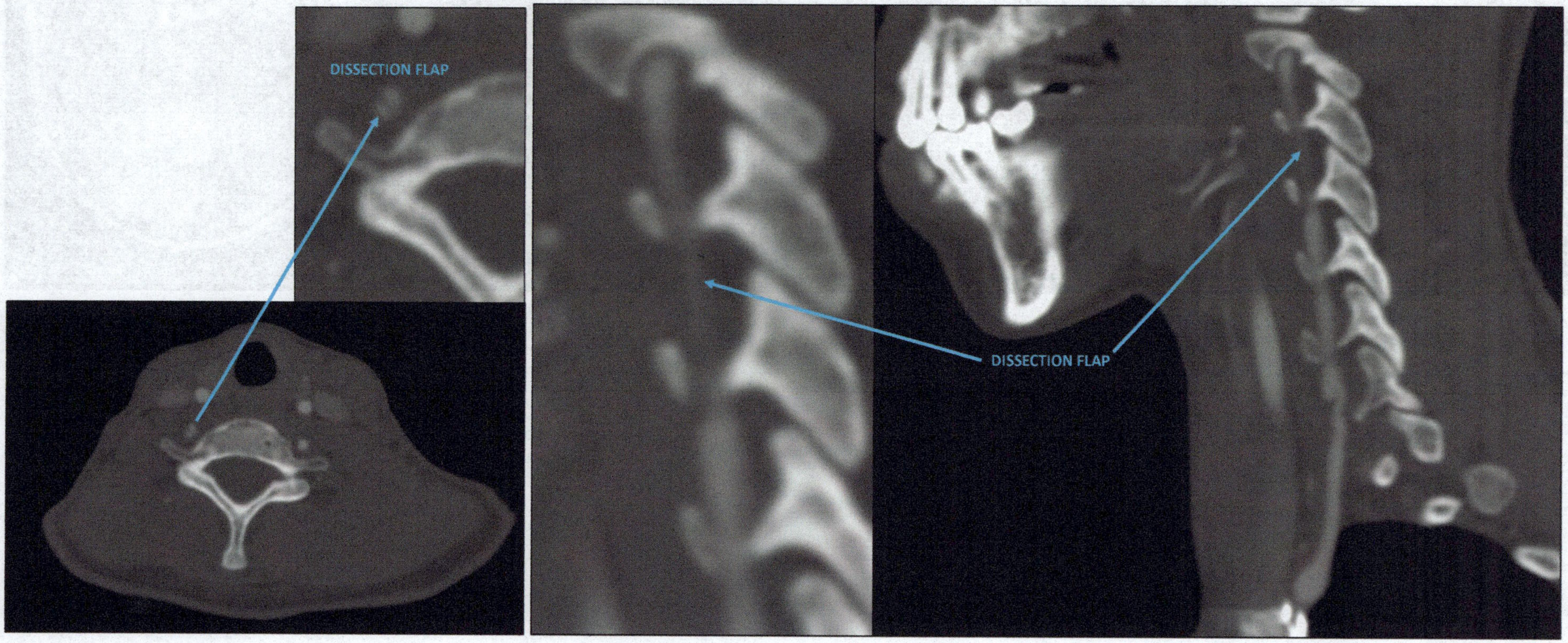

NEURORADIOLOGY

MENINGIOMA

IMAGING:
- **Broad based Dural attachment ("tail")**
- **Extra-axial tumor → mass effect on brain**
- **Vasogenic edema**

USMLE POINTS:
- Benign tumor of arachnoid cells
- **Most common primary benign CNS tumor in adults**
- Histology: Whorled pattern +/- psammoma bodies
- Associations: **NF2, MEN1**
- Treatment: Radiation therapy (non-accessible), Surgical resection depending on size and patient symptoms

MODALITIES: MRI WWO

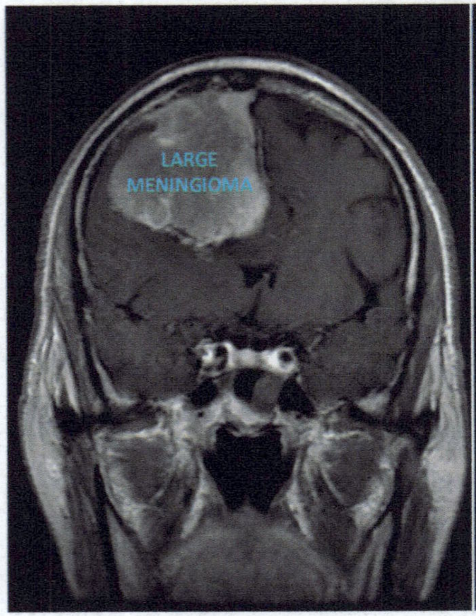

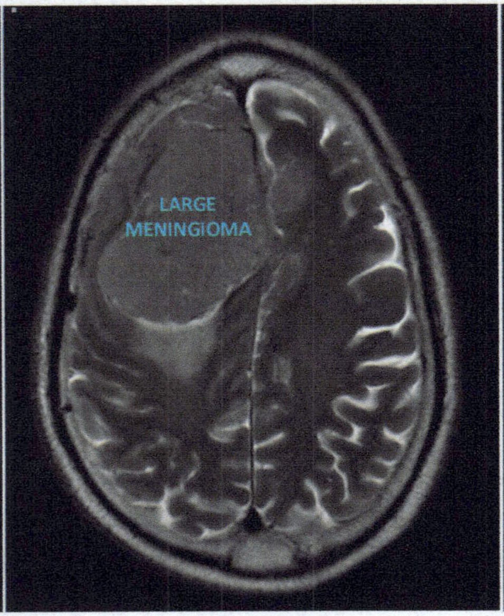

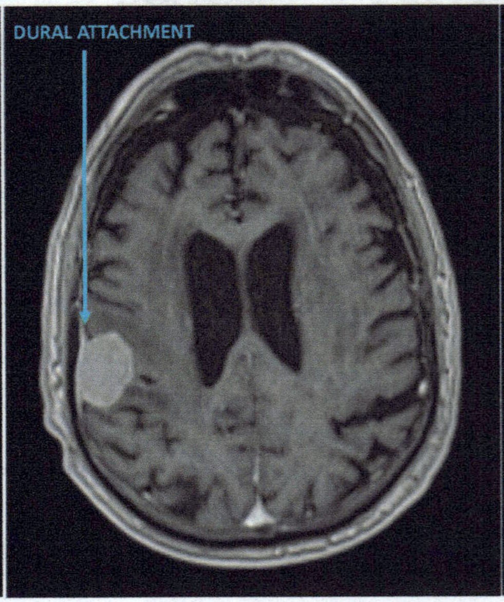

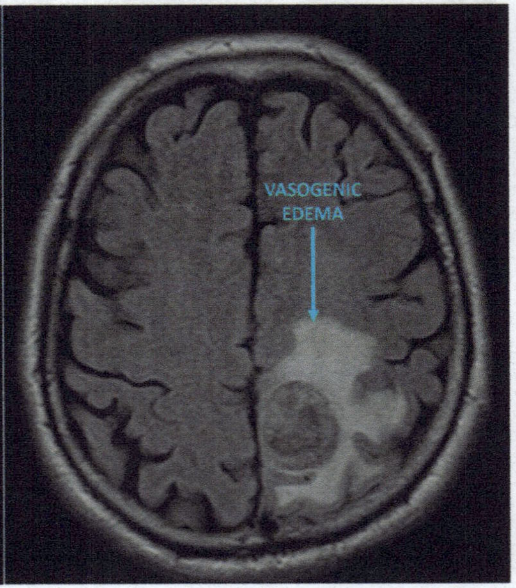

NEURORADIOLOGY

MENINGITIS

IMAGING: Inflammation of the subarachnoid space: Arachnoid mater & Pia mater

USMLE POINTS: Infectious or noninfectious process
Inflammation → cerebral edema → vasogenic intracranial hypertension → Herniation → Death

Waterhouse friderichsen syndrome

Petechial rash → Neisseria meningitidis

Associations: Neurosarcoidosis
Behcet syndrome (penile ulcers)

Medications: TMP-SMX
IVIG
Infliximab

Presentation: Nuchal rigidity, Kernig sign, Brudzinski sign
Hydrocephalus, hearing loss, and seizures, secondary to fibrosis

LP:

Bacterial:	**Increased opening pressure**	**Increased PMN**	**Decrease glucose**
Viral:	**Normal opening pressure**	**Increased lymphocytes**	**Normal glucose**
Fungal:	**Increased opening pressure**	**Increased lymphocytes**	**Decreased glucose**

MODALITIES: MRI WWO

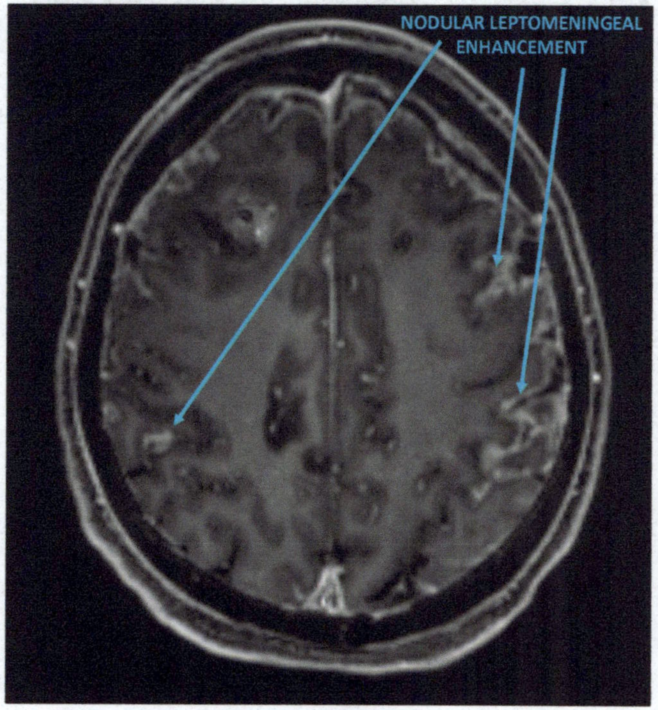

NEURORADIOLOGY

PITUITARY ADENOMA

IMAGING:

Microadenoma: **Low signal lesion in the pituitary**
Smaller than 1 cm

Macroadenoma: **Large lesion in the pituitary (suprasellar mass)**
Larger than 1 cm → Compresses optic chiasm

USMLE POINTS:

Microadenoma: Most commonly hormonally active → Most commonly prolactin secreting
No visual field defects
Octreotide, Bromocriptine, Cabergoline

Macroadenoma: **CN 3 Compression → Bitemporal hemianopsia (loss of peripheral vision)**
Not usually hormonally active (unlike microadenoma)
Transsphenoidal resection

Suprasellar Masses:
- S: Sarcoid
- A: Aneurysm, **Adenoma**
- T: Teratoma or tuberculosis (and other granulomatous diseases)
- C: **Craniopharyngioma**, cleft cyst (Rathke), chordoma
- H: Hypothalamic glioma, hamartoma of tuber cinereum, histiocytosis
- M: Meningioma, metastasis
- O: Optic nerve glioma

MODALITIES: MRI WWO

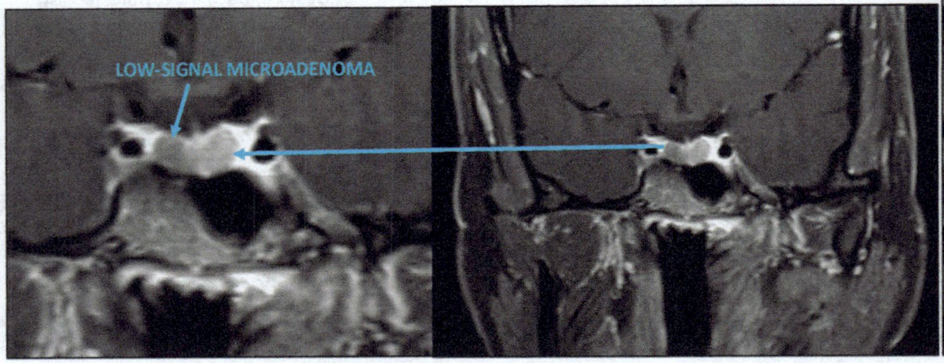

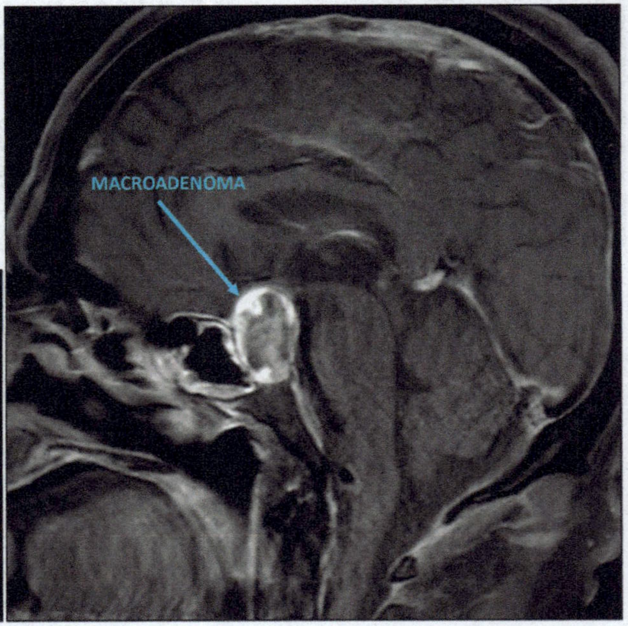

NEURORADIOLOGY

ORBITAL CELLULITIS

IMAGING: Pre- and post-septal infection
May extend into ethmoid air cells

USMLE POINTS: Bacterial spread from ethmoidal or maxillary sinusitis
May progress to subperiosteal abscess
Staphylococcus aureus and streptococci (most common)

Presentation: **Proptosis**
Ophthalmoplegia
Visual changes

Risk Factors: **Bacterial rhinosinusitis**

MODALITIES: CT W / MRI WWO

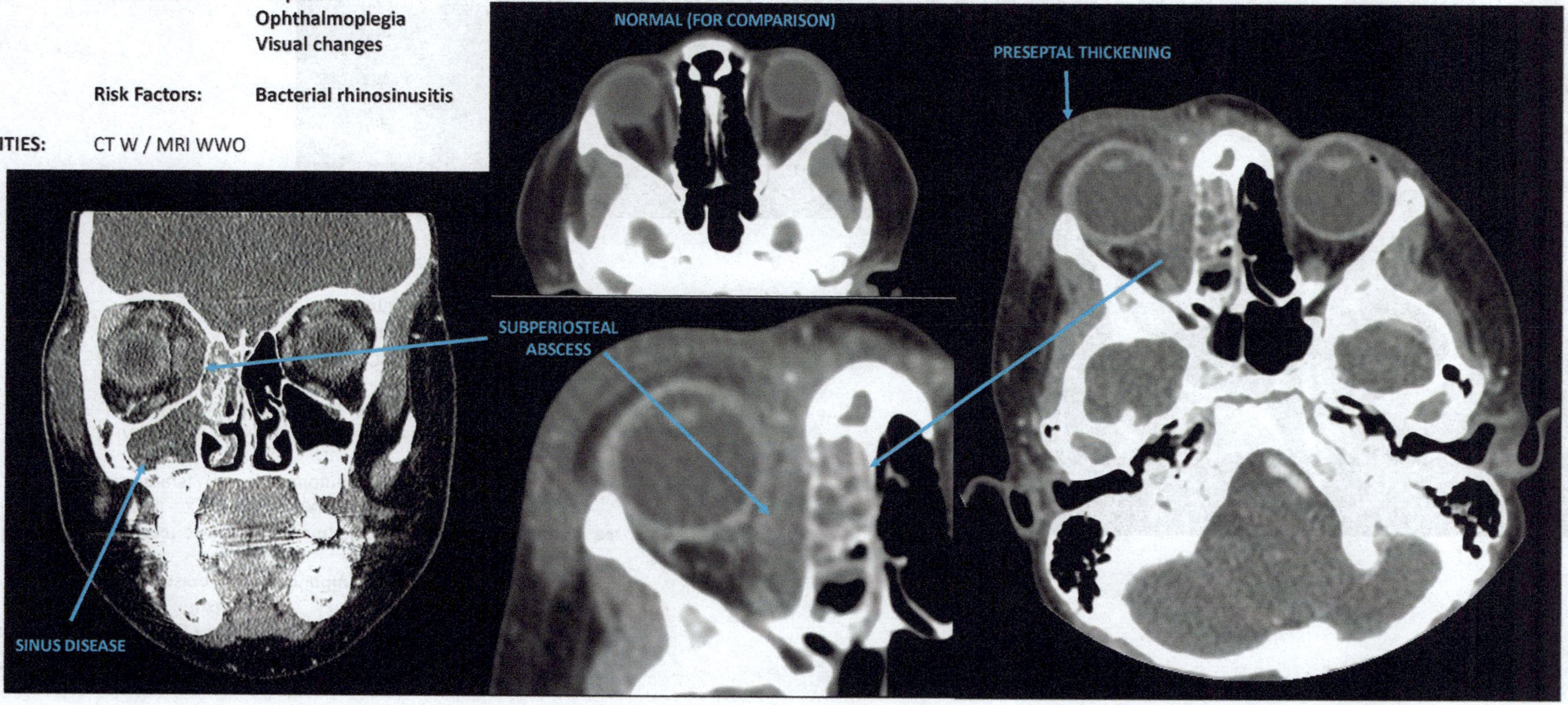

NEURORADIOLOGY

OTITIS EXTERNA

IMAGING:
Thickening / induration of the peri-auricular soft tissue
Mastoid effusions
No extension into the middle ear

USMLE POINTS:
Presentation: **Ear pain, discharge, erythema of outer ear**
Trauma: S. Aureus
Swimmers: Pseudomonas

Disruption of protective barriers in external auditory canal → Cellulitis
Uncomplicated otitis externa → Children

Malignant otitis externa: Otomastoiditis
Can spread to deeper tissues (seen with diabetic patients)
Immunocompromised patients

MODALITIES: CT W (TEMPORAL BONE STUDY)

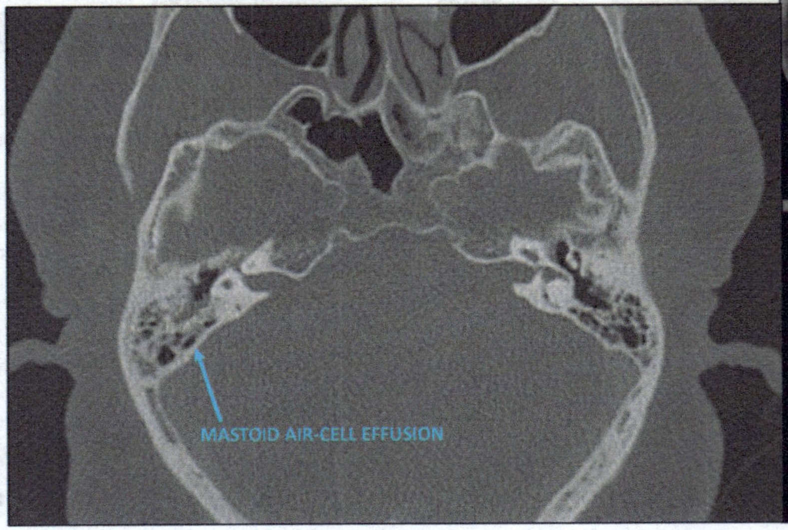

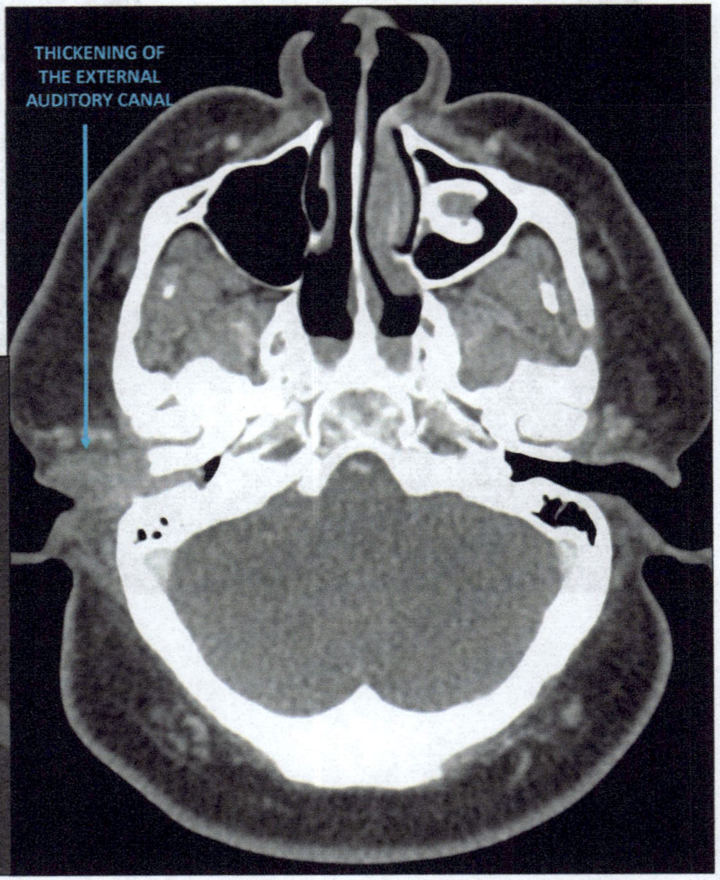

NEURORADIOLOGY

SIALOLITHIASIS

IMAGING: **Wharton's duct → Dilated submandibular gland**
Stenson's Duct → Dilated parotid gland

USMLE POINTS: Presents as recurrent pre/peri-prandial pain and swelling in affected gland
Submandibular duct obstruction more common
Edematous / inflamed salivary glands due to obstruction

MODALITIES: CT W

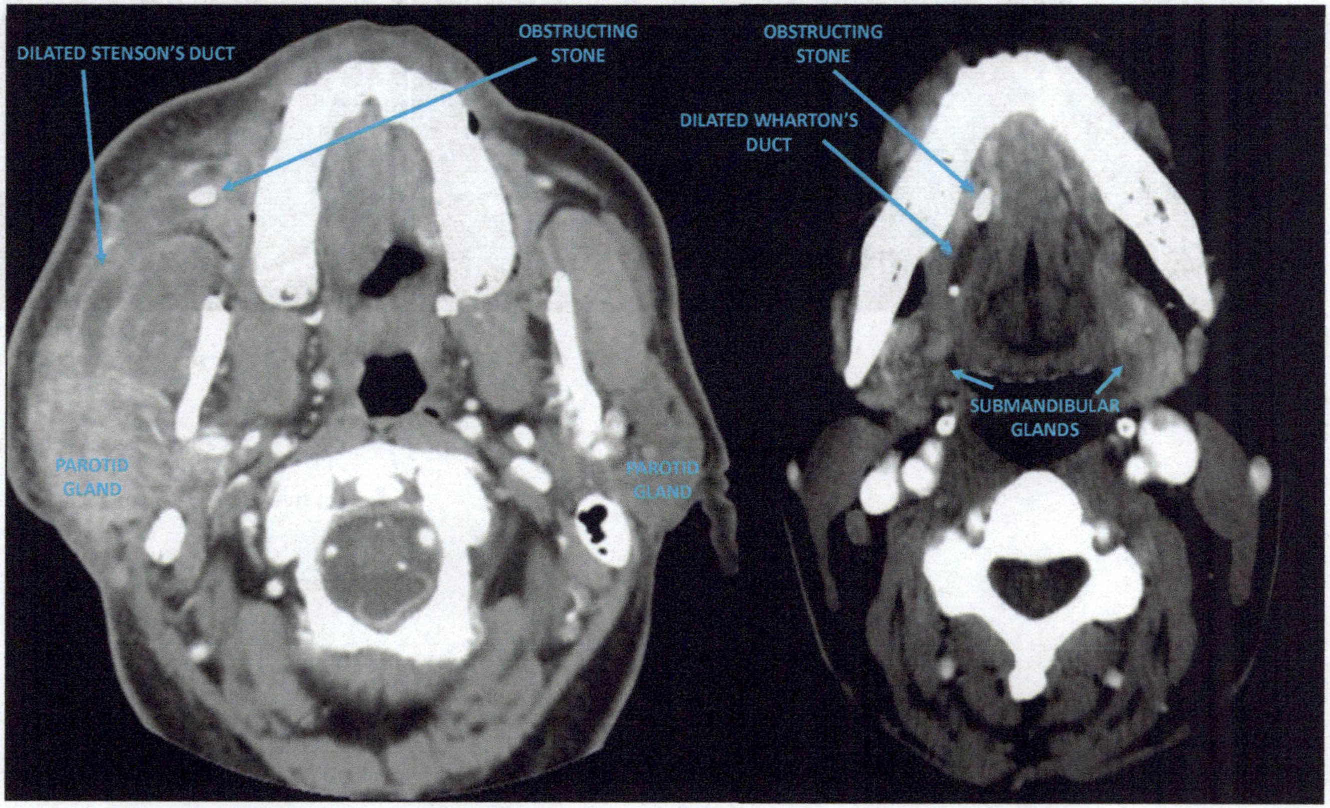

NEURORADIOLOGY

NEUROANATOMY

USMLE POINTS:

Putamen:
- **Striatum → Putamen + caudate**
- **Lentiform Nuclei → Putamen + globus pallidus**

Red Nucleus: **Midbrain**
- Contains cell bodies of upper motor neurons
- Control's flexors of the upper limb via the rubrospinal tract

Substantia Nigra: **Midbrain**
- Black/dark brown appearance due to melanin pigments
- Dopamine synthesis in the brain
- Decreased motor function in **Parkinson's disease**

Caudate nuclei:
- **Maintaining body and limb posture**
- **Controlling approach-attachment behaviors**
- **Atrophied in Huntington's disease**

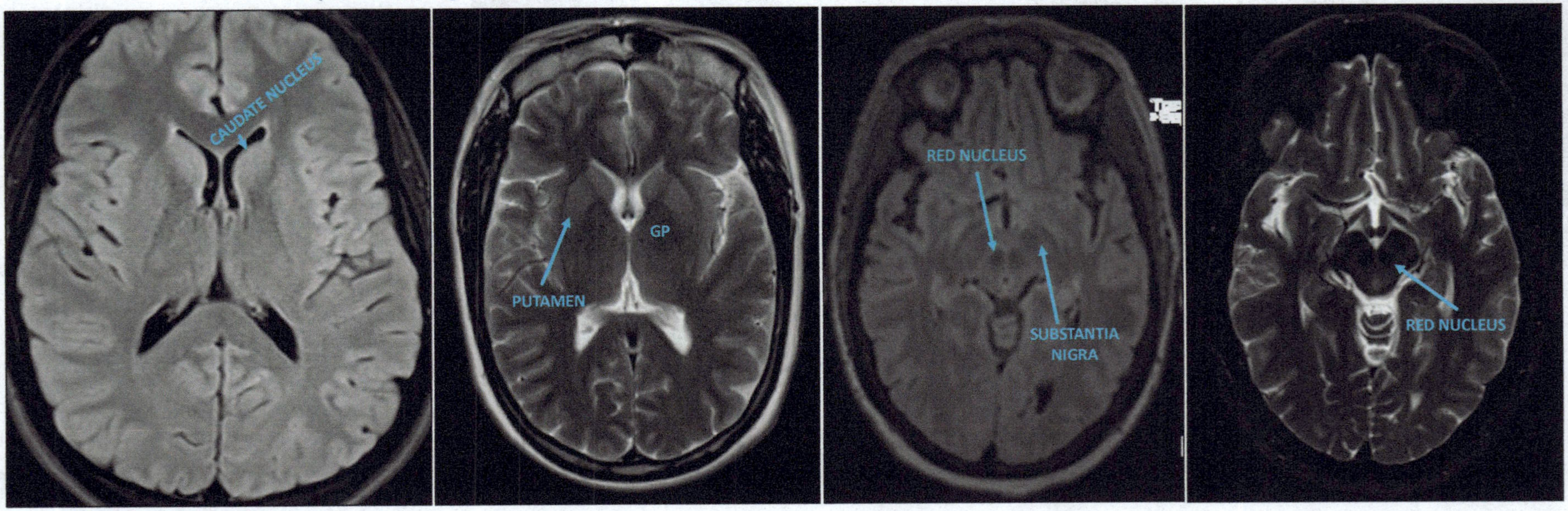

BRAIN HERNIATION

IMAGING:

Uncal: **Transtentorial displacement** of the temporal lobe uncus under the tentorium cerebelli

Subfalcine: **Medial herniation of the ipsilateral cingulate gyrus beneath the free edge of the falx cerebri**

USMLE POINTS:

Uncal: **Related to mass effect (IPH / Tumor) → Increased ICP**
Ipsilateral dilated pupil with a "down and out" gaze due to **compression of CN III**
Compression of the **PCA →** infarction of the occipital lobe **→ Contralateral homonymous hemianopsia with macular sparing**

Subfalcine: **Related to mass effect (IPH / Tumor) → Increased ICP**
Compression of the anterior cerebral artery, which causes infarction

MODALITIES: CT WO

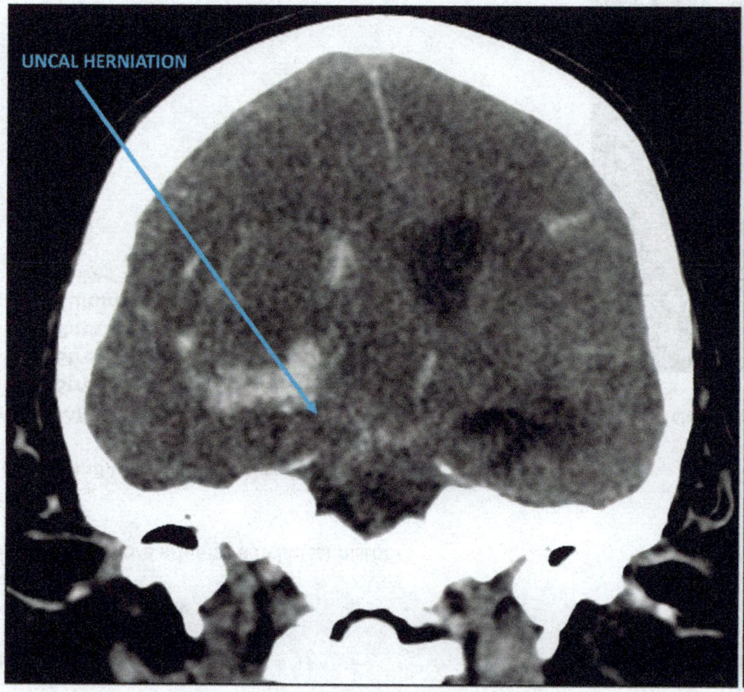

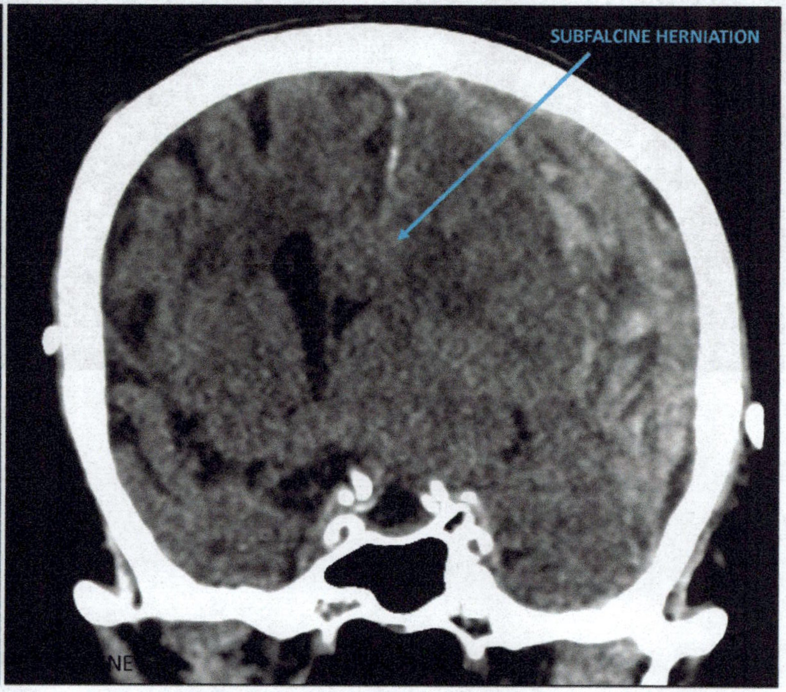

NEURORADIOLOGY

SEPTIC EMBOLI

IMAGING:

Multiple rim enhancing cavitary lesions
Gray-white junction
Differentiate from metastasis (more edema) w/ clinical history

USMLE POINTS:

Bacterial endocarditis
IVDA + Fever, AMS, cough, and tricuspid regurgitation (S. aureus)

Infective endocarditis:
Mitral valve > tricuspid valve (IVDA → S. aureus, Pseudomonas, Candida)
Strep gallolyticus → Colon cancer
Strep viridans → Dental procedures
Roth spots, Janeway lesions, Osler nodes
Culture negative endocarditis: HACEK
Dukes' criteria

MODALITIES: MR WWO

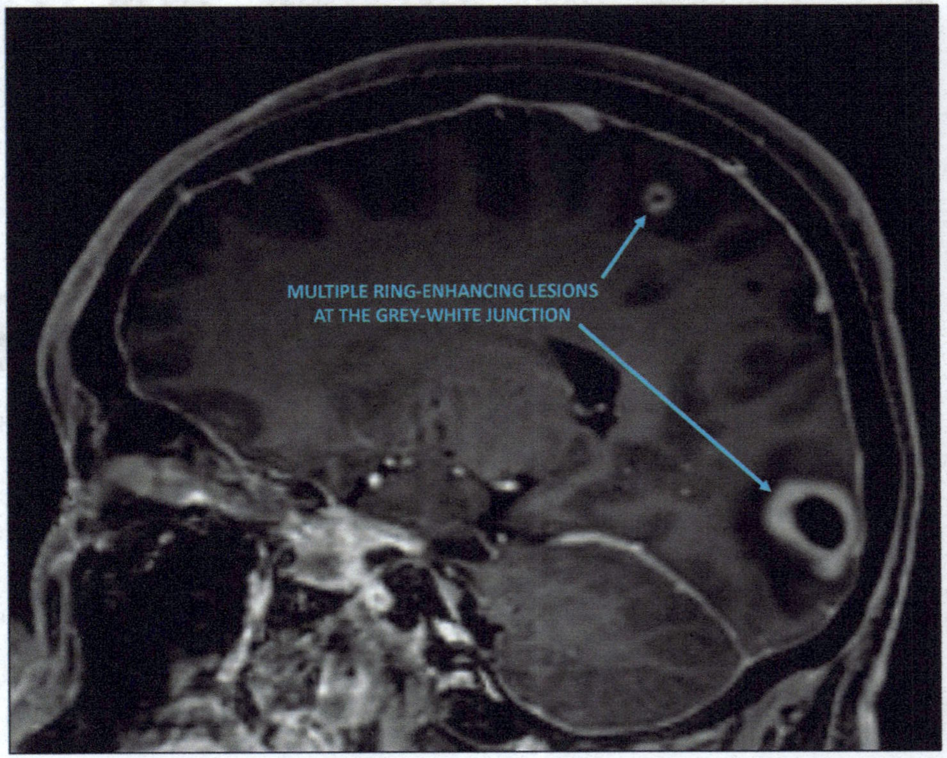

NEURORADIOLOGY

SINUSITIS

IMAGING:
Mucosal thickening
Aerosolized secretions
Air-fluid levels
OMU / SE Recess

USMLE POINTS:
Septal deviation are more prone
Patients with Infections in ethmoid or sphenoid sinus → Cavernous sinus

Organisms:
S. pneumoniae
H. influenzae
Moraxella cattarrhalis

Associations:
Kartagener disease
Cystic fibrosis
Wegener's granulomatosis

Invasive Fungal:
Immunosuppressed
Diabetes
Aspergillus (most common)
Mucormycosis

Treatment:
Amoxacillin-clavulanate for acute sinusiits
Amphotericin-B + deibreiment for invasive fungal rhinosinusitis

MODALITIES: CT WO

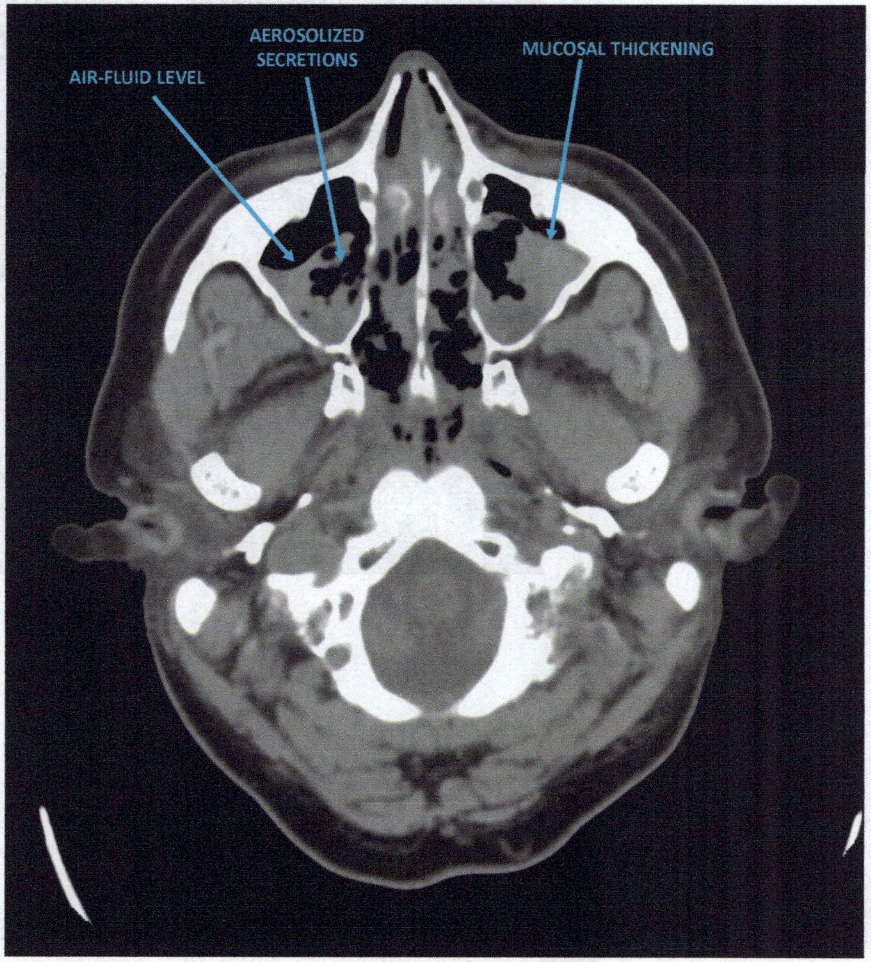

NEURORADIOLOGY

STURGE-WEBER SYNDROME

IMAGING:

CT: **"Tram-track" sign of cortical and subcortical calcification**

ANGIO: Absent superficial cortical veins with abnormal and enlarged deep venous drainage

USMLE POINTS:

Encephalotrigeminal angiomatosis
Developmental anomaly of **neural crest derivatives** due to somatic mosaicism
Activating mutation in one copy of the GNAQ gene
Port-wine stain of the face (nevus flammeus) – V1 V2 distribution
Ipsilateral leptomeningeal angiomas → **seizures or epilepsy / intellectual disability**
Episcleral hemangiomas→ IOP and early-onset glaucoma

MODALITIES: CT WO / MRI WO

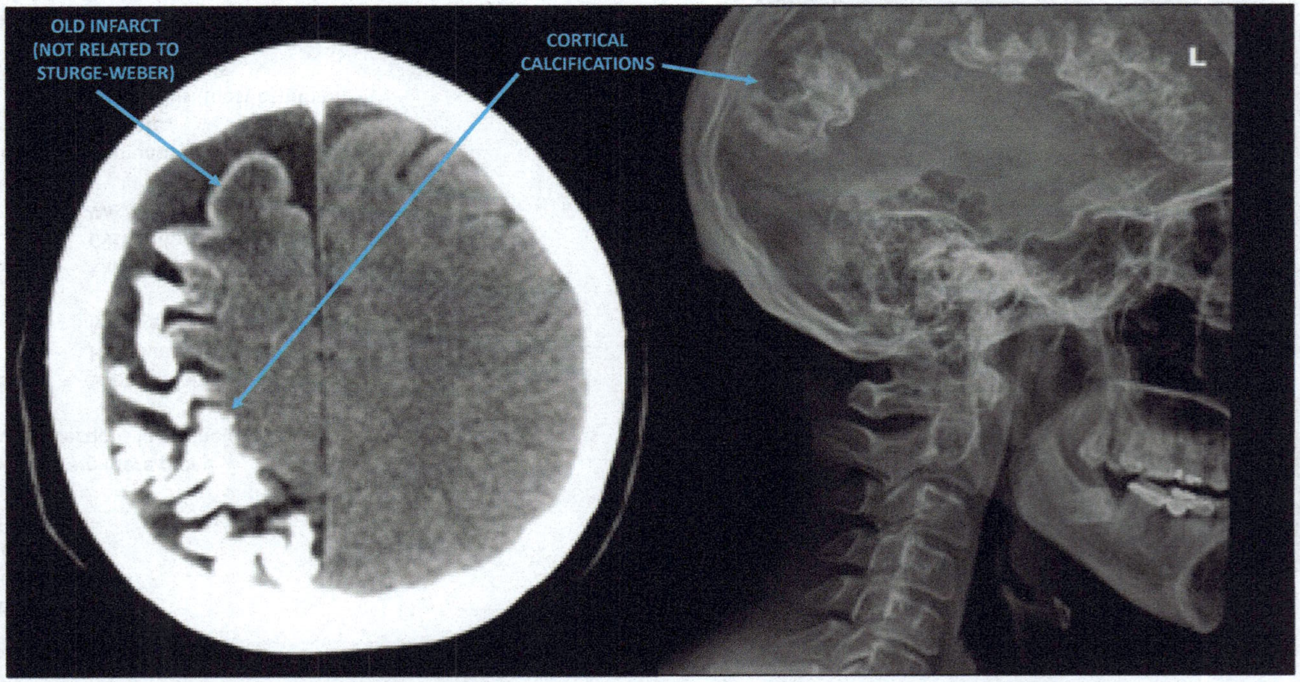

CHEST – THORACIC – PULMONARY

CHEST – THORACIC – PULMONARY

VAPING-ASSOCIATED LUNG DISEASE

IMAGING:
Bilateral ground glass
Basilar predominance + Sometimes subpleural or lobular sparing
Important to DDx from COVID-19 pneumonitis (more patchy and more peripheral + Clinical Hx)

USMLE POINTS:
Inhalational pulmonary injury induced by **electronic cigarettes**
Often **young** patient
Can progress to ARDS
Absence of pulmonary infection
Associated with vitamin-E acetate (thickening agent illegal tetrahydrocannabinol-containing vapes)

MODALITIES: XR → CT WO

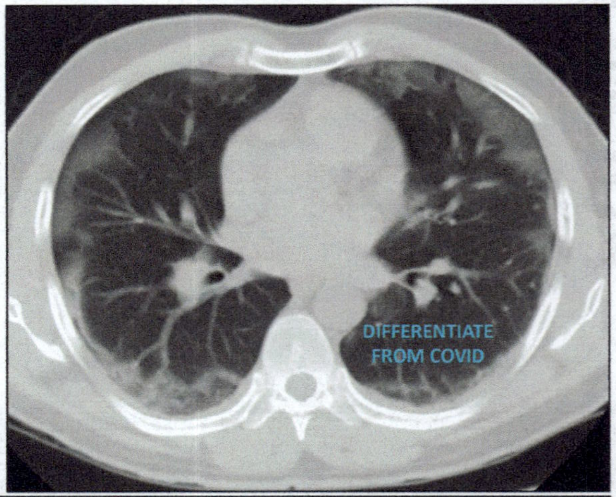

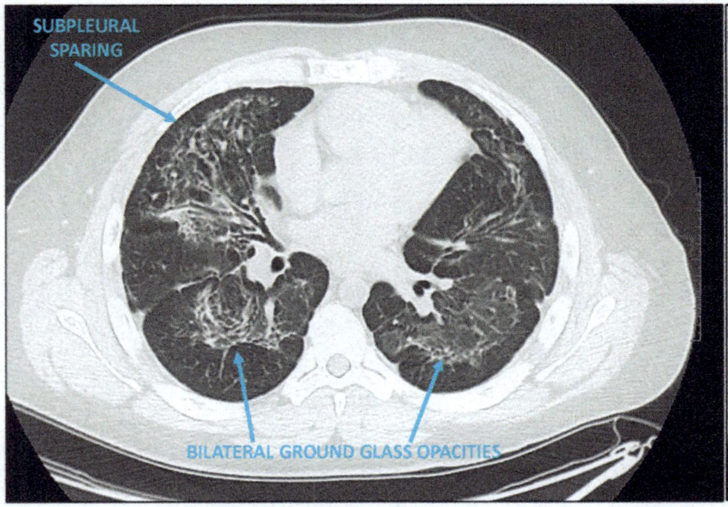

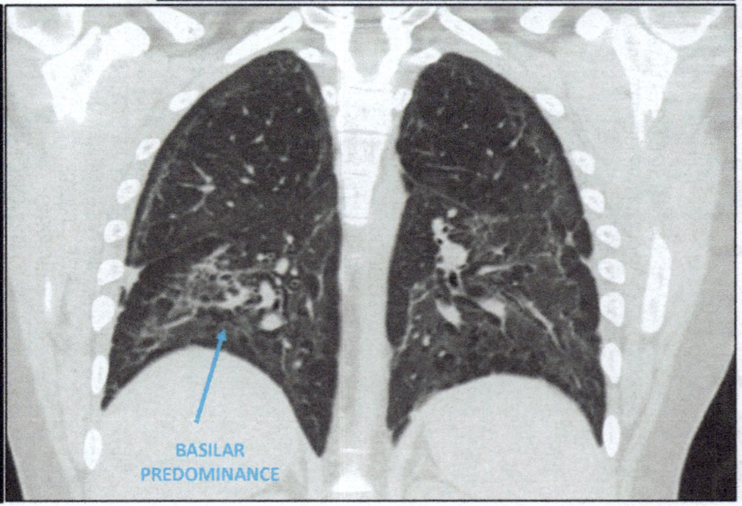

CHEST – THORACIC – PULMONARY

CONGESTIVE HEART FAILURE

IMAGING: **Cardiomegaly + Effusions + Pulmonary edema/congestion**

USMLE POINTS:
Decreased EF → Fluid banks up into lungs → Pulmonary edema and pleural effusions
S3 sound, JVD, and serum BNP (if negative excludes CHF) are used to distinguish CHF from ARDS
Systolic dysfunction as a result of dilated cardiomyopathy → Biventricular congestive heart failure
High output cardiac failure → AV Fistula, Thyrotoxicosis

Treatment: Diuretics / Thoracocentesis

Transudative effusion: Decreased protein content due to increased hydrostatic pressure
Due to decreased oncotic pressure (nephrotic syndrome, cirrhosis)

Exudative effusion : Increased protein content
Malignancy, pneumonia
Drained due to risk of infection

Lymphatic effusion: Due to thoracic duct injury from trauma or malignancy
Milky appearing fluid with increased triglycerides
Tuberous sclerosis

<u>Lights Criteria</u>

Pleural : Serum Protein	< 0.5	**Transudate**
	> 0.5	Exudate
Pleural : Serum LDH	< 0.6	**Transudate**
	> 0.6	Exudate
Pleural Fluid LDH	< 2/3 ULN	**Transudate**
	> 2/3 ULN	Exudate

MODALITIES: XR → CT WO

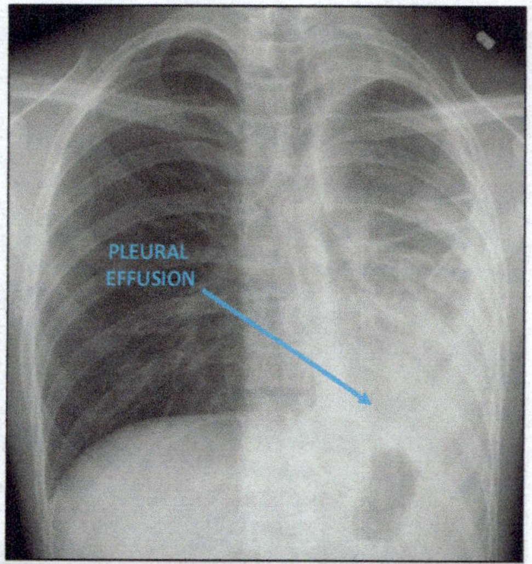

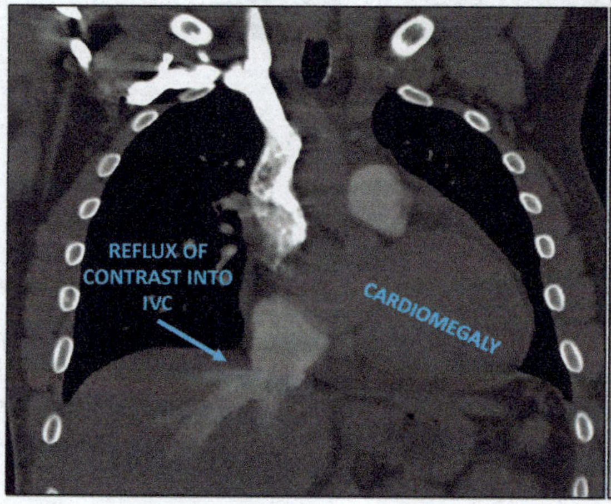

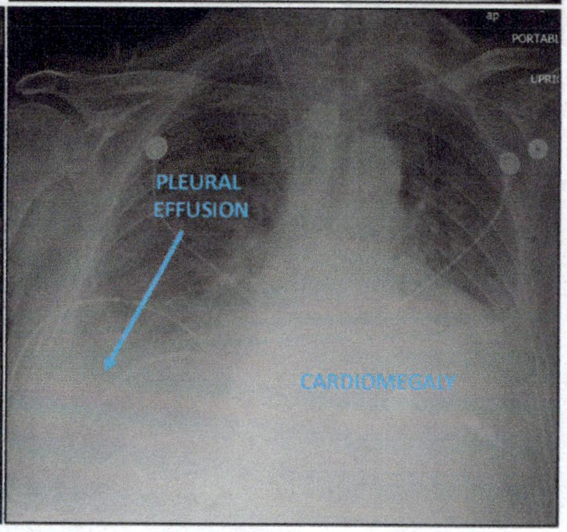

CHEST – THORACIC – PULMONARY

COVID-19

IMAGING: Ground-glass opacities: **Bilateral, peripheral, and basal predominant distribution**

USMLE POINTS: Infectious disease caused by severe acute respiratory syndrome coronavirus 2 **(SARS-CoV-2)**
Definitive diagnosis of COVID-19 requires a **positive RT-PCR test**
Cellular entry via **spike protein (S-protein) to the ACE-2 Receptors → Commonly found on alveolar cells**

Presentation: Fever, Cough, Soar throat, **Anosmia**

Complications: ARDS
DVT / PE
Stroke
Acute cardiac injury → Elevated troponins

Risk Factors: **Old age, Vitamin D deficiency,** Male, **Obesity**, DM, Cancer/chronic illness

MODALITIES: XR → CT WO

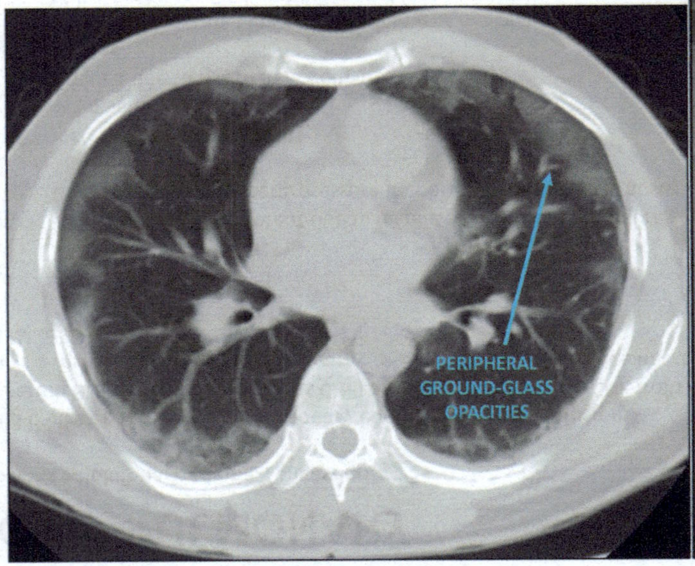

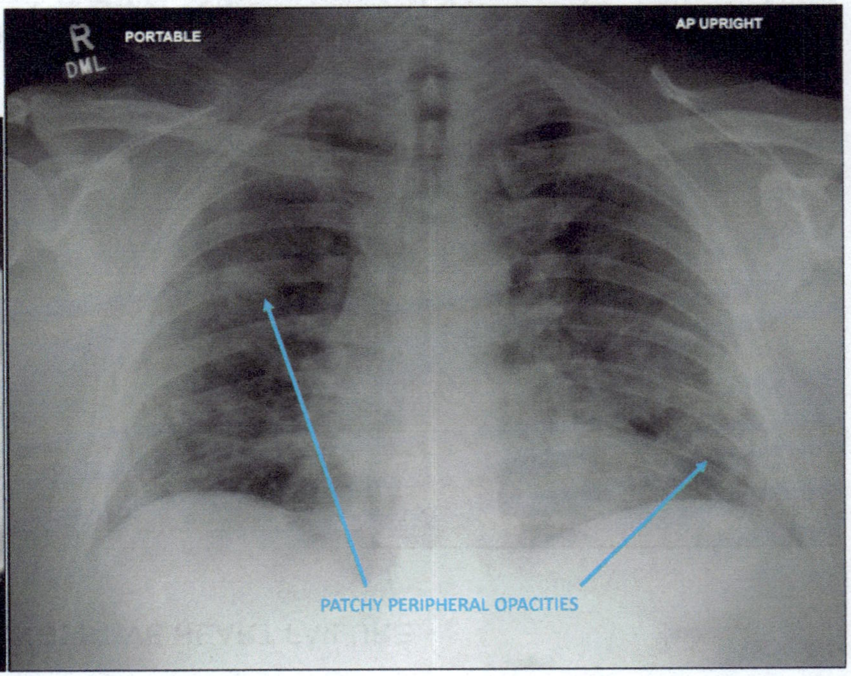

COVID-19

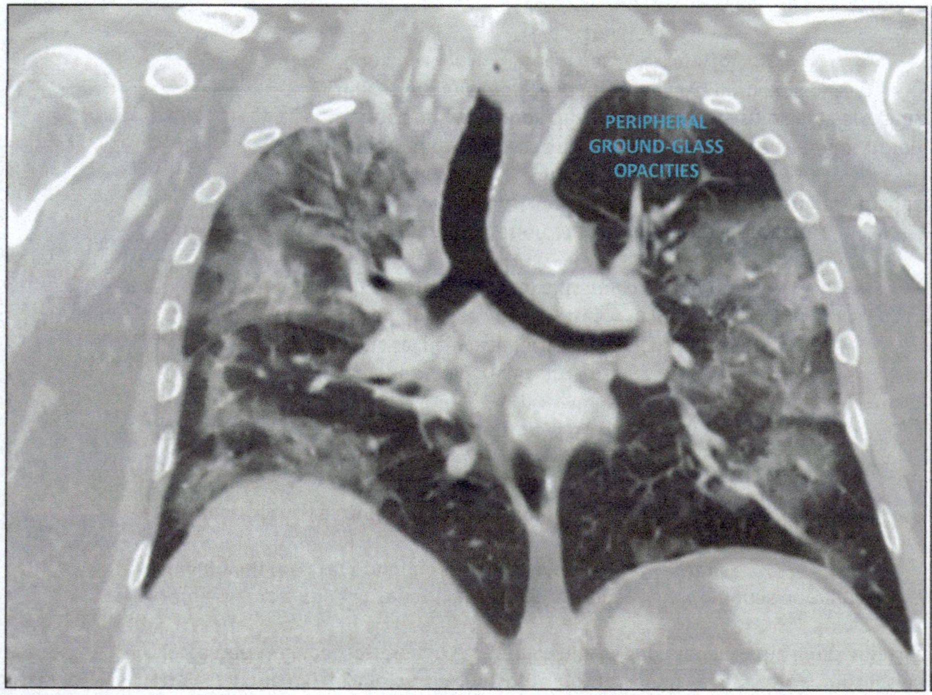
PERIPHERAL
GROUND-GLASS
OPACITIES

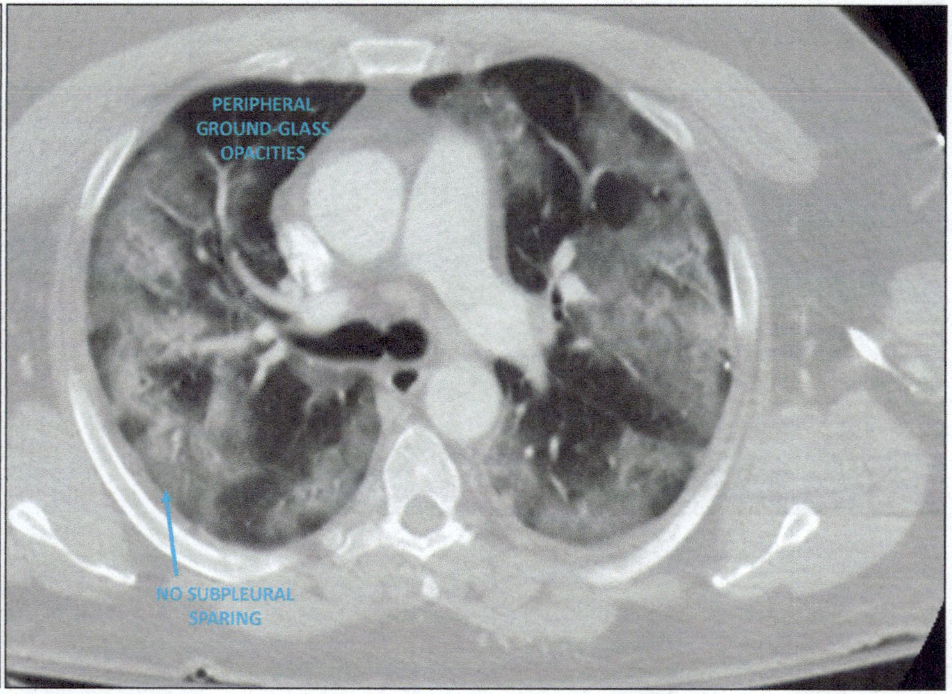
PERIPHERAL
GROUND-GLASS
OPACITIES
NO SUBPLEURAL
SPARING

CHEST – THORACIC – PULMONARY

CYSTIC FIBROSIS

IMAGING:
Child + Thick-walled bronchiectasis
Intervening lung is often densely fibrotic and retracted
Reticulonodular pattern on CXR

USMLE POINTS:
Defect in the **CFTR gene on chromosome 7** (Autosomal Recessive) → encodes an ATP-gated Cl- channel
Increased H_2O reabsorption in CF → thick mucus secreted into the lungs and GI tract

Adolescents with recurrent pulmonary infections: **Pseudomonas aeruginosa**
Infant with recurrent pulmonary infections: **S. aureus**

Absence of the vas deferens → Infertility
May cause biliary cirrhosis and/or liver disease

Diagnosis: **Increased Cl^- concentration (> 60 meQ/L) in sweat**

Treatment: Replacement of pancreatic enzymes
Hypertonic saline which facilitates mucus clearing
Aerosolized dornase alfa (DNase) → hydrolyzes DNA in mucus → Decreased viscosity
Chest physiotherapy which aids mucus clearance

Bronchiectasis: **Permanent dilatation of bronchioles and bronchi**
Due to chronic **obstruction which results in permanently dilated airways**
Tuberculosis / CF / Kartageners
Associated with bronchial obstruction, such as a tumor or foreign body
Associated with **poor ciliary motility** (e.g. smoking, Kartagener syndrome)
Recurrent infections and foul-smelling, purulent sputum
Complications: Secondary (AA) amyloidosis
Hypoxemia
Cor pulmonale

MODALITIES: **XR → CT WO**

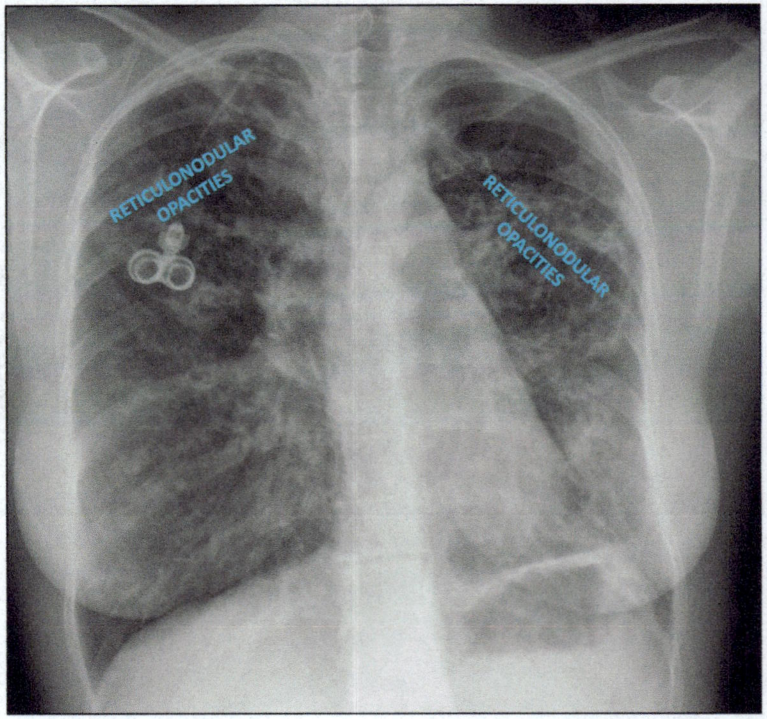

CYSTIC FIBROSIS

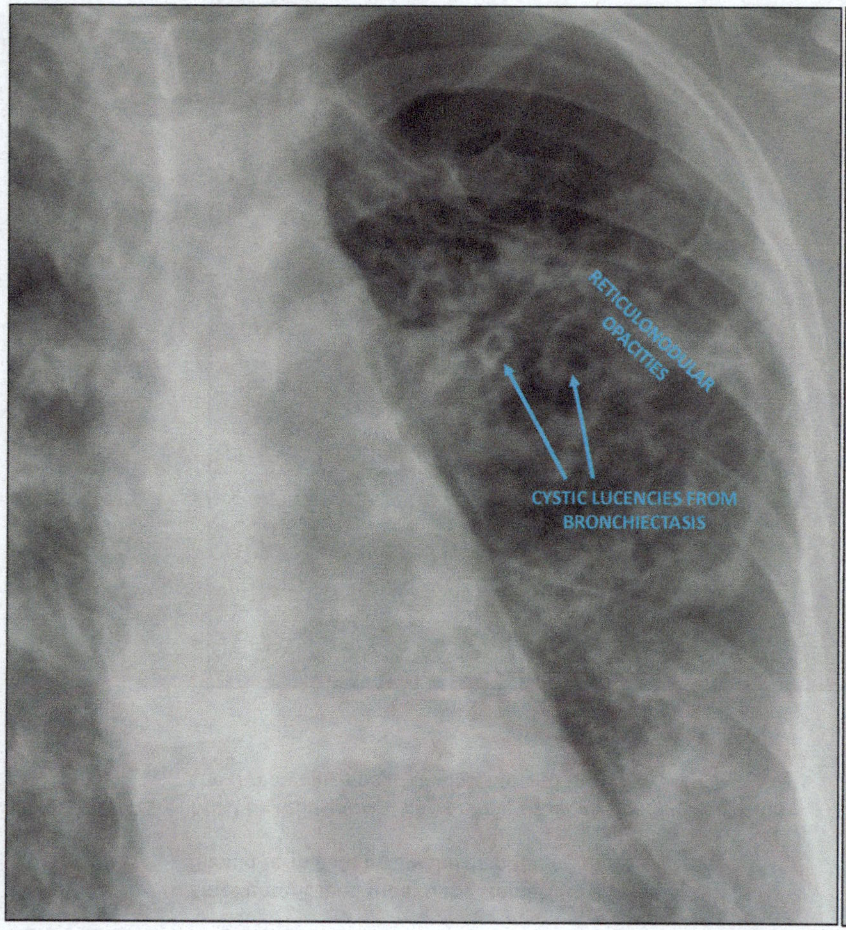

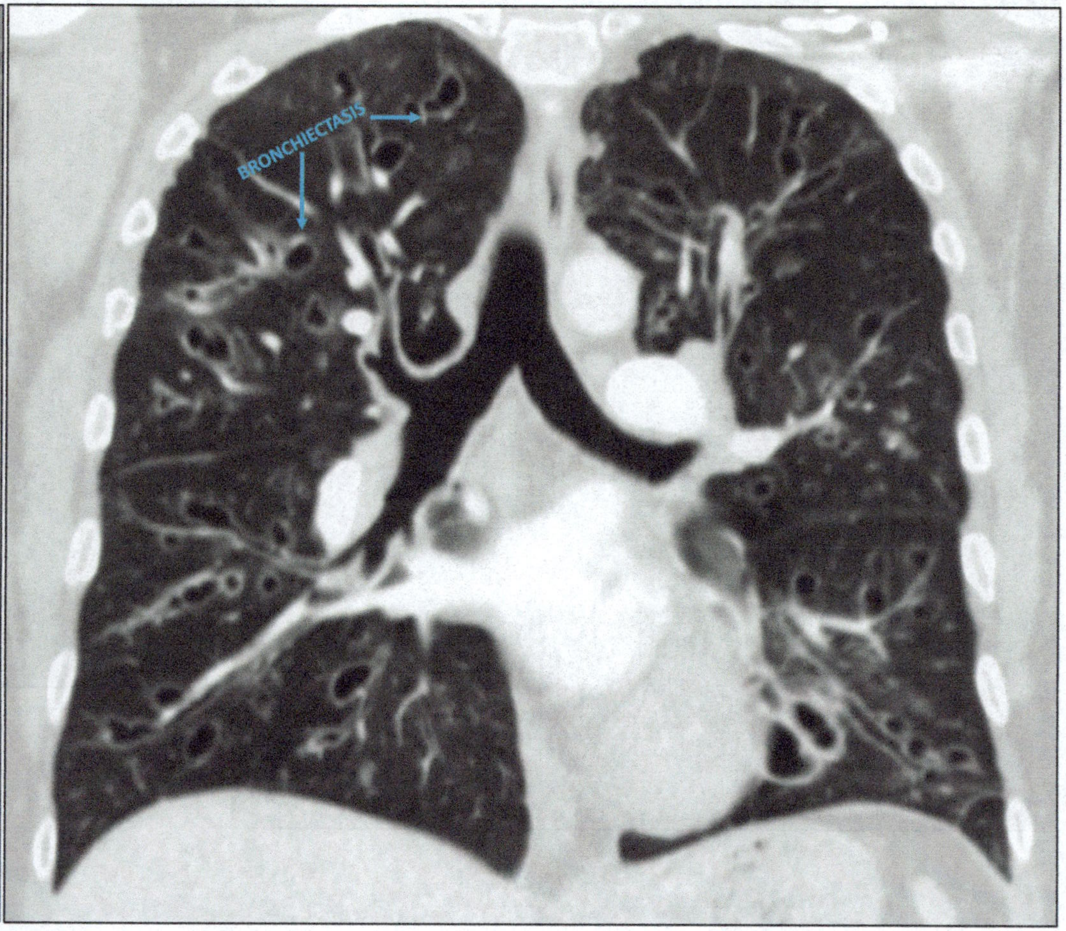

CHEST – THORACIC – PULMONARY

NG TUBE IN LUNG

IMAGING: **Trace enteric feed tube to the stomach on every CXR**
Should terminate below the diaphragm

USMLE POINTS: **Must be repositioned and re-imaged before feeding can begin**
Life threatening pneumonitis if fed into the lung

MODALITIES: XR

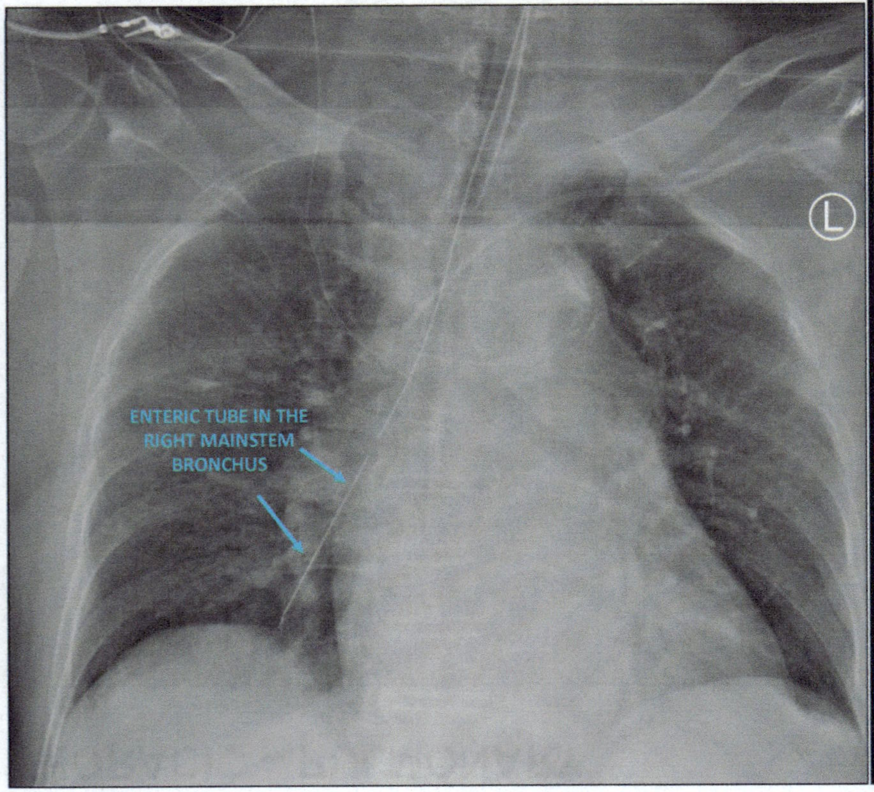

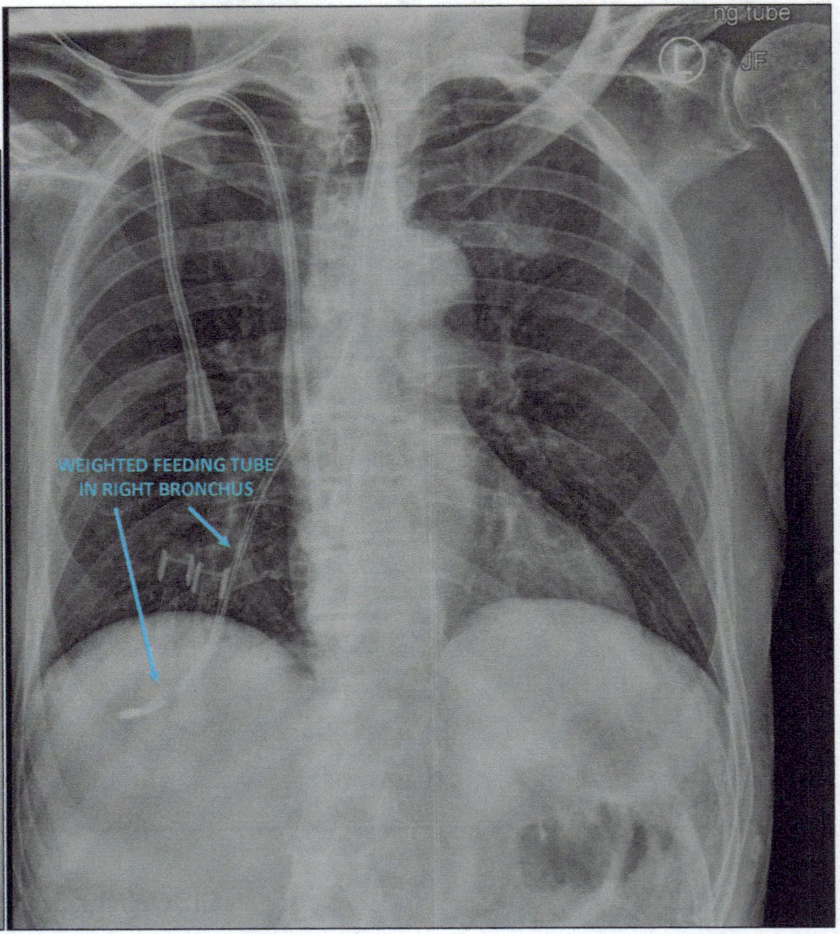

CHEST – THORACIC – PULMONARY

PNEUMONIA

IMAGING:

Lobar: **Consolidation** within entire lobe or lung
Interstitial/atypical: Diffuse interstitial infiltrates
Aspiration: **Dependent airspace consolidation + Risk factors. Look for debris in the tracheobronchial tree**

USMLE POINTS:

Atypical: **Mycoplasma pneumoniae** (living in close quarters) → Military, prisoners
No cell, No gram stain

Bacterial:

Streptococcus pneumoniae: Most common cause (95%) of community-acquired lobar pneumonia
Middle-aged adults and the elderly

Klebsiella pneumoniae: **Elderly, alcoholics, and diabetics (due to aspiration)**
Thick mucoid capsule that results in gelatinous, 'currant jelly' sputum

Actinomyces: Branching, filamentous bacteria is associated with dental carries and resultant aspiration pneumonia
Empyema neccessitans

Staphylococcus aureus: **Abscess** formation or empyema (pus in the pleural space)

Aspiration: **Anaerobes**
Presents as cough/fever days after aspiration event
CXR infiltrate in dependent lung segment (classically in RLL)
Pneumonitis: Inflammation due to aspiration of gastric acid with direct tissue injury
Supine during aspiration → Involves superior segment of the right lower lobe

ARDS: Resemble those of **typical pulmonary edema or pulmonary hemorrhage**
Diffuse bilateral coalescent opacities → **"White-out" appearance of CXR**
Respiratory failure with bilateral lung opacities and no evidence of HF/fluid overload
Diffuse alveolar damage with impairment of the alveolar-capillary interface

PaO2 / FiO2:		
	<100	**Severe**
	100 – 200	**Moderate**
	200 – 300	**Mild**

MODALITIES: XR → CT WO

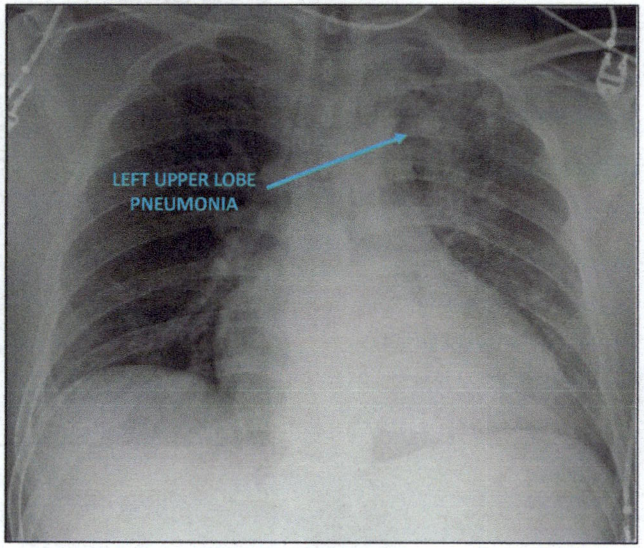

CHEST – THORACIC – PULMONARY

PNEUMONIA

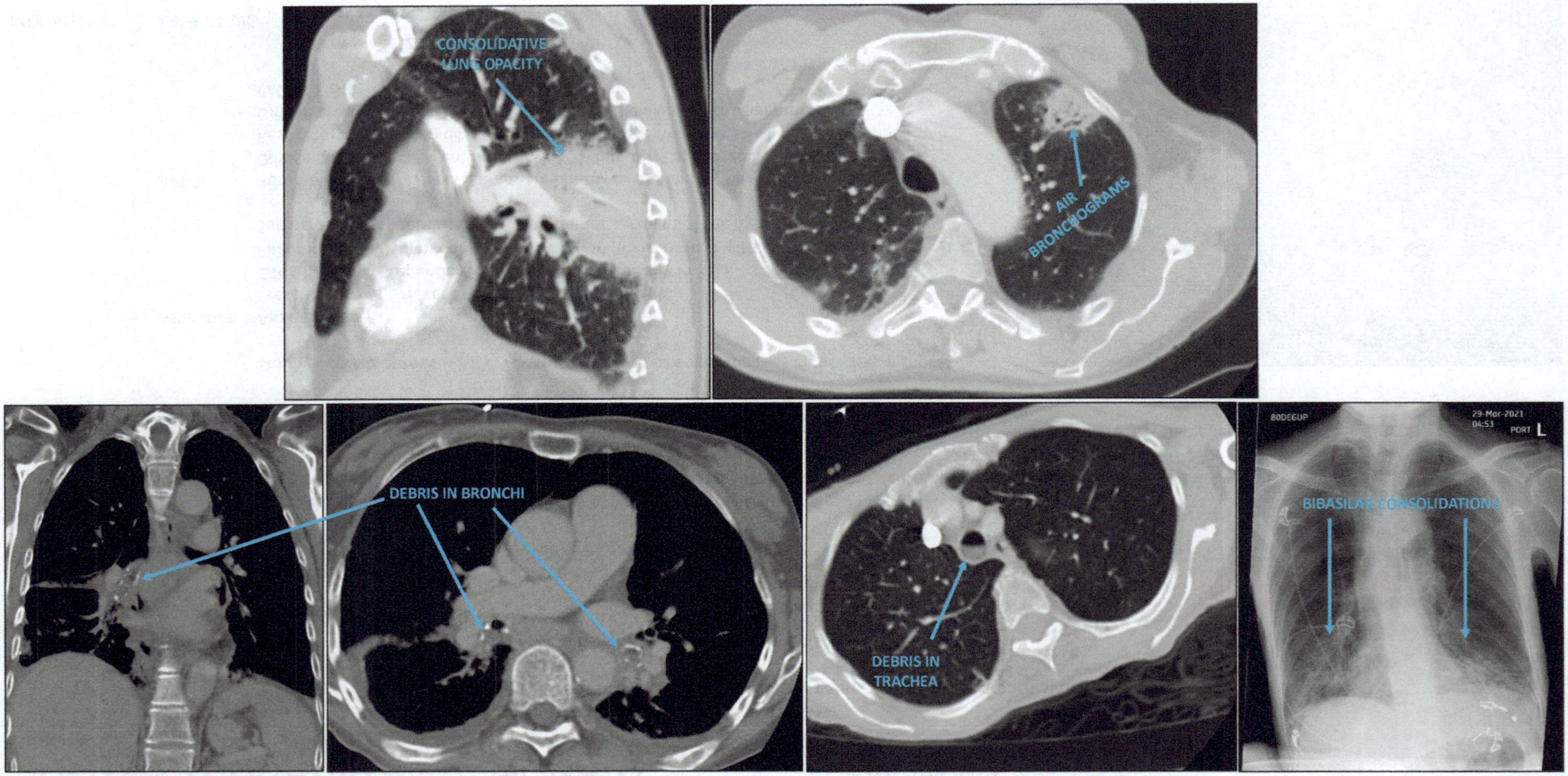

CHEST – THORACIC – PULMONARY

PNEUMONIA

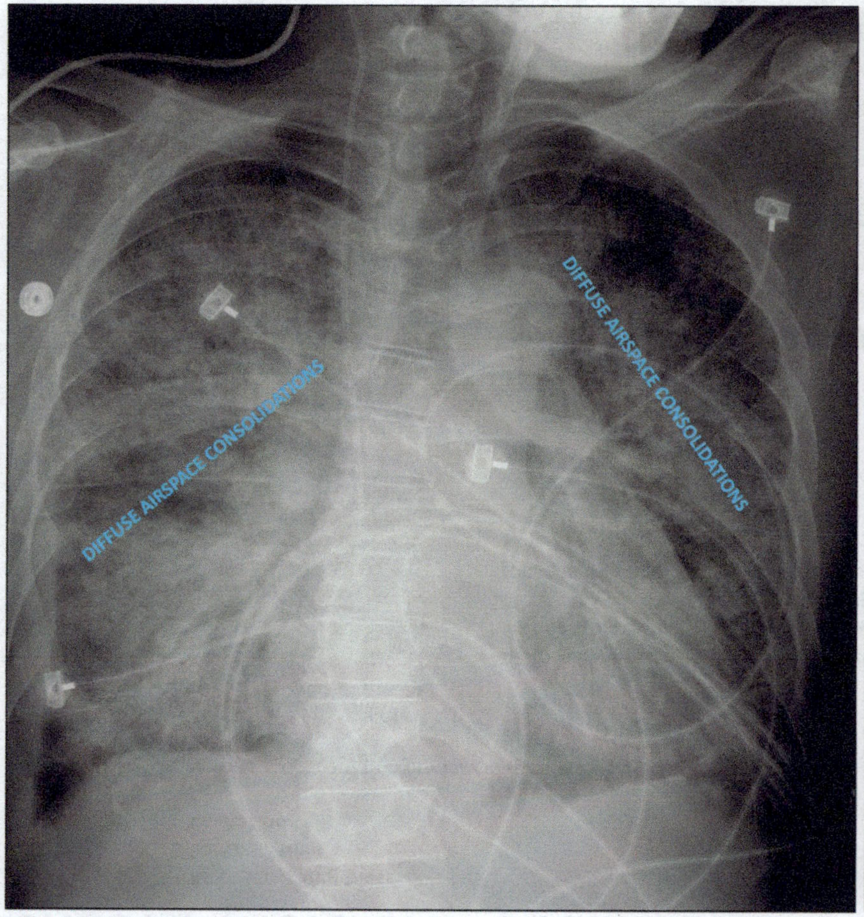

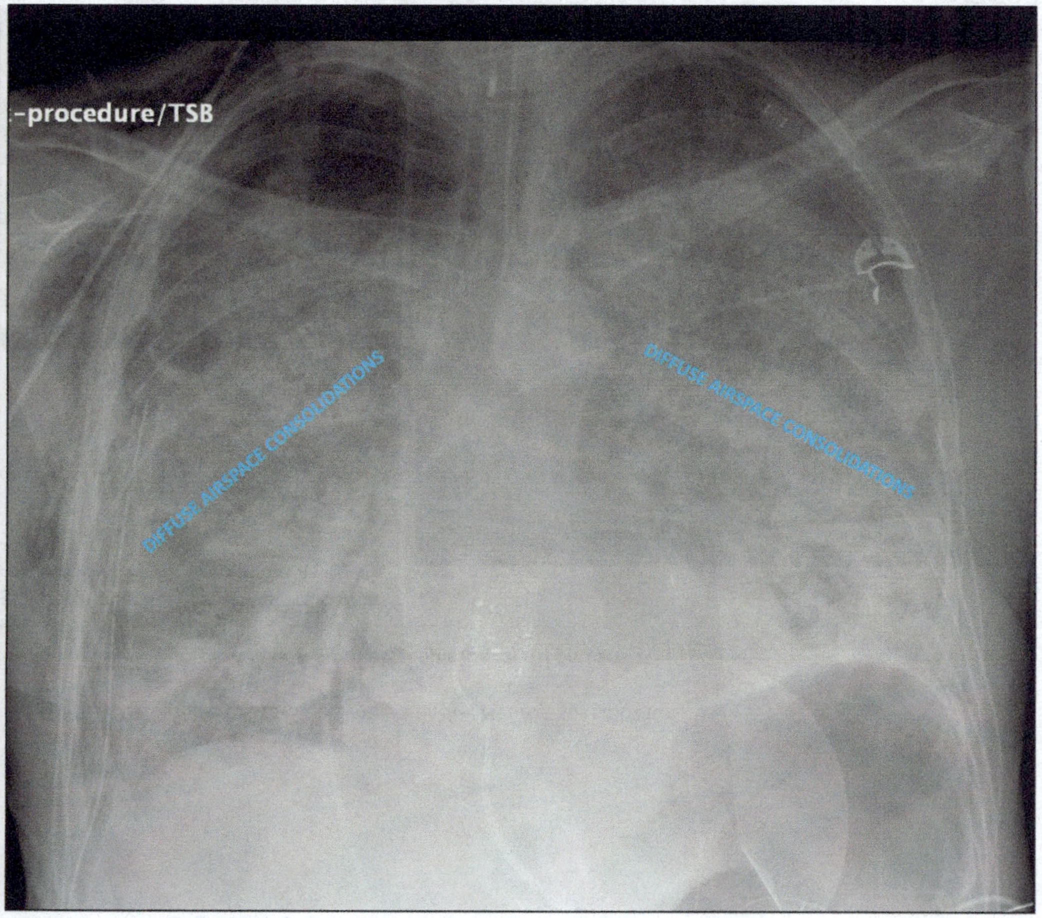

CHEST – THORACIC – PULMONARY

SQUAMOUS CELL CARCINOMA

IMAGING:
Aggressive lung Mass
Central / Hilar
Cavitation

USMLE POINTS: Second most common primary lung carcinoma (30%) (adenocarcinoma most common)

Classification:	SCLC	SCLC	MYC gene, **ACTH, ADH, Lambert Eaton,** Chromogranin A+, Neuron-specific enolase+
	NSCLC	Adenocarcinoma	**Mucin producing, Most common in non-smokers, Lepidic growth pattern**
		Large cell carcinoma	Smoking
		SCC	**Smoking, Keratin pearls, PTHrP (hypercalcemia)**
		Bronchial carcinoid tumor	Neuroendocrine tumor, Chromogranin A+

MODALITIES: XR → CT W

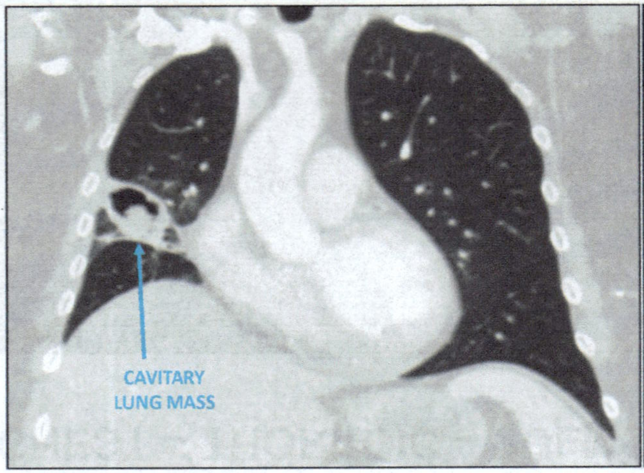

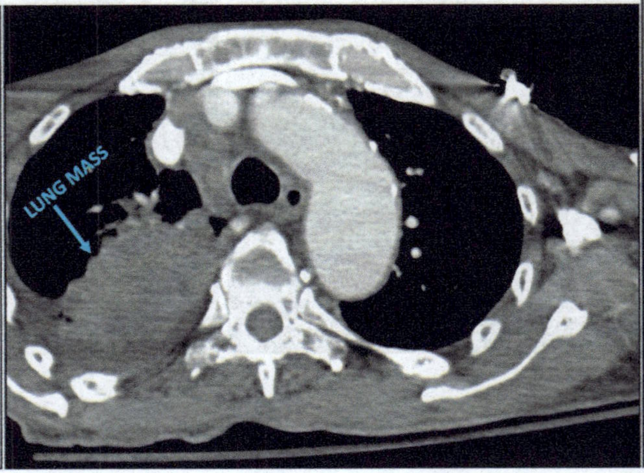

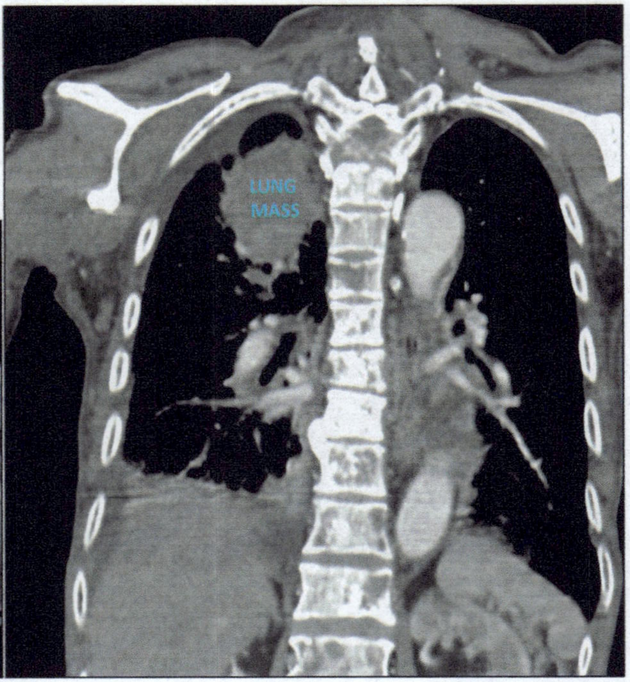

CHEST – THORACIC – PULMONARY

PANCOAST TUMOR

IMAGING: **Apical lung mass**
Occasionally rib involvement or extension into the supraclavicular fossa

USMLE POINTS: Brachial plexus may be involved (C7, T1, T2)
Shoulder pain → Scapula and axilla

Horner syndrome: **Ipsilateral ptosis**
Miosis
Anhidrosis (denervation of sympathetic chain)

AKA Superior sulcus tumor (most commonly bronchogenic carcinoma → SCC)

MODALITIES: XR → CT W

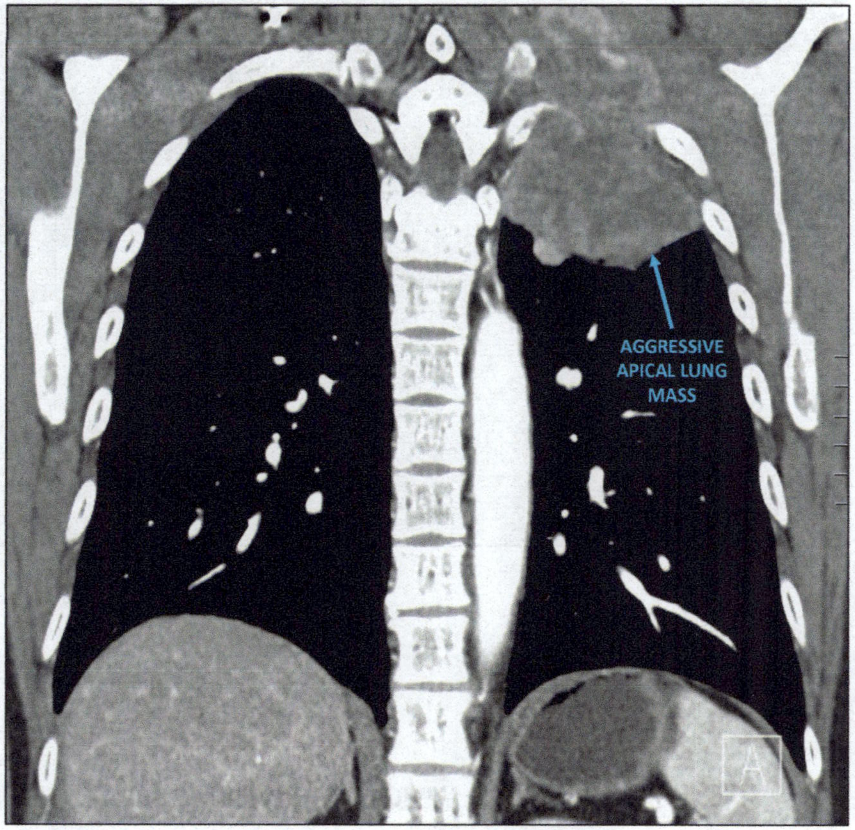

CHEST – THORACIC – PULMONARY

RIGHT MAINSTEM INTUBATION

IMAGING: **Ideal position of an ETT is 5 ± 2 cm above the carina**

USMLE POINTS: Decreased ventilation of contralateral lung → subsequent reduction in respiratory reserve
Hyperinflation of involved side
Right mainstem bronchus is more straight

MODALITIES: XR

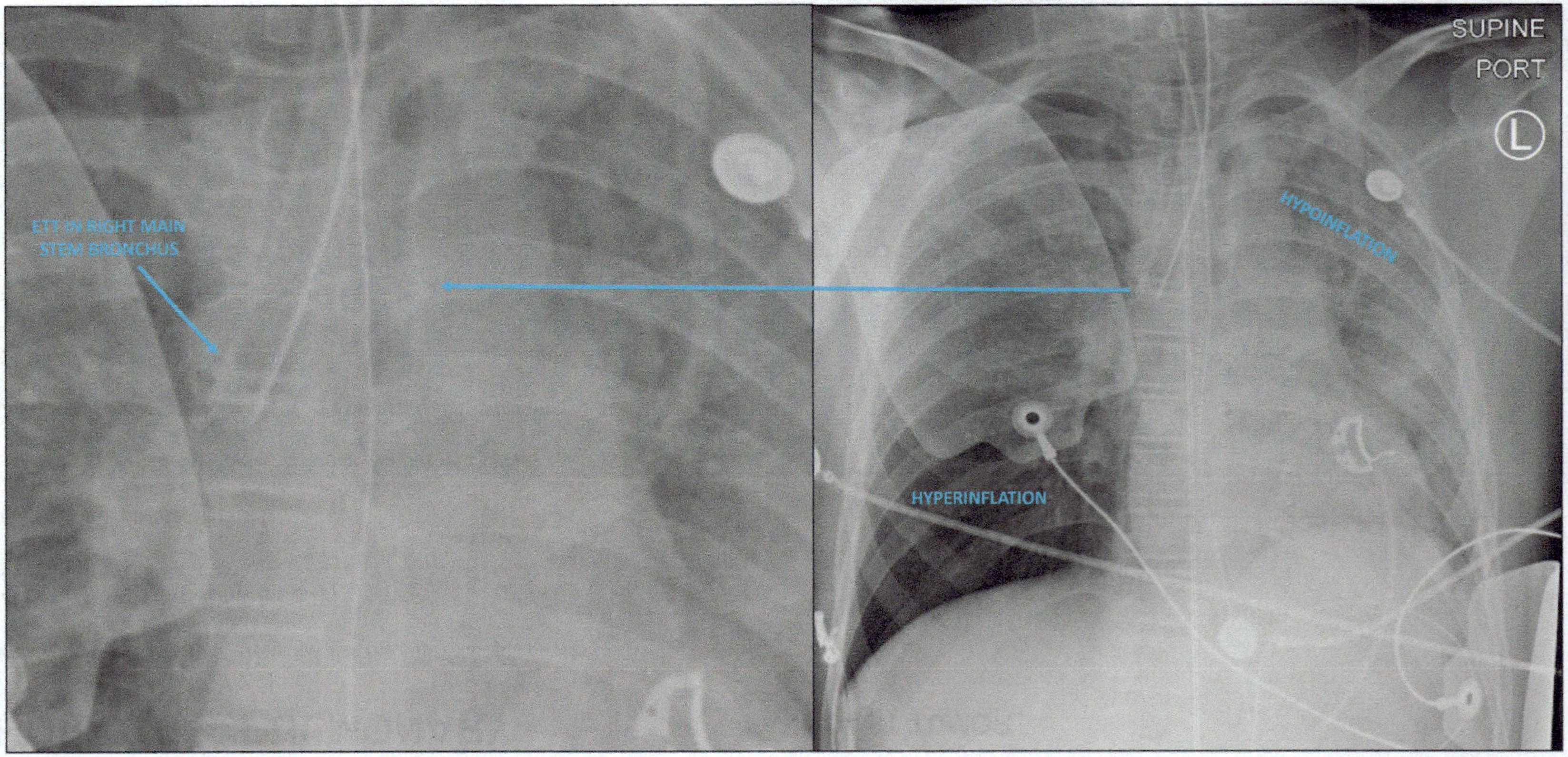

CHEST – THORACIC – PULMONARY

PULMONARY EMBOLISM

IMAGING:

CTA: **Filling defect within the pulmonary arteries**
RLL most common
Pulmonary infarcts
RV Dilation (strain) → Echocardiography

VQ: Ventilation – Perfusion **Mismatch**
Matched defects are not pulmonary emboli

USMLE POINTS:

Saddle PE → Electromechanical dissociation → **Sudden Death from PEA (pulseless electrical activity)**
Spiral CTA is the imaging test of choice for pulmonary embolism

VQ scan: **Renal insufficiency (GFR <30)**
Contrast allergies
Pregnancy

MODALITIES: CTA / VQ

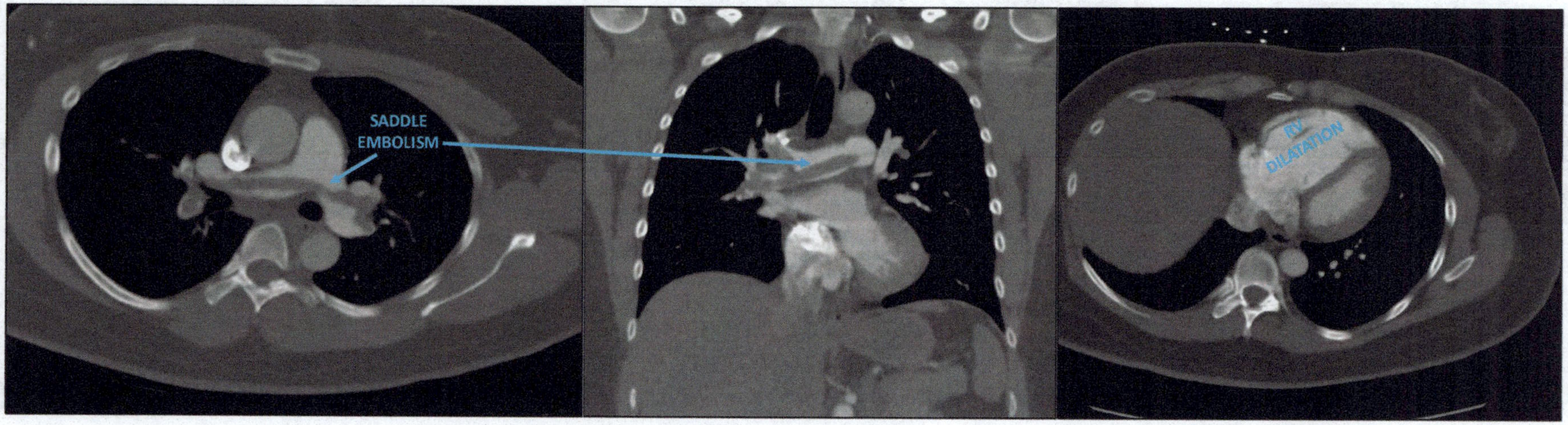

CHEST – THORACIC – PULMONARY

PULMONARY EMBOLISM

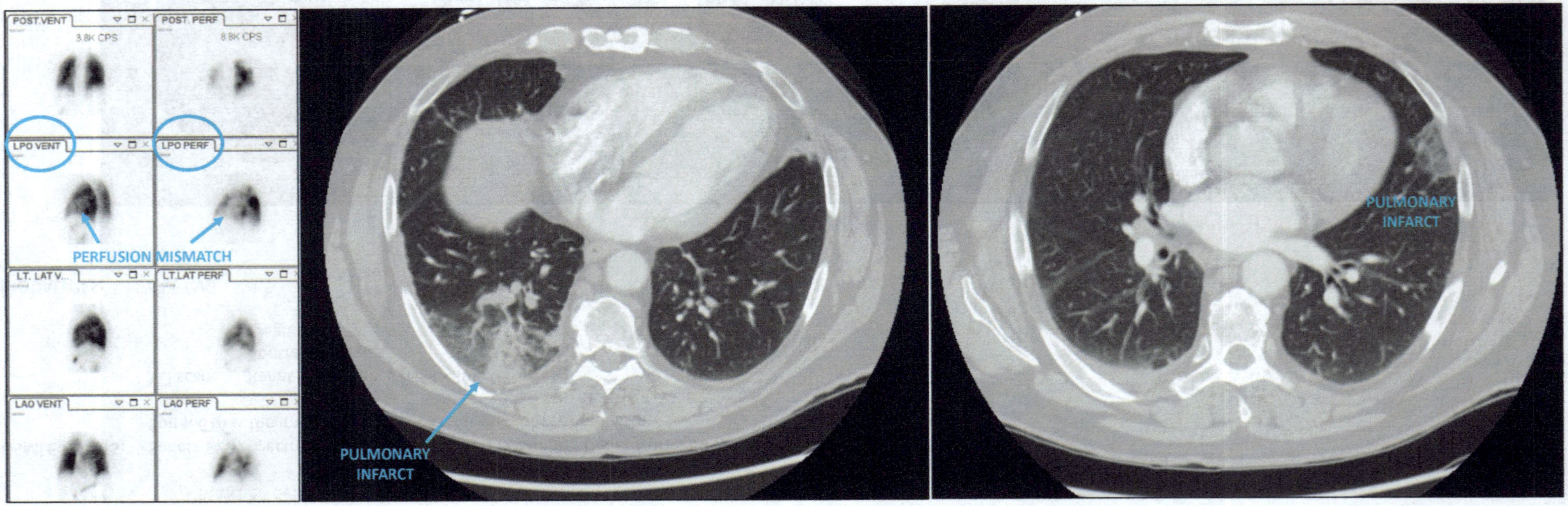

CHEST – THORACIC – PULMONARY

SARCOIDOSIS

IMAGING:
Bilateral hilar adenopathy
Coarse reticular opacities
Don't need to know stages

USMLE POINTS:
African American female
Interstitial restrictive lung disease → Decreased diffusion capacity
Schaumann bodies, which are calcium and protein inclusions inside of giant cells

Associations:
- Neurosarcoidosis
- Myocarditis
- **Hypercalcemia (renal stones)**
- **Uveitis**
- **Erythema nodosum**
- Rheumatoid-like arthropathy

Labs: **Elevated ACE levels**

Treatment: **Oral corticosteroids**

MODALITIES: XR → CT WO

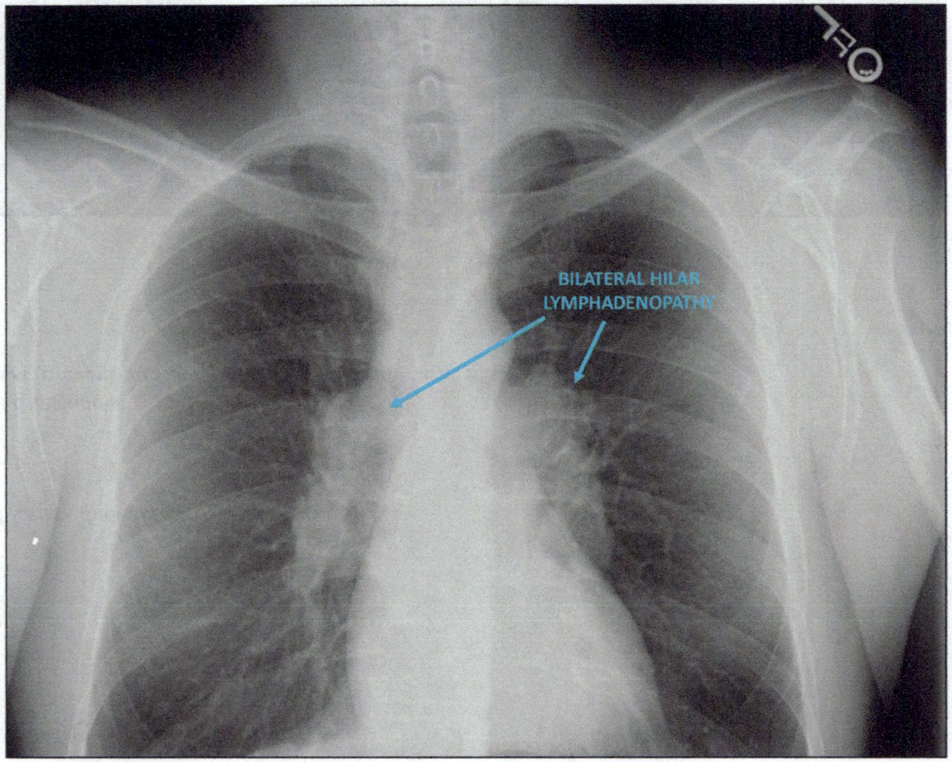

CHEST – THORACIC – PULMONARY

COPD

IMAGING:

Emphysema (hyperlucent lungs)
Increased AP diameter of chest
Flattening of the diaphragms

USMLE POINTS:

Irreversible bronchial obstruction
Most common cause of secondary spontaneous pneumothorax
Administered excessive oxygen can develop hypercapnia (reversal of hypoxia induced pulmonary vasoconstriction)
Long-standing COPD → Decreased sensitivity to $PaCO_2$
Main contributor to respiratory drive is arterial PaO_2 levels

Superimposed pneumonia: **Haemophilus influenzae, Moraxella** catarrhalis, and Legionella
Treatment: **Ipratropium → competitive M3 receptor antagonist (prevent** bronchoconstriction in asthmatic and COPD patients)

MODALITIES: XR → CT WO

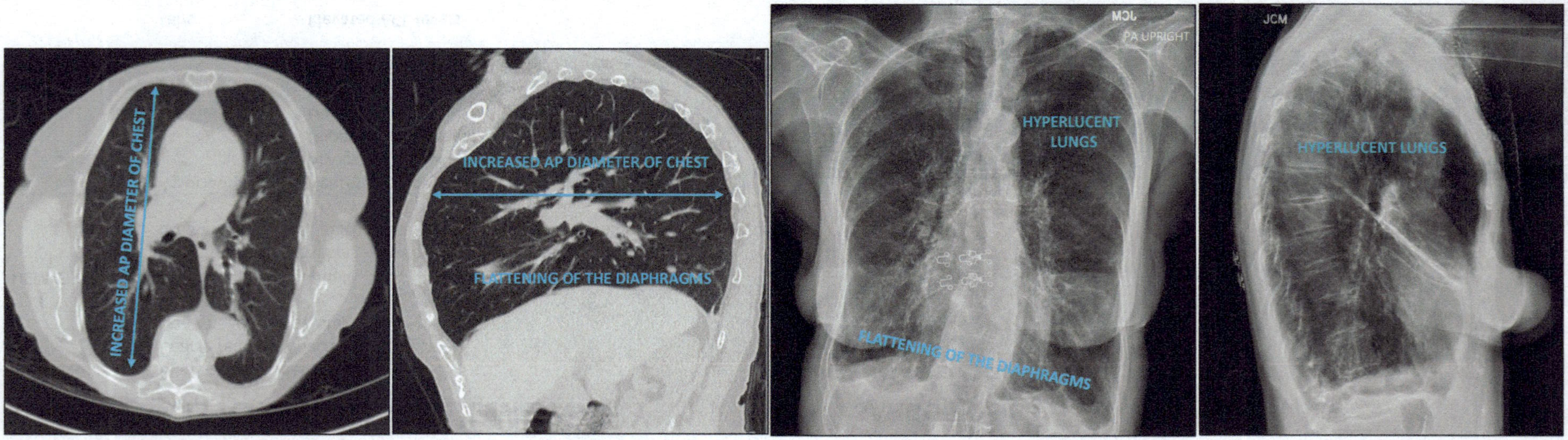

CHEST – THORACIC – PULMONARY

PNEUMOTHORAX

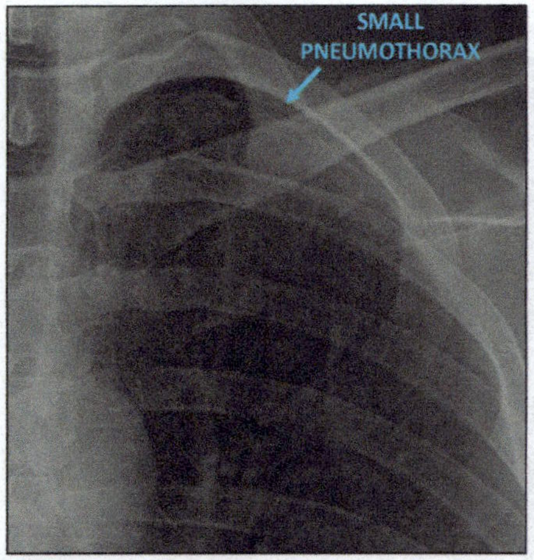

IMAGING:
Apical lucency
Be able to differentiate from **skin fold** (lung markings extend beyond skin fold)
Mediastinal shift

USMLE POINTS:
Unilateral chest pain and expansion
Hyperresonance and decreased lung sounds

Spontaneous pneumothorax: Due to rupture of apical subpleural bleb or cysts (Tall, thin, young)

Tension physiology: **Kinking of IVC → Decreased CO**
Requires chest tube

MODALITIES: XR → CT WO

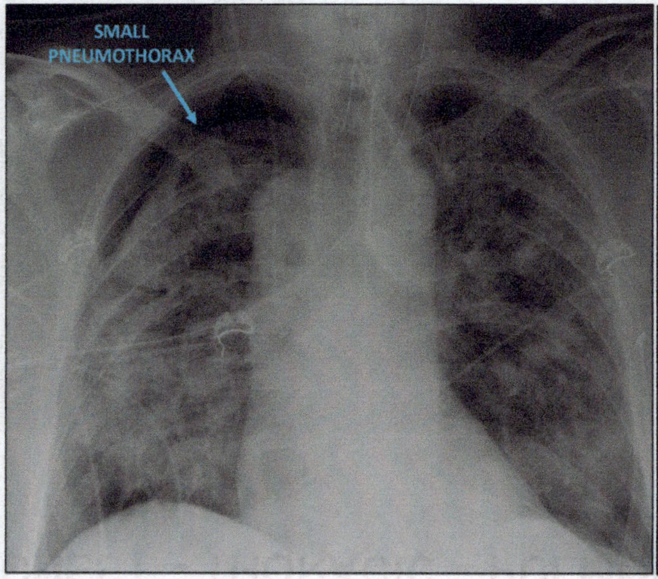

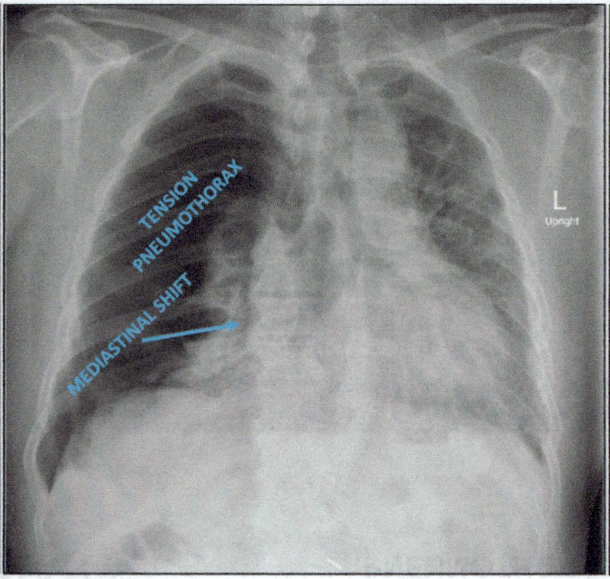

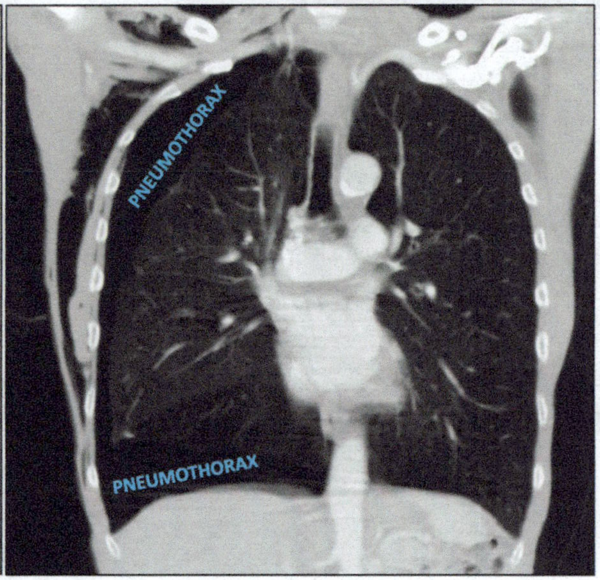

PNEUMOTHORAX

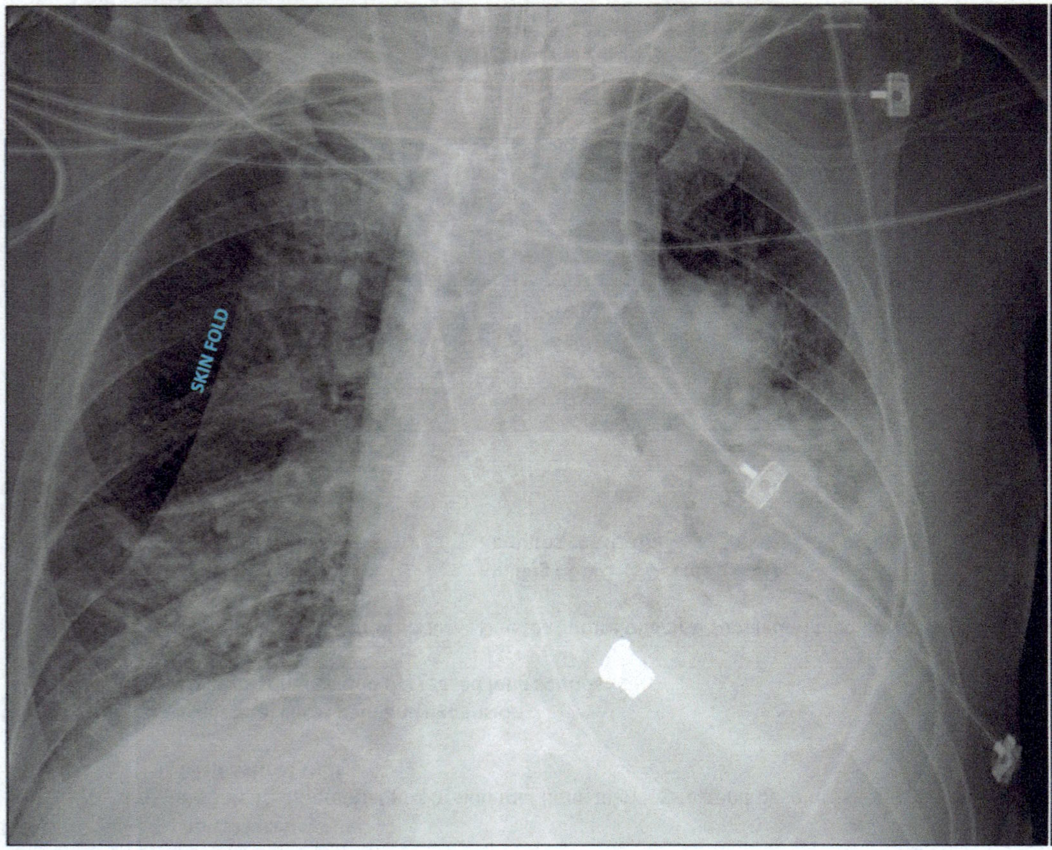

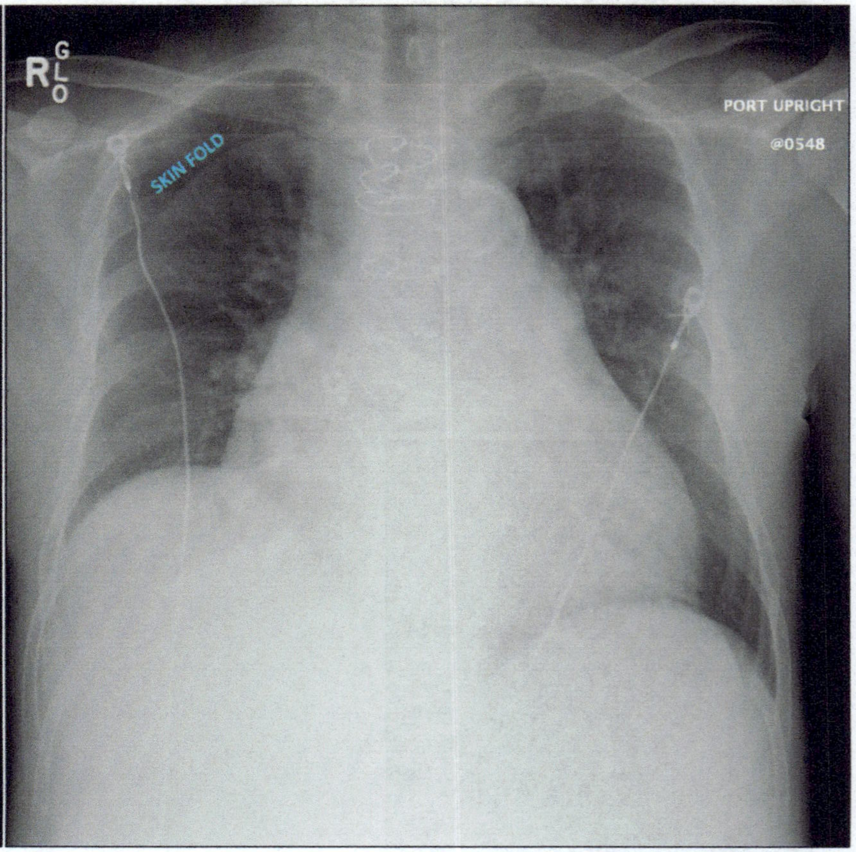

CHEST – THORACIC – PULMONARY

IMAGING: Nonspecific: **Upper lobe consolidation + Clinical history (immigrant)**
Cavitation rare in primary TB

USMLE POINTS: Mycobacteria tuberculosis primarily resides and **proliferates in macrophages**
Transmitted via inhalation of airborne particles
Acid fast positive / Lowenstein-Jensen agar

Primary: **Ghon complex (Hilar nodes + ghon focus)**
Healing fibrosis and calcification → latent (positive PPD+)

Reactivated: **Upper lobes, cough, night sweats, and hemoptysis**
Aspergilloma

Miliary: Disseminated into the blood (bacteremia) → Poor prognosis

Treatment:
- Rifampin
- Isoniazid
- Pyrazinamide
- Ethambutol

Aspergilloma:
Ball-like consolidation within old cavity (gravity dependent)
DDx: Squamous cell carcinoma (also cavitates)
Grow in old lung cavities formed by previous infection → TB & Klebsiella
Will not form in a SCC cavity

MODALITIES: XR → CT WO

TUBERCULOSIS

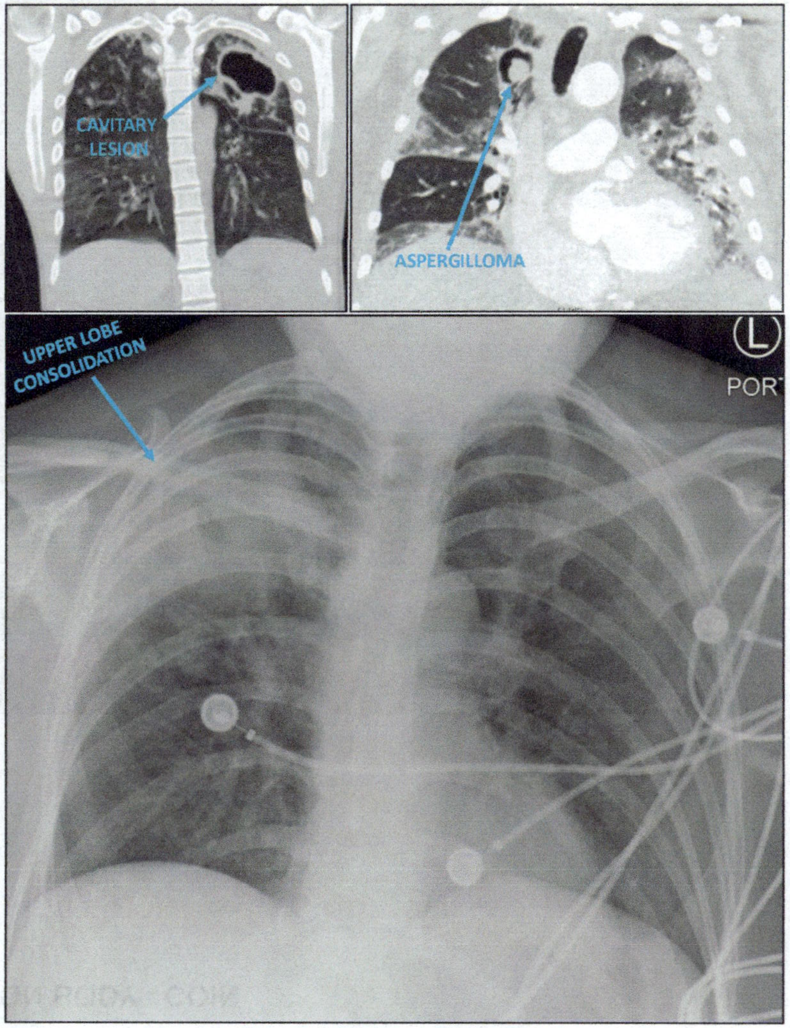

CHEST – THORACIC – PULMONARY

IMAGING:
- Esophagus: **En fosse (coronal)**
- Trachea: **Profile (sagittal plane)**

USMLE POINTS:
Sudden-onset respiratory distress in a child
Most aspirated foreign bodies end up in the **right mainstem bronchus**
Treatment: **Endoscopic retrieval**

DDX: Disc-battery (double edge)

MODALITIES: XR → CT WO / FLX

FOREIGN BODY - COIN

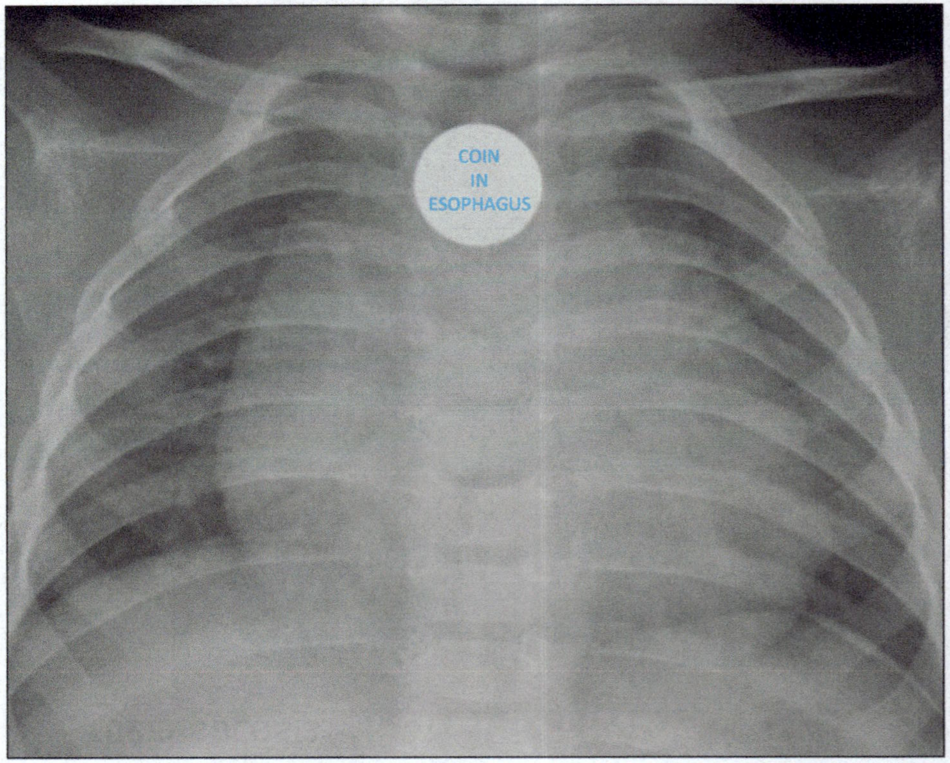

CHEST – THORACIC – PULMONARY

PCP PNEUMONIA

IMAGING: **Predominantly perihilar in distribution + Clinical History**
Fine reticular interstitial changes

USMLE POINTS: **AIDS-defining illness that** presents with a CD4+ count < 200
Bronchoalveolar lavage: Disc-shaped yeast or dark oval bodies
Respiratory transmission
Treatment: **TMP-SMX**
Dapsone & Pyrimethamine (prophylaxis)

Decreased diffusion capacity of CO

MODALITIES: XR → CT WO

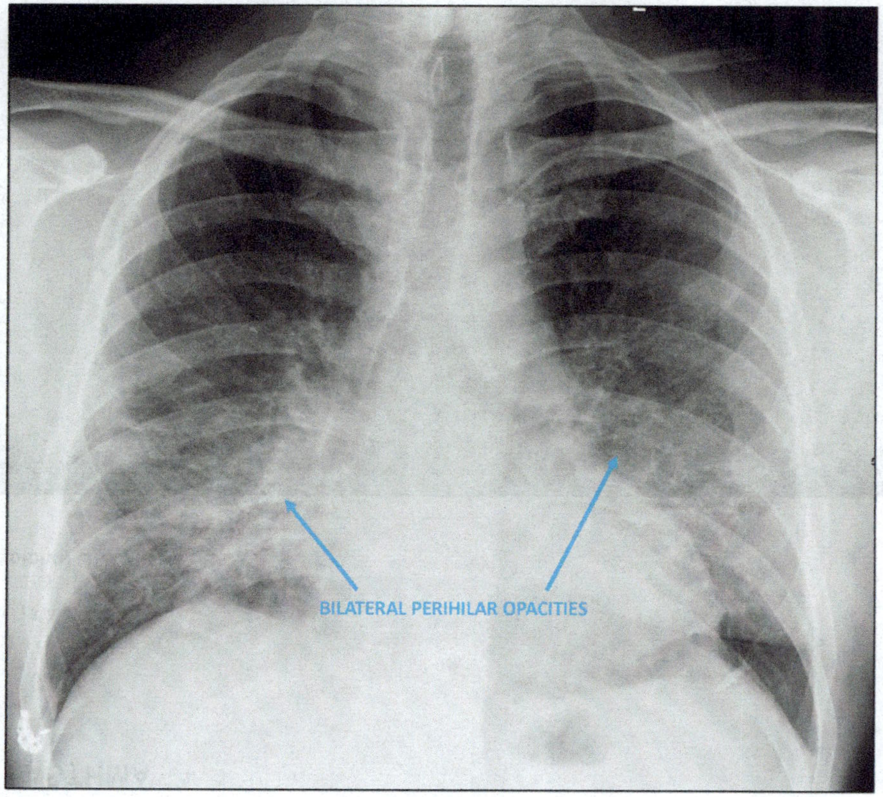

CHEST – THORACIC – PULMONARY

ASTHMA

IMAGING: Hyperinflation
Bronchial wall thickening: **Peribronchial cuffing**

USMLE POINTS:

Presentation: **Wheezing / Episodic cough**
Productive cough with eosinophil-derived crystals (Charcot-Leyden crystals)

Treatment: Short-acting **$\beta 2$ agonist +/- systemic corticosteroids (methylprednisolone) OR Epinephrine**

PFTs:

Intermittent:	FEV1 > 80% predicted
Mild persistent:	FEV1 ≥ 80% predicted
Moderate persistent:	FEV1 60 – 80% predicted
Severe persistent:	FEV1 < 60%
Obstructive patters:	**FEV1/FVC < 70%**

MODALITIES: XR → CT WO

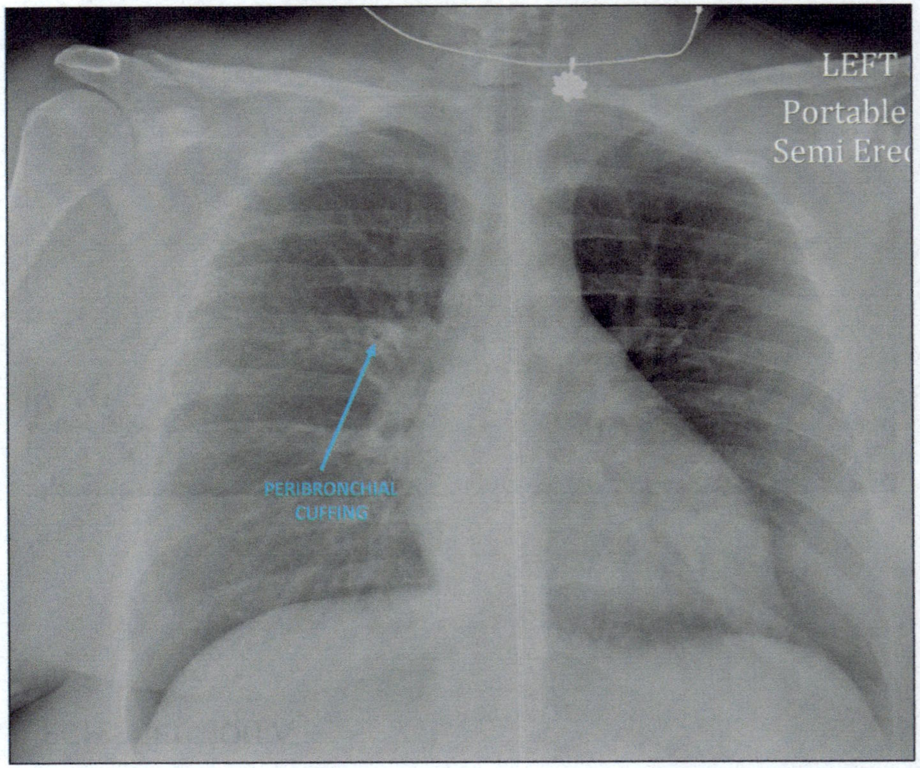

CHEST – THORACIC – PULMONARY

IMAGING: Solitary pulmonary nodule (look for it)
Mass: >3 cm / Nodule: <3 cm

USMLE POINTS: Followed-up as per Fleishner Society Guidelines (beyond scope of USMLE / COMLEX)

Low Risk:	Size	< 0.8 cm	Age < 40	Smoking cessation for > 15 years (or never smoked)
Intermediate Risk:	Size	0.8 - 2 cm	Age 40 - 60	Smoking cessation within the last 5 - 15 years (or current smoker)
High Risk:	Size	> 2 cm	Age > 60	Smoking cessation within the last 5 years (or current smoker)

MODALITIES: XR → CT WO / PET-CT

SOLITARY PULMONARY NODULE

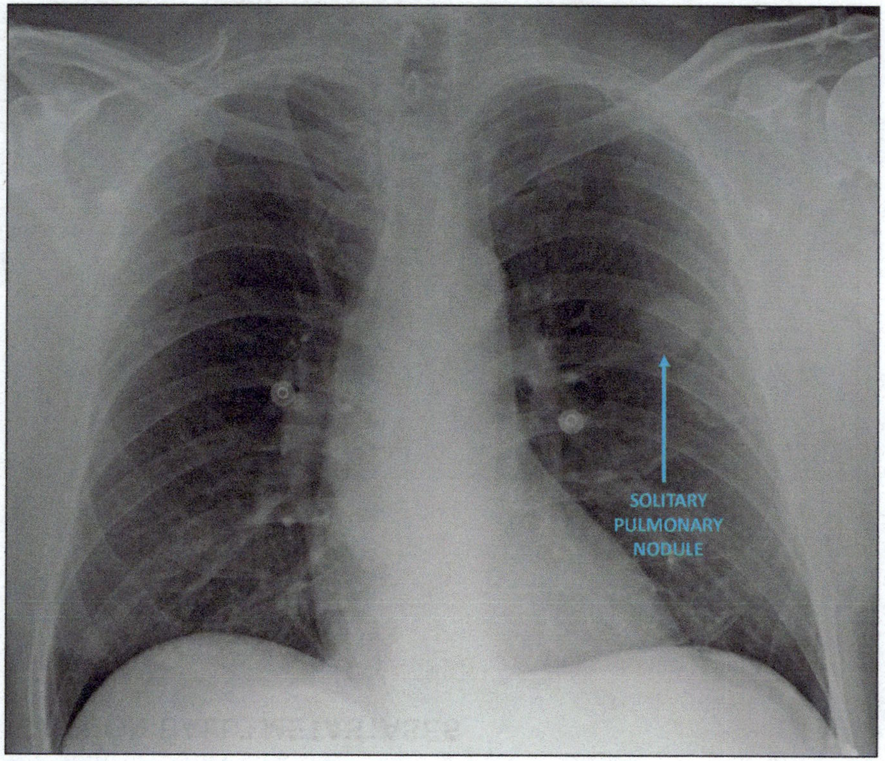

CHEST – THORACIC – PULMONARY

"CANNON-BALL" METASTASES

IMAGING: Multiple large, well-circumscribed, round pulmonary metastases

USMLE POINTS: Choriocarcinoma (female)
Renal cell carcinoma
Testicular cancer (male)

MODALITIES: XR → CT WO

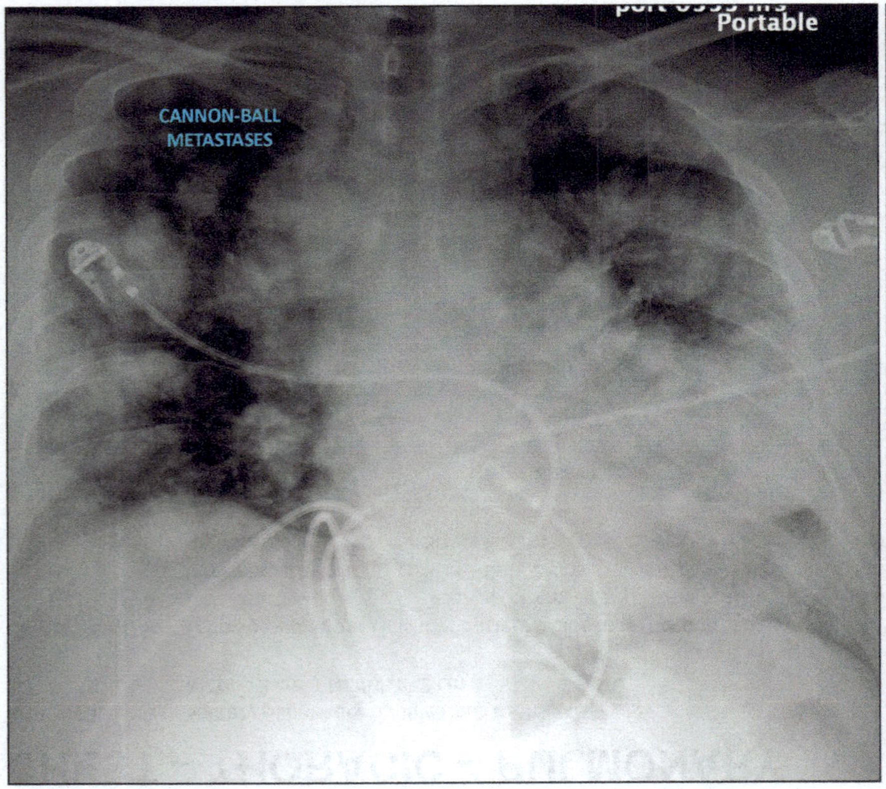

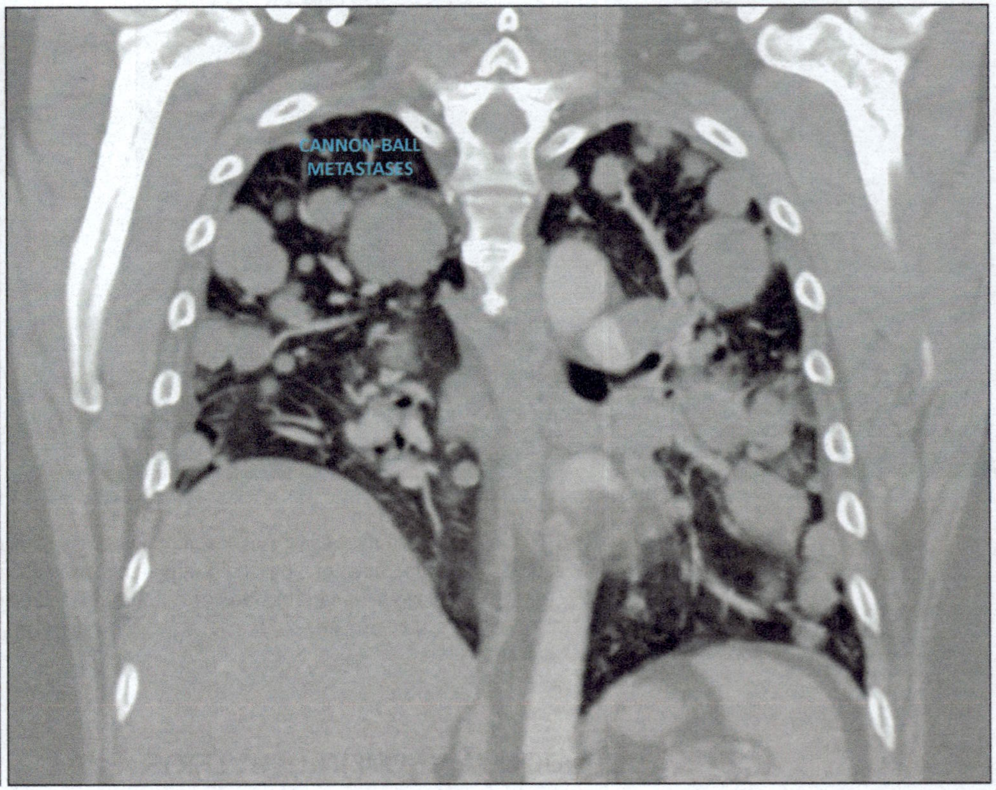

CHEST – THORACIC – PULMONARY

EMPYEMA

IMAGING:
Pleural effusion + Thick pleura
Effusion may contain locules of air
Loculated effusions do not necessarily mean empyema

USMLE POINTS:
Pus in the pleural space
Low pH, low glucose,
Neutrophilia + positive gram stain / culture
S. aureus pneumonia
Requires tube thoracostomy

Lights Criteria:

Pleural : Serum Protein	< 0.5	Transudate
	> 0.5	**Exudate**
Pleural : Serum LDH	< 0.6	Transudate
	> 0.6	**Exudate**
Pleural Fluid LDH	< 2/3 ULN	Transudate
	> 2/3 ULN	**Exudate**

MODALITIES: CT W

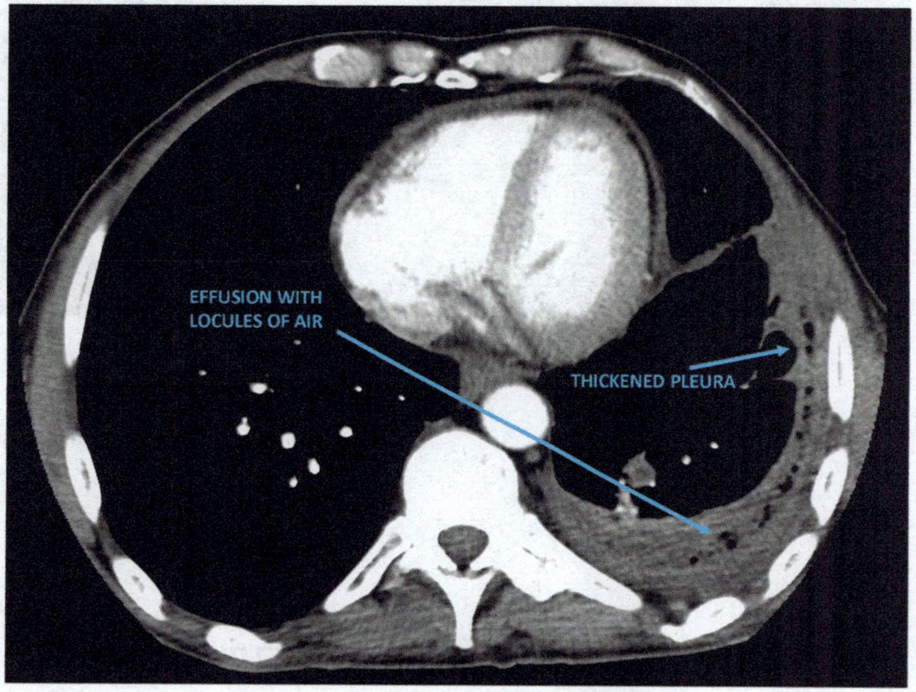

CHEST – THORACIC – PULMONARY

INTERSTITIAL LUNG DISEASE (UIP/IPF)

IMAGING: **Honeycombing: Walls of the stacked cysts are well-defined and often thick (1-3 mm)**
Subpleural, peripheral, and basal in distribution

USMLE POINTS: **Irreversible finding commonly seen in diffuse pulmonary fibrosis (UIP)**
Decreased diffusing capacity and increased A-a gradients
Inflammation to lung parenchyma → Secondary pulmonary hypertension
Associations: Granulomatosis with polyangiitis (Wegener), GP, sarcoidosis, pneumoconiosis, pulmonary LCH
Bleomycin, busulfan, methotrexate, and procarbazine

MODALITIES: XR → CT WO

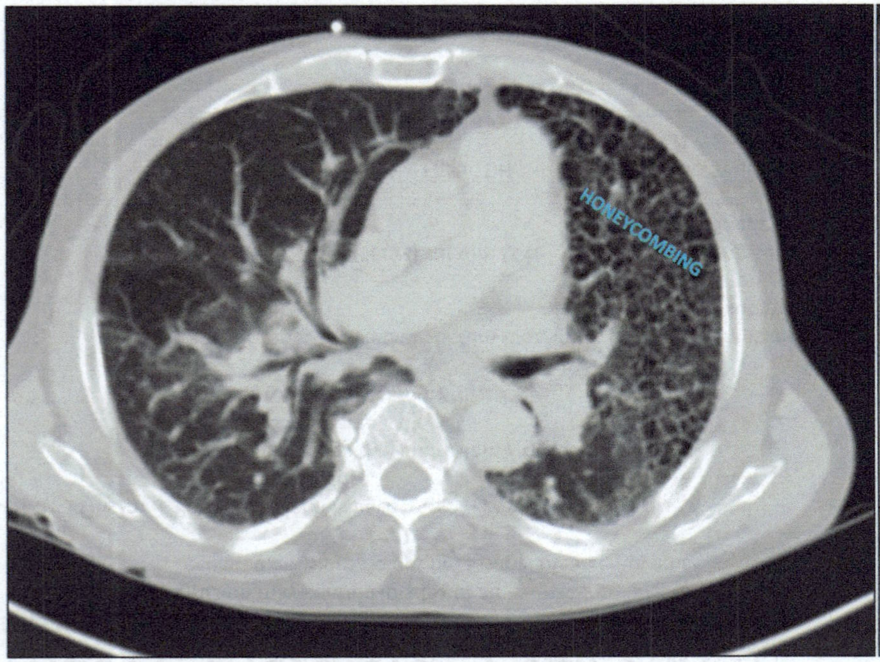

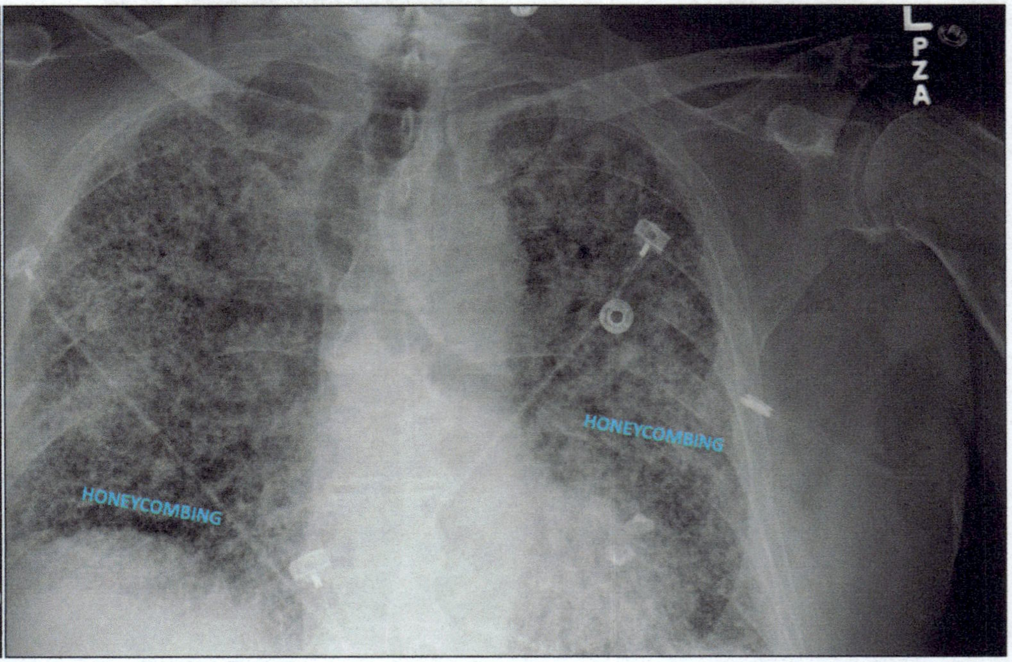

CHEST – THORACIC – PULMONARY

PULMONARY ABSCESS

IMAGING: **Cavitary lesion with air fluid level + Thick, irregular wall**

USMLE POINTS: Most commonly from **aspiration**

Anaerobic bacteria: **Bacteroides, Fusobacterium, Peptostreptococcus, and Prevotella**
Aerobic bacteria: **S. aureus and klebsiella**

Treatment: **Clindamycin, Carbapenem, Ampicillin-Sulbactam**
Associations: **Hyponatremia** (infection-induced ADH secretion)
Risk factors: Patients with bronchial obstruction/cancer
Aspiration

MODALITIES: XR → CT W

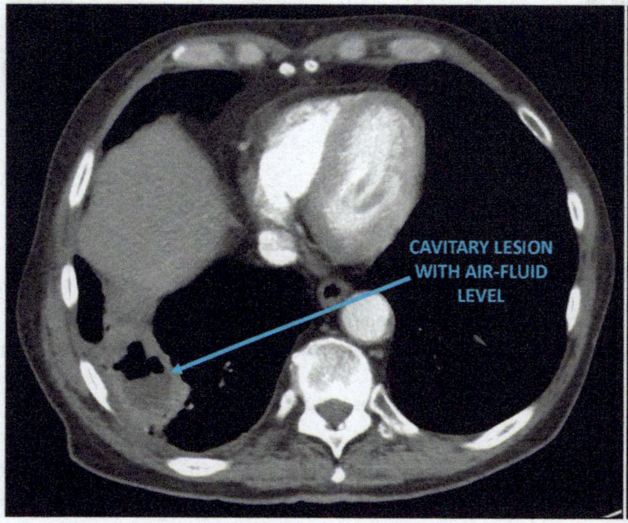

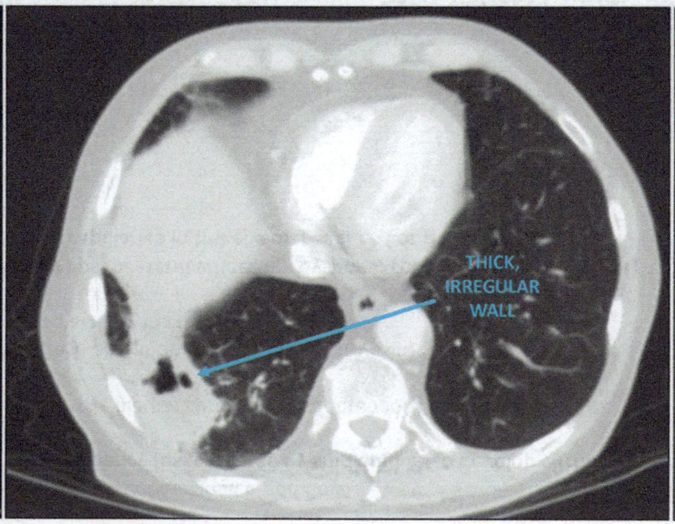

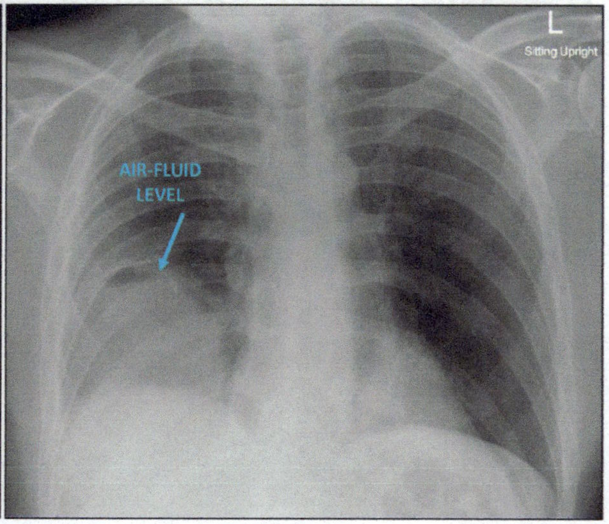

CHEST – THORACIC – PULMONARY

EMPHYSEMA

IMAGING:

Centrilobular emphysema: Most common. Upper lung zones. Smoking

Panacinar emphysema: Lower zones, matching areas of maximal blood flow.
Alpha-1-antitrypsin deficiency (exacerbated by smoking). Also develop cirrhosis.

Paraseptal emphysema: Peripheral, adjacent to the pleural surfaces → spontaneous pneumothorax

USMLE POINTS: Destruction of alveolar air sacs → Imbalance of elastase and antiproteases (α1-antitrypsin)
α1-antitrypsin deficiency, resulting in excess elastase activity in alveoli

Presentation: **Prolonged expiration with pursed lips, bilateral wheezing, dyspnea, cough**
Complications: **Hypoxemia (due to destruction of capillaries in the alveolar sac) → Cor pulmonale**

PFTs:
Decreased FEV1sec / FVC
Increased TLC and RV
Decreased diffusion capacity

MODALITIES: XR → CT WO

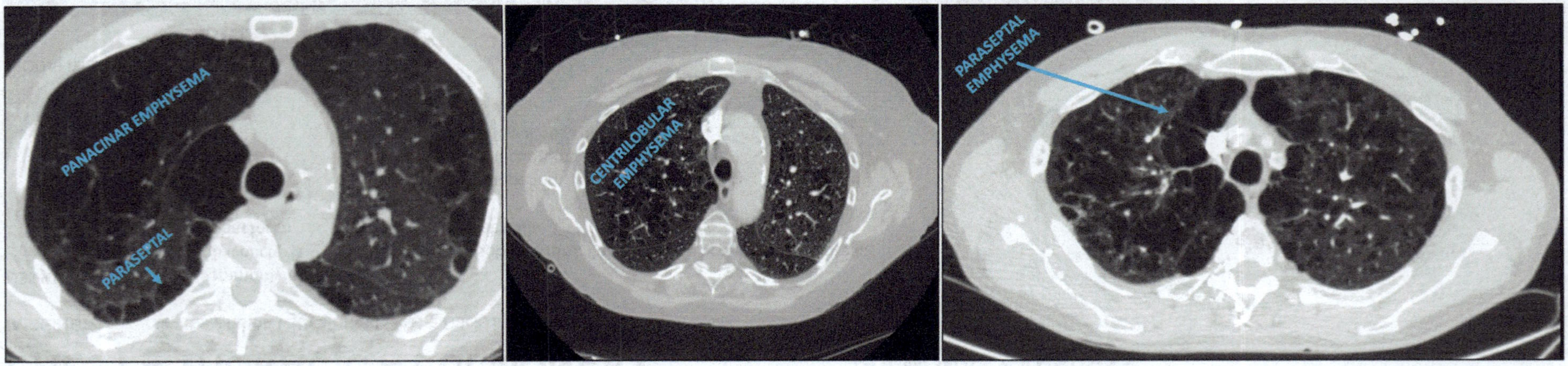

CHEST – THORACIC – PULMONARY

ASBESTOSIS

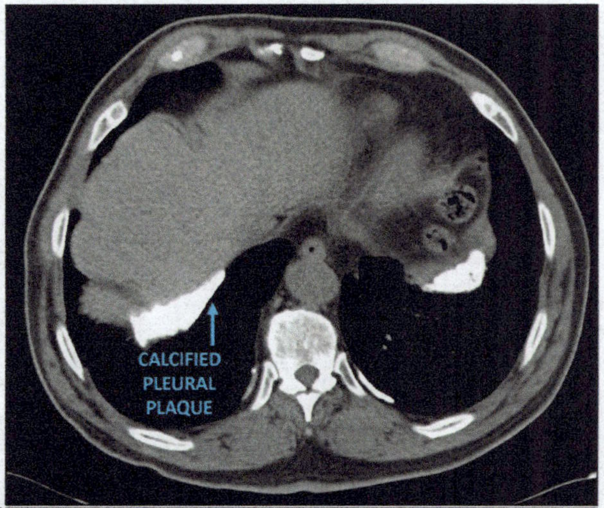

IMAGING:
Pleural effusions + pleural plaques are common manifestations of asbestos-related disease
No pathognomonic radiological features specific for asbestosis
Irregular opacities with a fine reticular pattern
Calcified or noncalcified pleural plaques may be evident
"Ivory white" calcified supradiaphragmatic and pleural plaques

USMLE POINTS:
Shipbuilding, roofing, plumbing
Dumb-bell fusiform golden-brown rods
Increased risk of bronchogenic carcinoma (more common) and mesothelioma (takes 20-40 years to develop)
No association with TB

MODALITIES: XR → CT WO

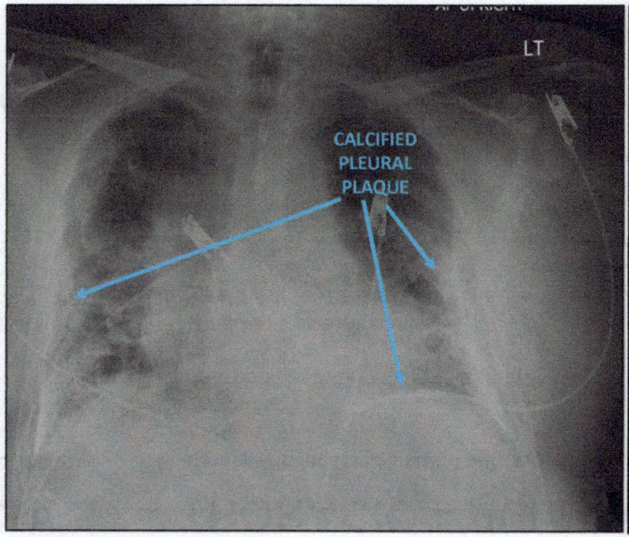

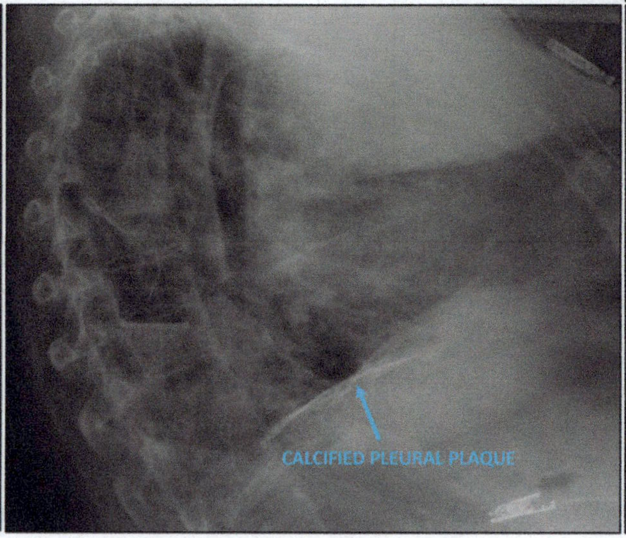

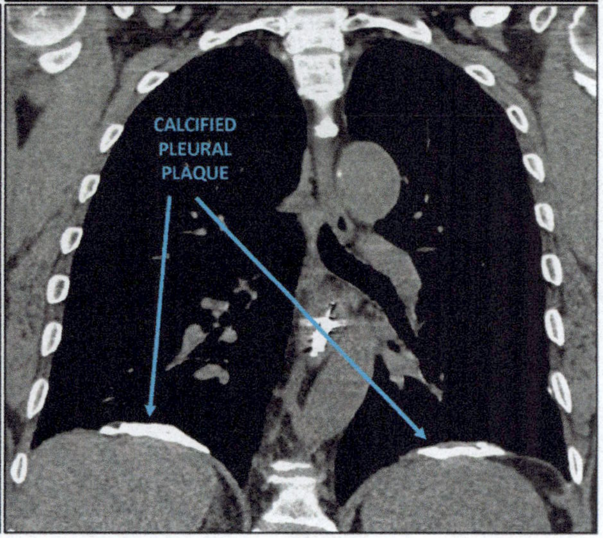

CHEST – THORACIC – PULMONARY

SILICOSIS

IMAGING:

Bilateral perihilar consolidation and/or ground-glass opacities + Clinical history
Progressive massive fibrosis
Upper lobes
Fibrotic nodules in the upper lobes of the lung + **"eggshell" calcification** of the hilar lymph nodes

USMLE POINTS:

Classified as a **pneumoconiosis**
Increases **risk for TB infection**, cor pulmonale, and Caplan syndrome
Prolonged silica exposure → **Sandblasters**, **Silica miners**, **Foundries**

Berylliosis: **Aerospace or nuclear industry worker**

MODALITIES:

XR → CT WO

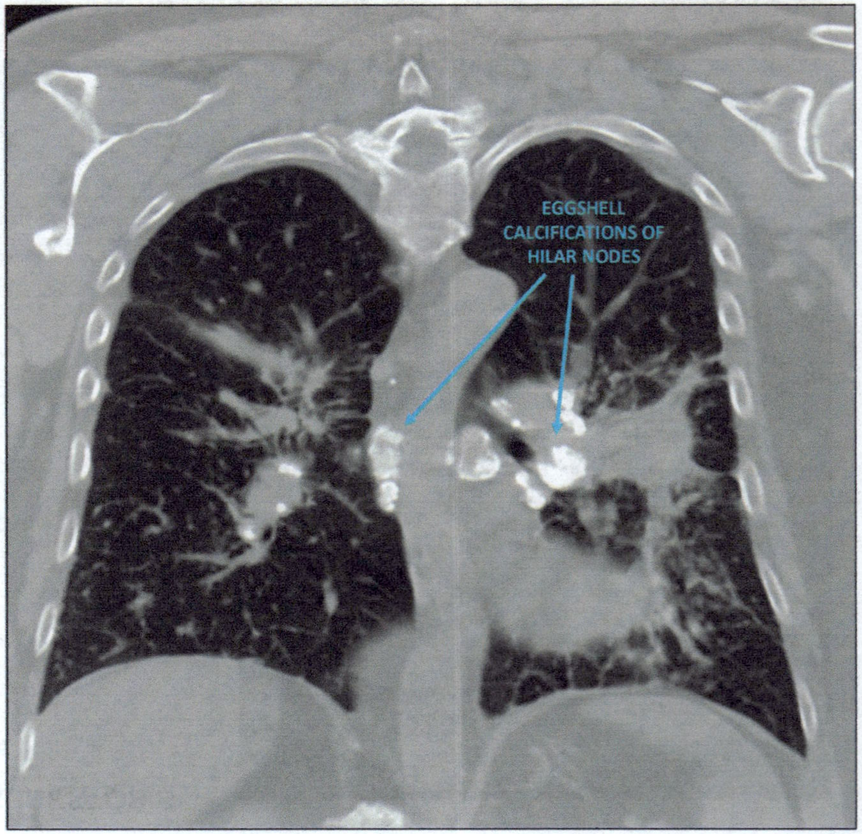

CHEST – THORACIC – PULMONARY

SVC SYNDROME

IMAGING:
Extrinsic compression
Intrinsic stenosis
Thrombosis of the superior vena cava

USMLE POINTS:
Most commonly from malignancy → **Mediastinal mass or Pancoast (superior sulcus) tumor**
Thromboembolic from indwelling central venous catheters
Impaired drainage of the upper extremities, neck, and head → **Facial edema** and dilated collateral veins in the upper torso, jugular vein, and head
Surgical intervention / Stent often required

MODALITIES: CTA

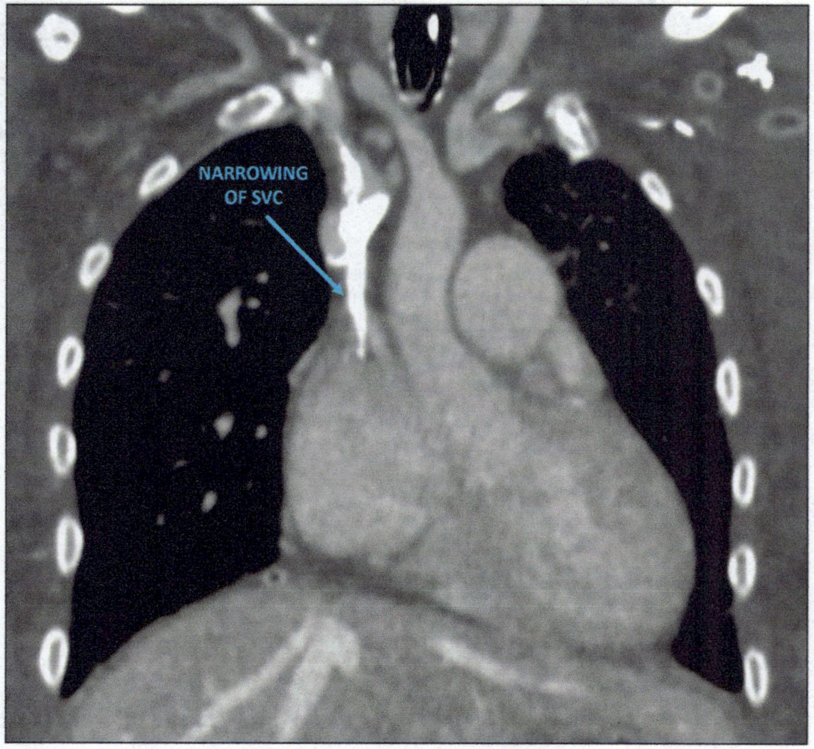

CHEST – THORACIC – PULMONARY

THYROID SCINTIGRAPHY

IMAGING:

Normal:	**Uniform distribution**
Graves:	**Diffusely increased radiotracer**
Multinodular:	**Patchy areas (increased trace in a nodule and the rest suppressed)**

USMLE POINTS:

Exogenous hyperthyroidism (or factitious hyperthyroidism) can cause **low RAI uptake** in scintigraphy

Painless thyroiditis, thyroid scintigraphy shows decreased radioiodine uptake

Hot nodules:	**Likely benign**
Cold nodules:	**Perform FNA**

MODALITIES: US / NUC

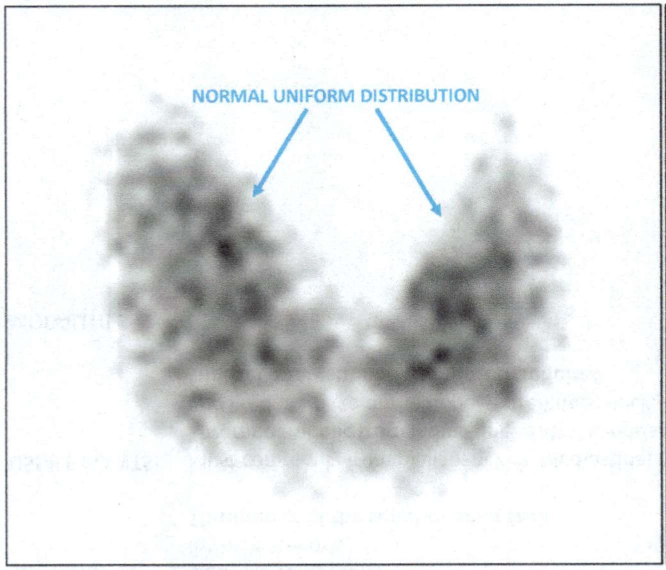

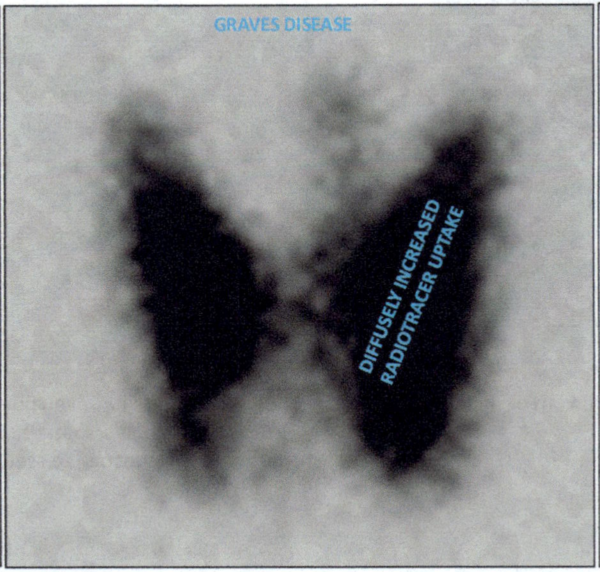

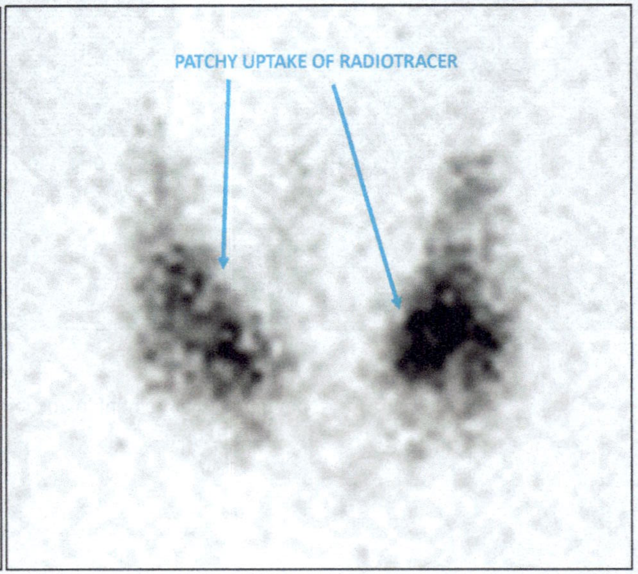

CHEST – THORACIC – PULMONARY

THYROGLOSSAL DUCT CYST

IMAGING: **Midline cystic lesion**
Most commonly infrahyoid

USMLE POINTS: **Anterior, midline neck mass**
Moves with swallowing or protrusion of the tongue
Most common cause of a midline neck mass
Along the course of the thyroglossal duct (foramen cecum to the thyroid gland)
Treatment: Surgical excision

MODALITIES: US / CT WO

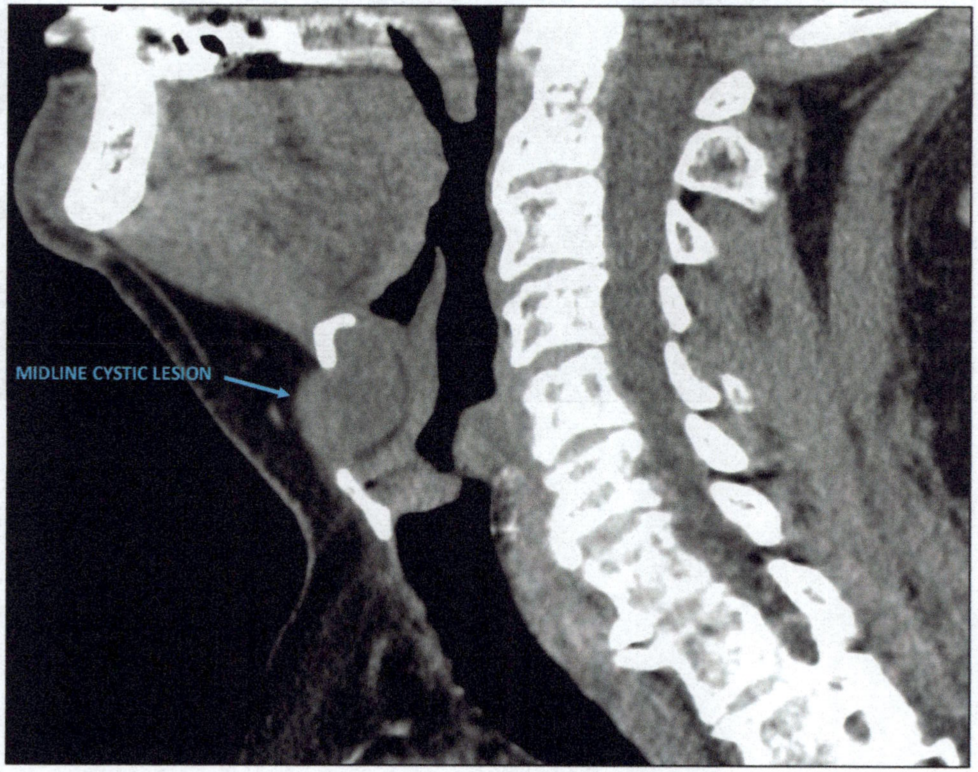

CHEST – THORACIC – PULMONARY

PNEUMOMEDIASTINUM

IMAGING: **Extraluminal air** within the mediastinum
Etiology: Lungs, trachea, central bronchi, esophagus, and peritoneal cavity
Pneumopericardium
Air outlining bronchial wall
"Continuous diaphragm sign"

USMLE POINTS: **Boerhaave syndrome** presents as esophageal rupture + pneumomediastinum + subcutaneous emphysema
Presentation: **Severe retrosternal pain**

MODALITIES: XR → CT WO

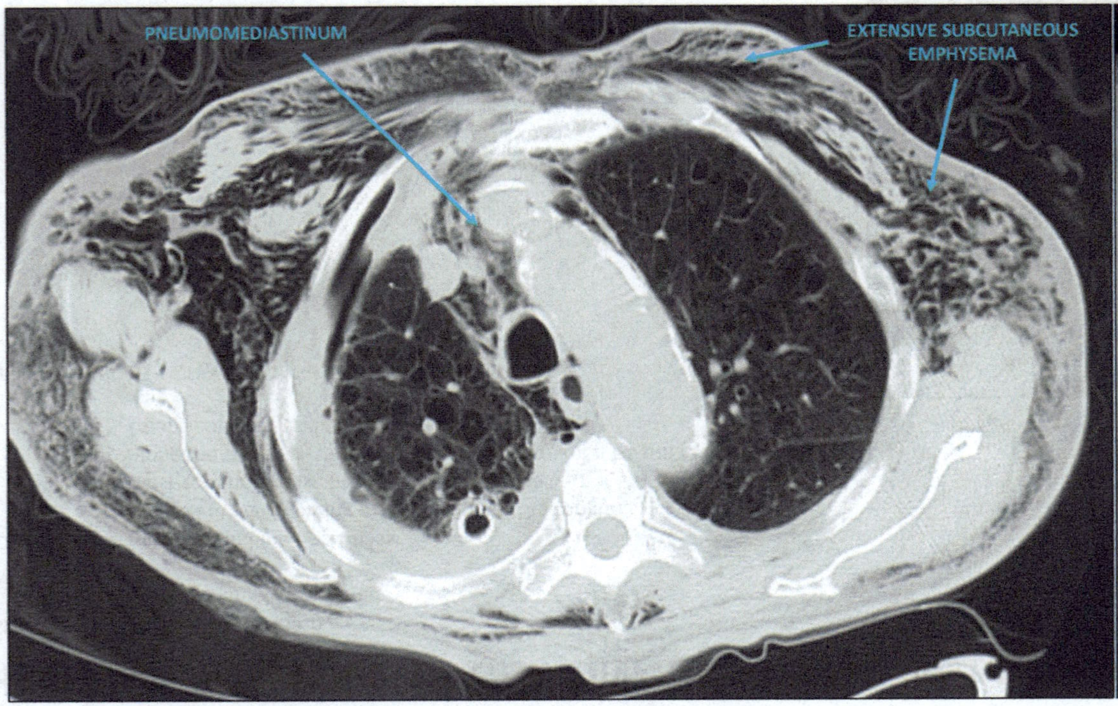

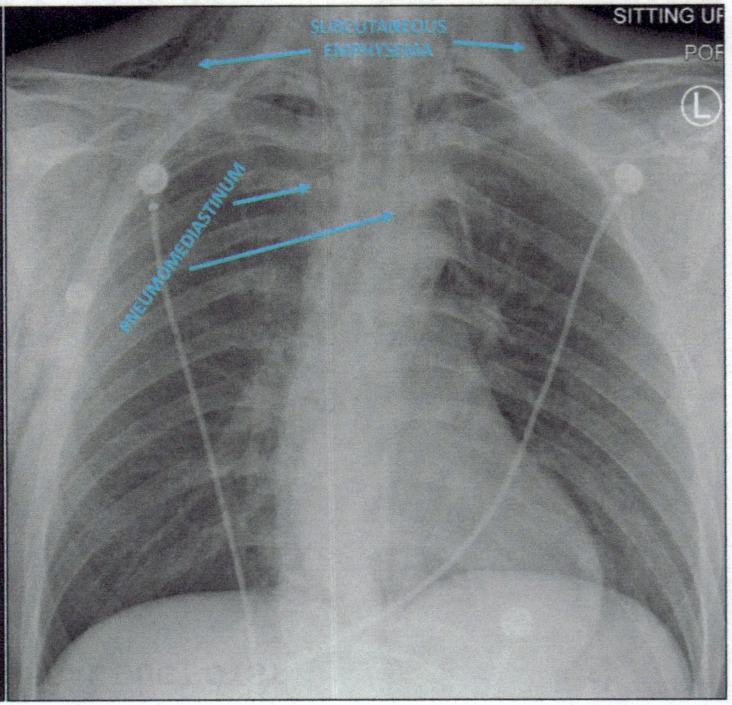

CARDIAC - VASCULAR

CARDIAC – VASCULAR

AORTIC RUPTURE

IMAGING:

Pending rupture: Induration / Stranding surrounding an aortic aneurysm
"Draped aorta sign" - Posterior wall of the aorta indistinct from adjacent structures
→ Contour of the aorta follows that of adjacent vertebrae

USMLE POINTS:

Hemorrhagic shock / Cardiac tamponade
Retroperitoneal hemorrhage adjacent the aneurysm

Triad:
- **Severe pain**
- **Hypotension**
- **Pulsatile mass**

Risk factors:
- Age
- **Hypertension**
- Male gender
- Smoking
- Family history
- **Marfan syndrome**
- **Ehlers Danlos Syndrome**

Treatment: **EVAR**

MODALITIES: CTA

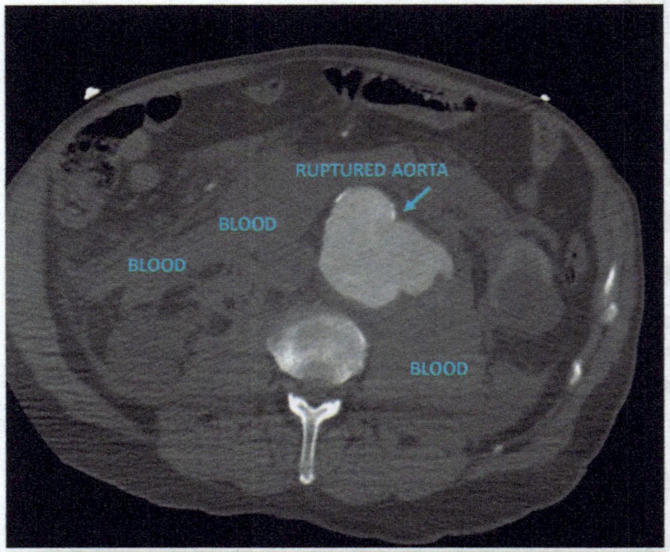

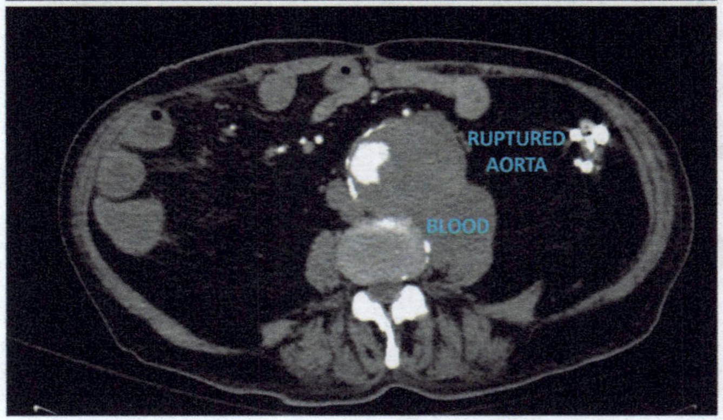

CARDIAC – VASCULAR

IMAGING: Blood entering the media through a tear in the intima → Intimal flap

Type A: **Before the takeoff of the Left subclavian artery (3rd branch vessel)**
Type B: **After the takeoff of the Left subclavian artery (3rd branch vessel)**

USMLE POINTS: Tearing of aortic intima which forms a false, blood-filled lumen

Risk factors:
- **Hypertension**
- Bicuspid aortic valve
- Connective tissue disorders (eg, Marfan syndrome)

Presentation:
- **Sudden-onset chest pain radiating to back**
- **Unequal BP in arms**
- **Weak and/or absent pulses**

Stanford Type B: **ONLY involves descending aorta**

Treatment:
- **Type-B:** **B-blockers**
- **Type-A:** **Surgery**

MODALITIES: CTA WWO (WO portion to look for IMH)

TYPE-B AORTIC DISSECTION

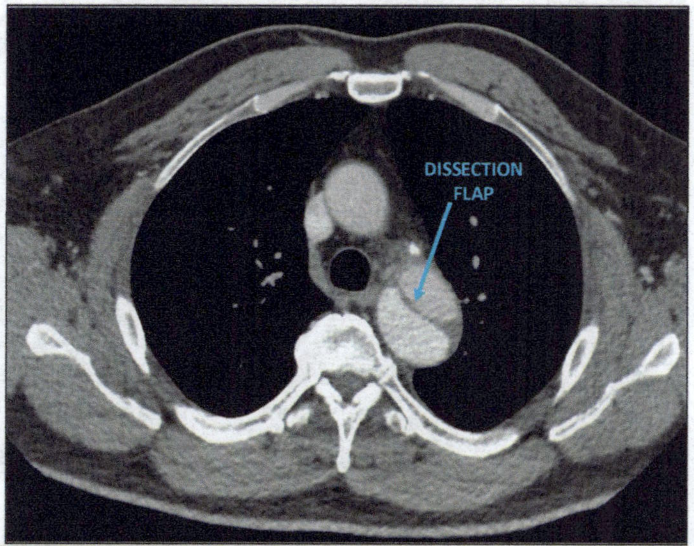

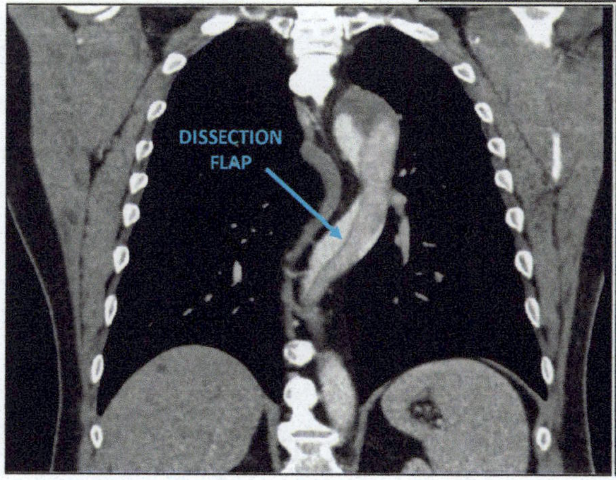

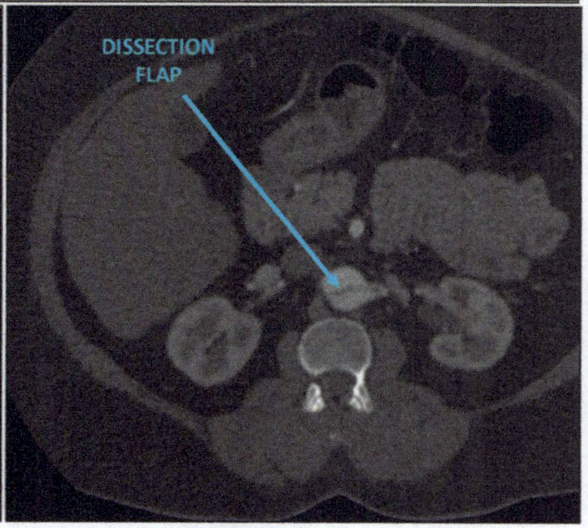

CARDIAC – VASCULAR

AORTIC INTRAMURAL HEMATOMA

IMAGING:
Blood in the intima of the aortic wall
Look for penetrating atherosclerotic ulcer
Should be assessed for on **NON-contract images**
Classified as Type A and B like Aortic dissections

USMLE POINTS:
Atypical type of aortic dissection
Contained hemorrhage **(usually from vasa vasorum) that does not result in intimal tear**

Presentation: **Chest pain radiating to back**

Risk Factors: **Hypertension**
Generally seen in descending aorta

Complications: Aortic rupture
Aortic dissection
Aortic aneurysm

Type A requires surgical treatment

MODALITIES: CT **WO (BETTER SEEN WITHOUT CONTRAST)**

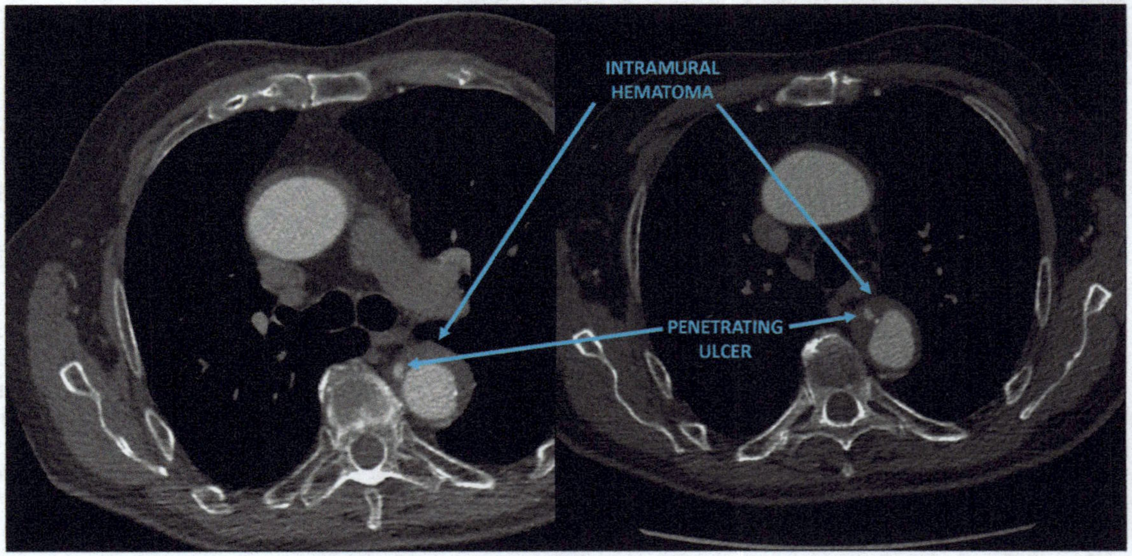

CARDIAC – VASCULAR

AORTIC COARCTATION

IMAGING:
Narrowing of aorta from distal to the brachiocephalic artery → the level of ductus arteriosus
Inferior rib notching
Blood supply to the descending aorta is via the patent ductus arteriosus
"3-sign" on CXR

USMLE POINTS:
Aortic narrowing near ductus arteriosus
Decreased blood flow across aorta in utero

Post-ductal: Adult
Pre-ductal: Infantile

Treatment: **Prostaglandin E1**

Associations: **Bicuspid aortic valve**
Turner syndrome

Presentation: Hypertension in upper extremities
Weak and/or delayed pulse in lower extremities
Harsh systolic murmur
Femoral pulse < Brachial pulses
Bounding pulses in upper extremities & carotids

MODALITIES: CTA

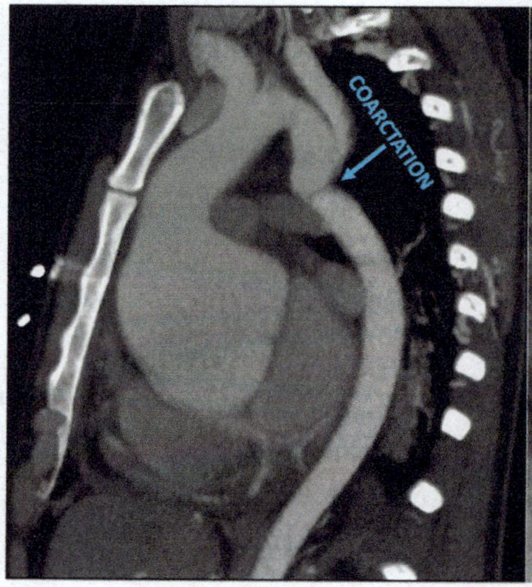

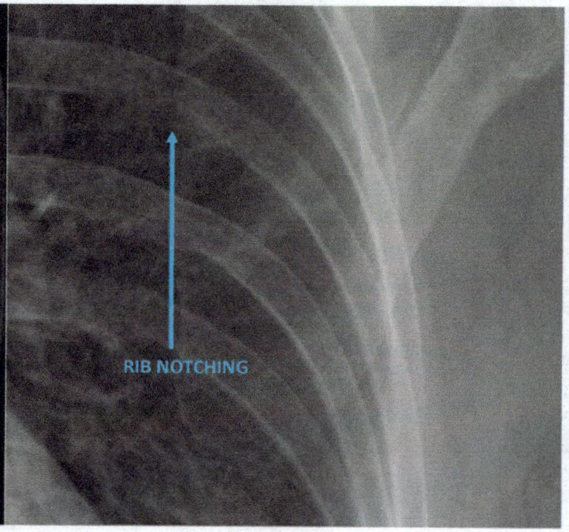

CARDIAC – VASCULAR

PERICARDIAL EFFUSION

IMAGING: CXR: "Water-bottle" Shape on CXR
CT: Fluid within the pericardium

USMLE POINTS: **Accumulation of fluid in the pericardial sac → Restricts ventricular filling**
Pulsus pardoxus
Risk factors: Pericardititis
Malignancy
SLE
TB
Uremia

Cardiac tamponade: Beck Triad: **Muffled heart sounds**
JVD
Hypotension

EKG: **Low voltage**
Electrical alternans

Cath: **Equalization of pressure in all chambers during diastole**

MODALITIES: XR / ECHO

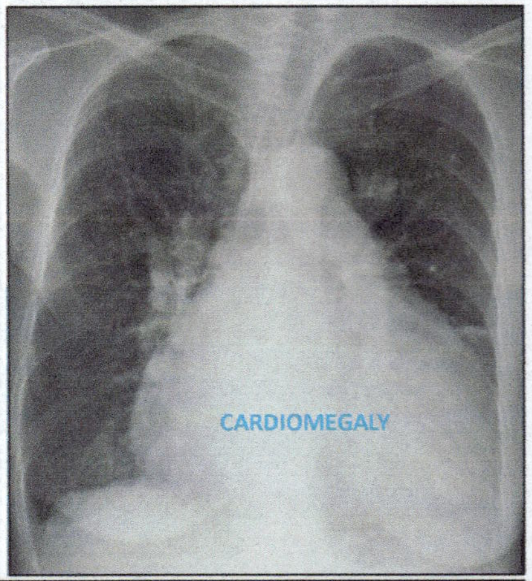

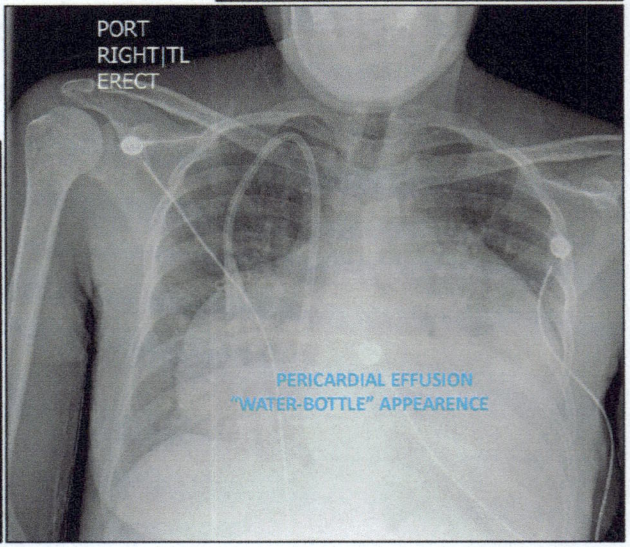

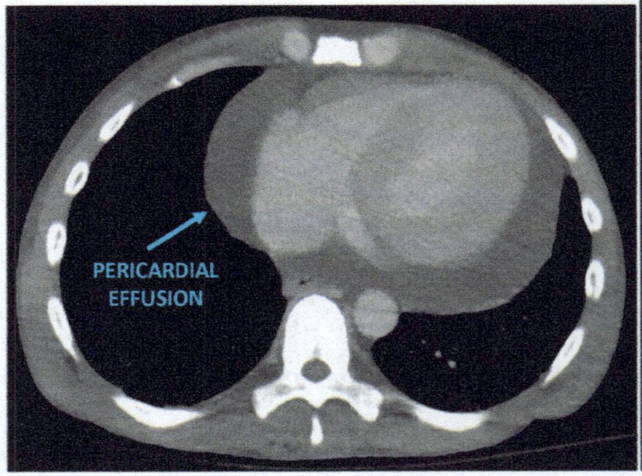

CARDIAC – VASCULAR

ATRIAL MYXOMA

IMAGING: **Most commonly in the left atrium**
Attached to the interatrial septum
in the fossa ovalis of the atrial septum

USMLE POINTS: Most common primary cardiac tumor in adults
Benign

Presentation: Fever, weight loss, fatigue **from IL-6 production**
May crumble and cause systemic embolization
Can result in **stroke**
Diastolic "pop"

Treatment: Surgery

MODALITIES: MR WWO

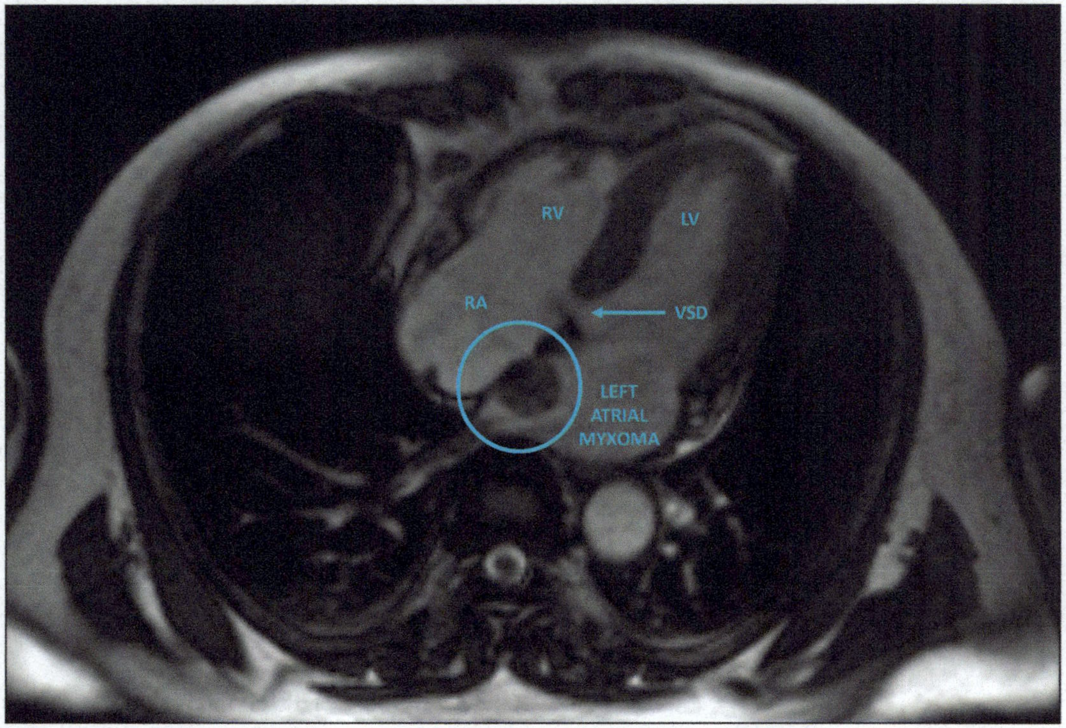

CARDIAC – VASCULAR

BEURGERS DISEASE

IMAGING: **Extensive arterial occlusive disease → corkscrew collateral vessels**
Will show on angiogram

USMLE POINTS: Smoking history + Painful (claudication)
Medium-vessel vasculitis
Males 25-40 years old with heavy smoking history

Presentation: **Intermittent claudication (pain → important to distinguish from other vasculitides)**
Ulceration
May lead to gangrene and autoamputation of digits

Treatment: **Smoking cessation**

MODALITIES: ANGIO / CTA

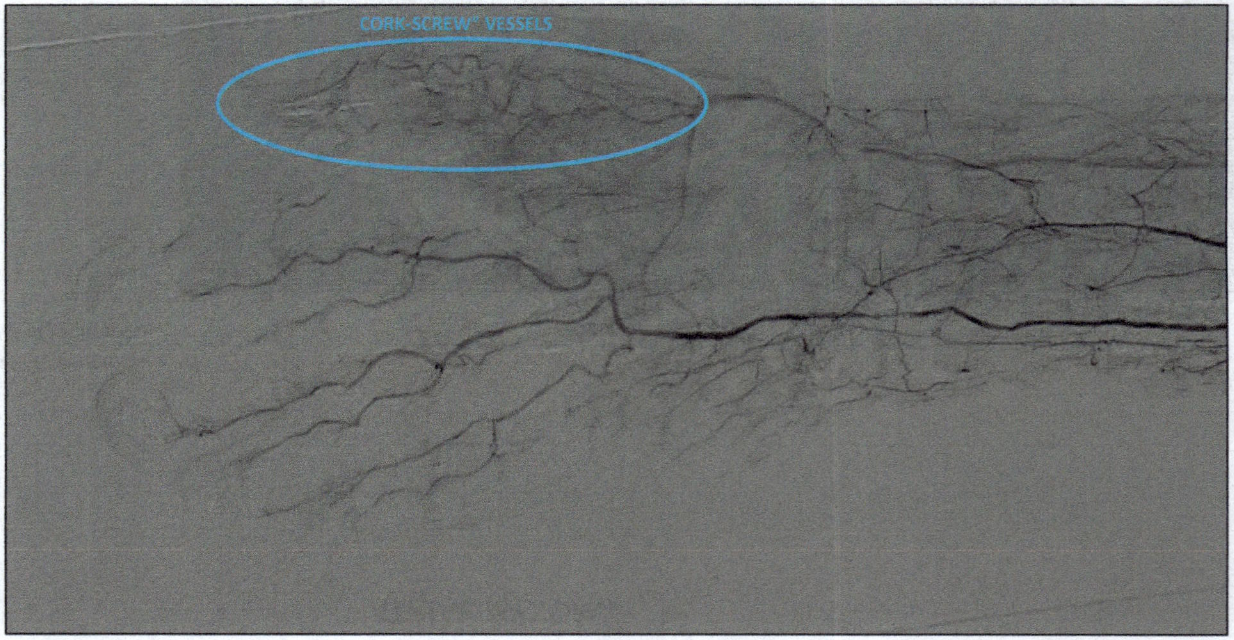

CARDIAC – VASCULAR

EBSTEIN ANOMALY

IMAGING:

CXR: **Severe right-sided cardiomegaly due to an elongated and enlarged right atrium**
Decreased pulmonary vasculature

CT: Apical displacement of the septal and posterior leaflets of the tricuspid valve
"Atrialization" of the right ventricle

USMLE POINTS:

Cyanotic congenital heart defect
Increased RA pressure → blood to left heart via foramen ovale or ASD (Tx: Prostoglandins)
Displacement of tricuspid valve leaflets downward toward apex of right ventricle
Holosystolic murmur

Associations:
Tricuspid regurgitation
Right-sided heart failure
May result from lithium exposure in-utero

MODALITIES: ECHO / CXR / CARDAIC MRI

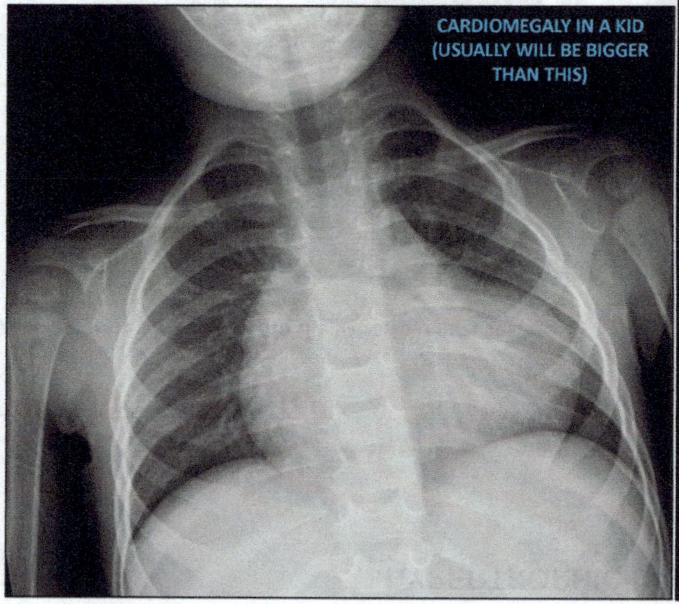

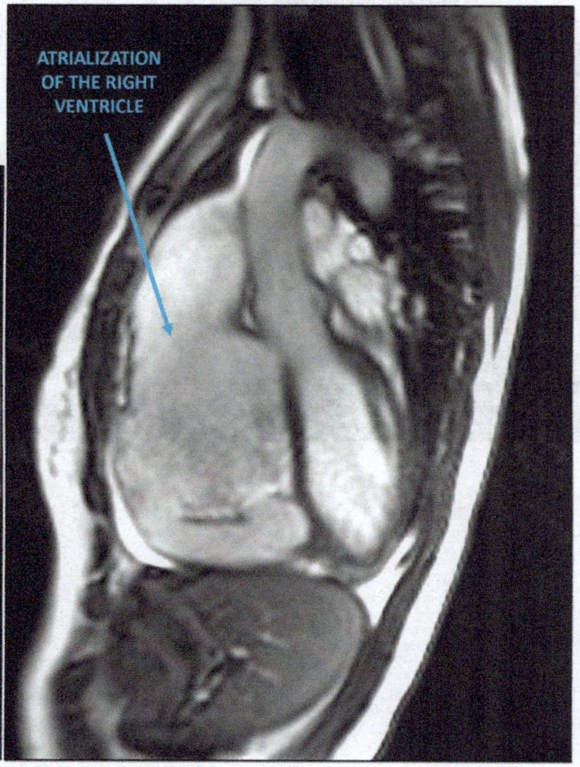

CARDIAC – VASCULAR

HYPERTROPHIC CARDIOMYOPATHY

IMAGING: **Hypertrophied and non-dilated left ventricle**
Thickening interventricular septum

USMLE POINTS: **Death is from arrythmias (after exercise)**
Familial (autosomal dominant) mutation in genes encoding sarcomeric proteins

Presentation: **S4**
LVOT obstruction: Ejection systolic murmur → Louder with the Valsalva maneuver
Mitral regurgitation

Treatment: B-blocker
Ca2+ channel blockers

MODALITIES: ECHO / CARDIAC MRI

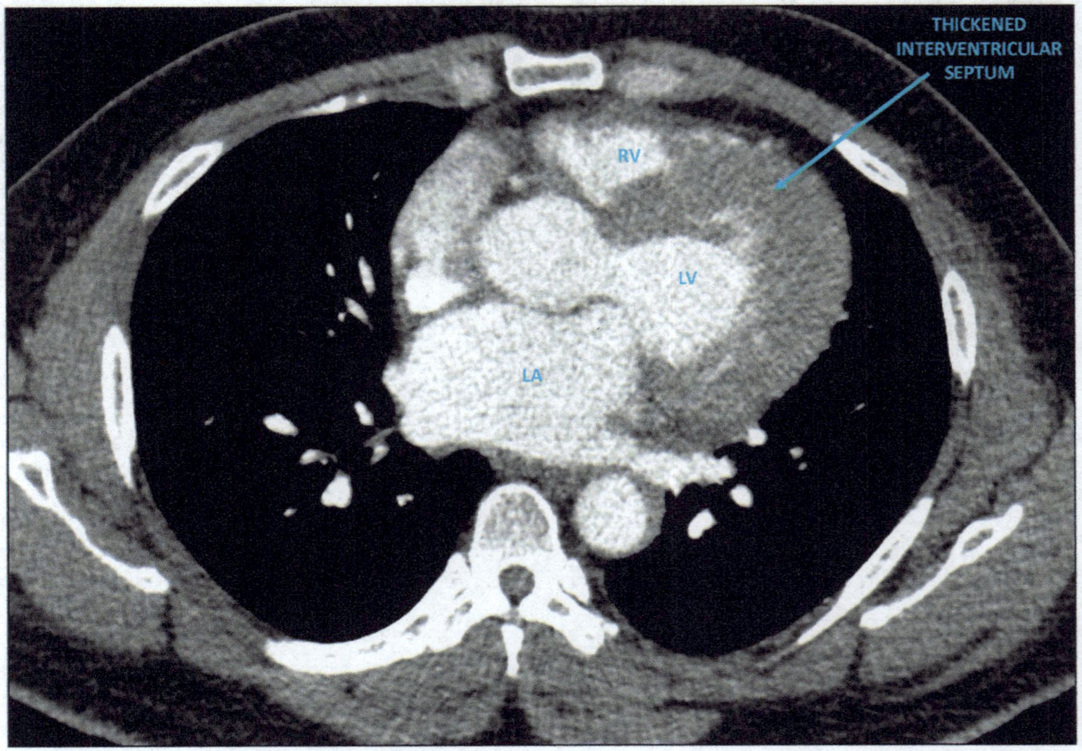

CARDIAC – VASCULAR

IMAGING: **Coronary artery aneurysm in a child**

USMLE POINTS: **Asian** children <4 years old

CRASH and BURN:
- **C**onjunctival injection
- **R**ash
- **A**denopathy
- **S**trawberry tongue
- **H**and-foot changes (edema, erythema
- **Burn**: fever >5 days

Myocardial infarctions or arrythmias and cause death

Treatment: **IV immunoglobulin**
Aspirin

MODALITIES: CARDIAC CT / CARDIAC MRI / ANGIO

KAWASAKI DISEASE

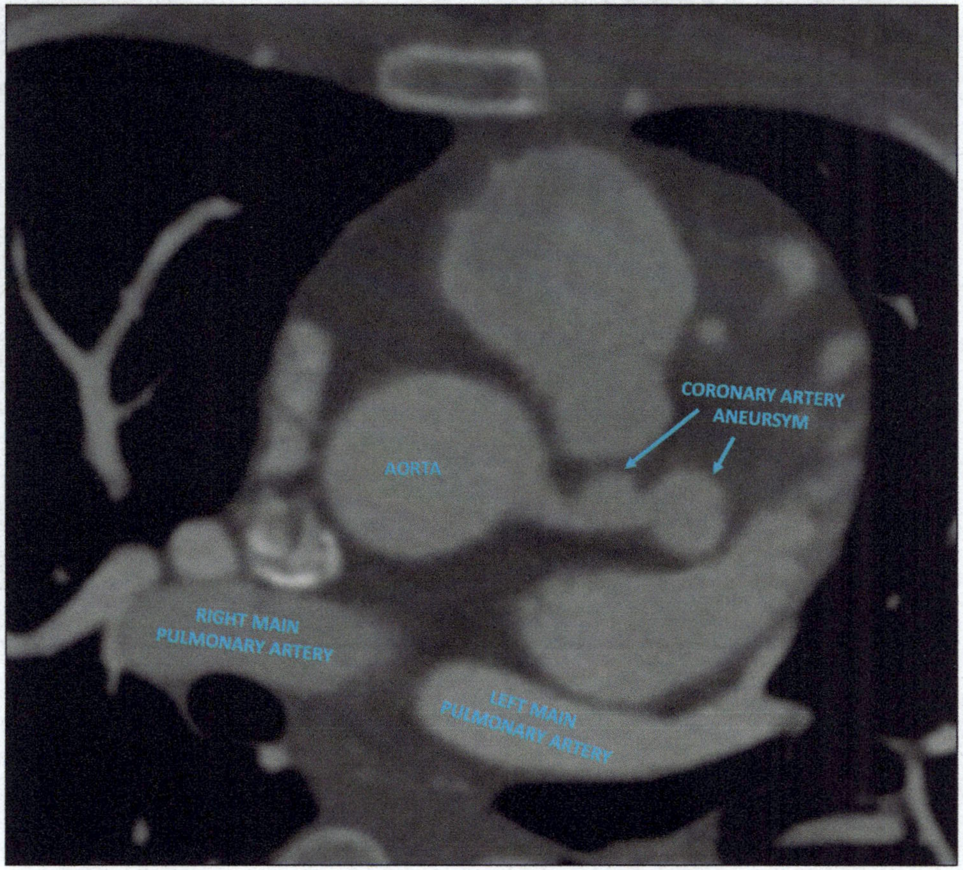

CARDIAC – VASCULAR

IMAGING: **Congenital defect → Opening in the interatrial septum of the heart**
Right atrial enlargement

USMLE POINTS: Congenital heart defect of the interatrial septum
Ostium secundum: **Most common**
Primum ASD: **Associated with other cardiac defects**

Pulmonary hypertension and **Eisenmenger** syndrome

Can result in "paradoxical emboli" from DVT

Associations: Fetal EtOH Sx
Trisomy 21

Auscultation: Loud S1
Wide, fixed split S2
Systolic ejection murmur

Surgery: **Shunt ratio: > 1.5:1**
Primum ASD
RH failure

MODALITIES: ECHO / CARDIAC CT / CARDAIC MRI

ATRIAL SEPTAL DEFECT

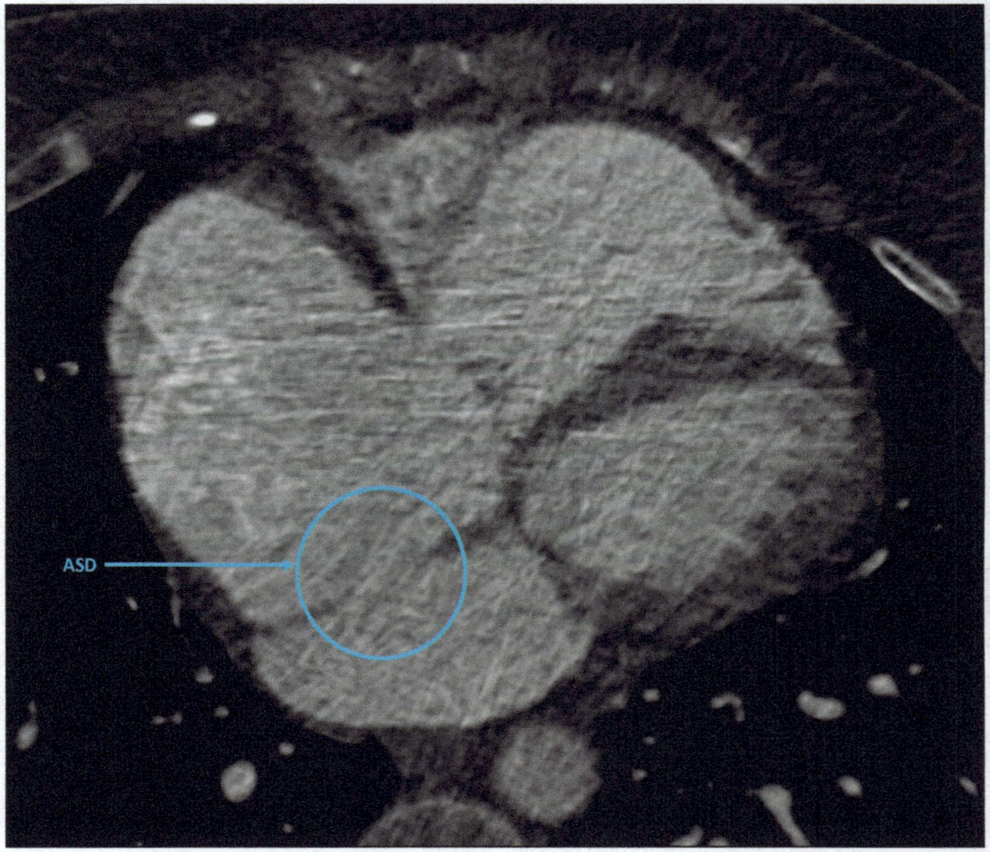

CARDIAC – VASCULAR

VENTRICULAR SEPTAL DEFECT

IMAGING: Opening in the interventricular septum of the heart

USMLE POINTS: Most common congenital heart defect
Left-to-right shunting in the heart → increased pulmonary blood flow to the pulmonary vasculature
Pulmonary hypertension and Eisenmenger syndrome

Associations:
Trisomy 21
DiGeorge Syndrome
Turner Syndrome

Auscultation:
High-pitched and harsh holosystolic murmur
Decreases with Valsalva & amyl nitrate
Increased with handgrip, squatting, and leg raise

Surgery:
Large defect
Heart failure
Pulmonary hypertension
Aortic insufficiency

MODALITIES: ECHO / CARDIAC CT / CARDAIC MRI

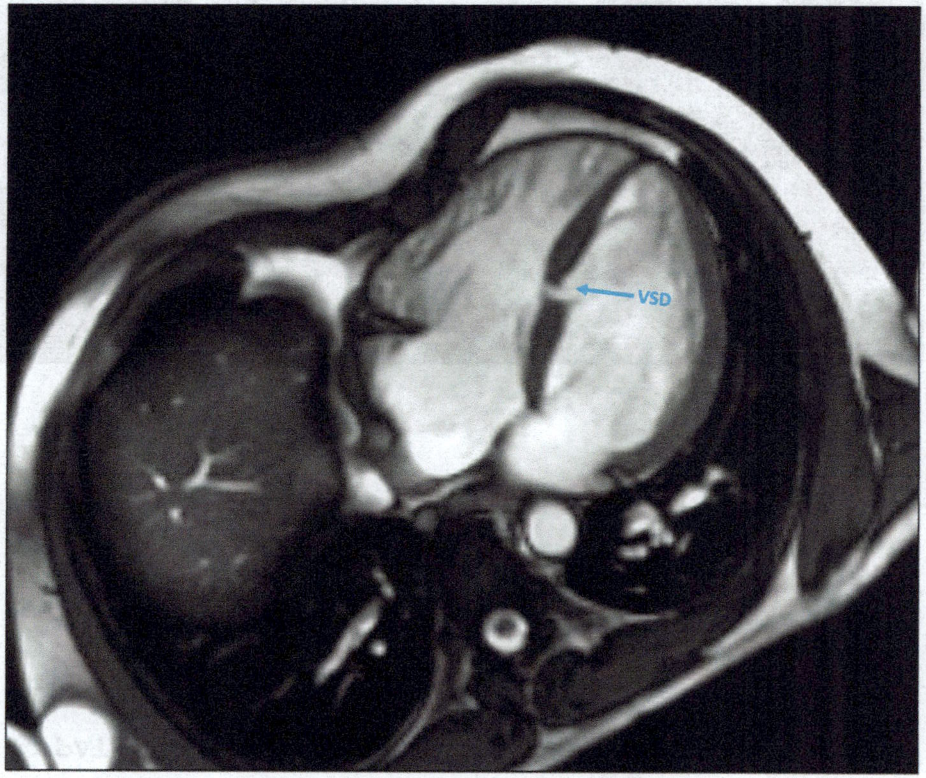

CARDIAC – VASCULAR

PATENT DUCTUS ARTERIOSUS

IMAGING: Fetal circulation between the aorta and the pulmonary arterial system
CXR: Increased pulmonary markings
Cardiomegaly

USMLE POINTS: Develops from 6th arch
Patency is maintained by prostaglandins and low oxygen tension
Closure can be obtained with Indomethacin
"Machine-like" or "to-and-fro" murmur
May eventually result in late cyanosis in lower extremities
B-type natriuretic peptide is a biomarker for PDA

Associations: **Maternal rubella**
Fetal EtOH syndrome
VSD

MODALITIES: ECHO (most specific)
CARDIAC CT / CARDAIC MRI

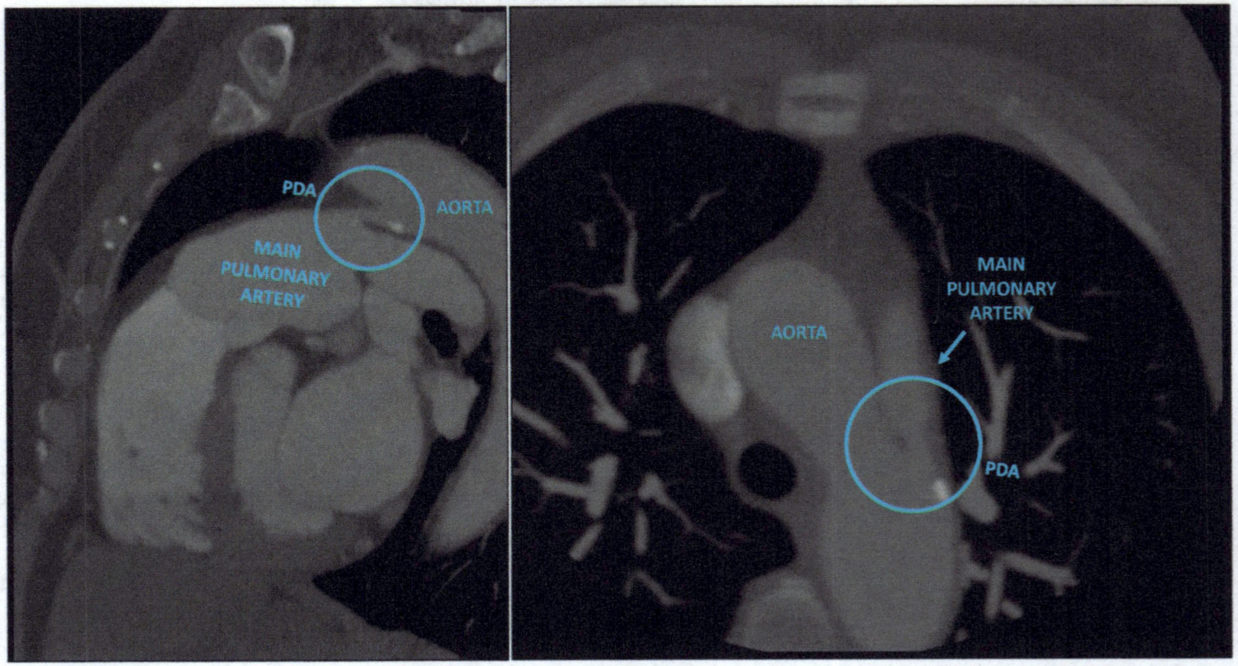

CARDIAC – VASCULAR

SMA OCCLUSION

IMAGING: **Occlusion of the SMA**
Leads to mesenteric ischemia → Look for edematous bowel
Look for pneumatosis / Portal Venous gas (sign of dead bowel)

USMLE POINTS: Most common cause of acute arterial embolism in acute mesenteric ischemia
SMA supplies distal duodenum, jejunum, ileum, and right colon from cecum to splenic flexure

Presentation:
- **Acute onset of severe abdominal pain**
- **Worst after eating (chronic mesenteric ischemia)**
- N/V/D
- > 60 years old

Treatment:
- Nonocclusive: IV Fluids, Anticoagulation, Vasodilators
- Occlusive: **Surgical revascularization with angioplasty**
  Thrombolytic therapy

Surgery: Laparotomy if bowel infarction / peritonitis

MODALITIES: CTA (best initial) → ANGIOGRAPHY

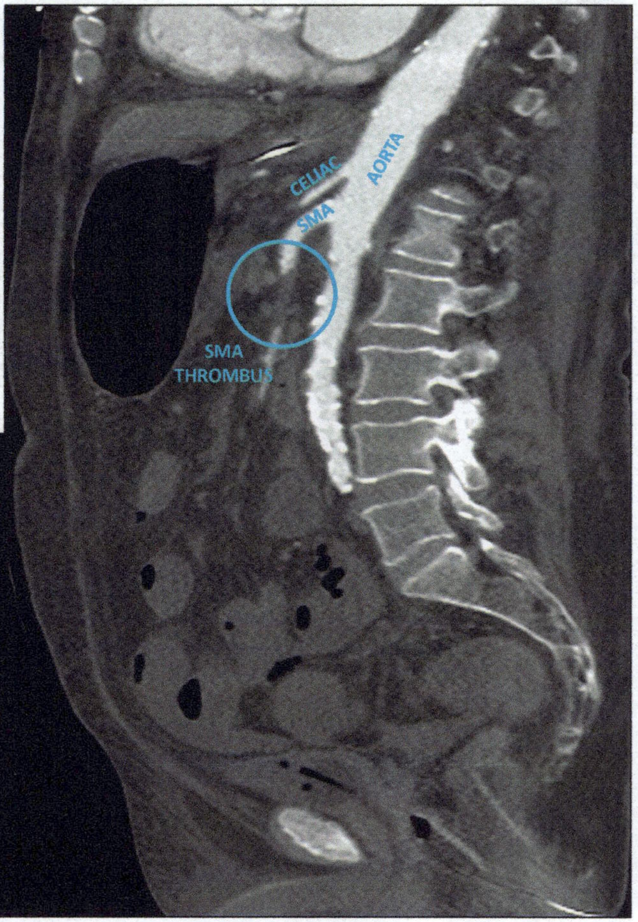

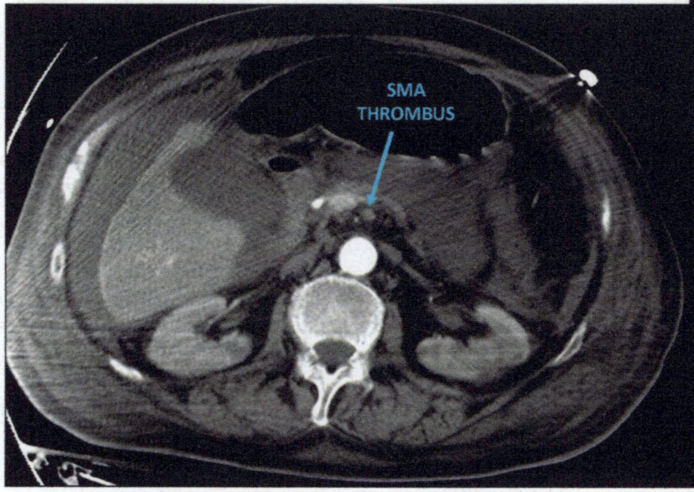

CARDIAC – VASCULAR

TAKAYASU ARTERITIS

IMAGING: **Wall thickening + Enhancement + occlusion of major branches**
Aorta may be diffusely narrowed, distally

USMLE POINTS: **Granulomatous, transmural fibrous thickening and narrowing of aortic arch and proximal great vessels**
Predominantly affects the aorta and its major branches
Type of large-vessel vasculitis
Asian females < 40 years old

Presentation: Weak pulse in upper extremities
Decreased blood pressure in upper extremities
Fever
Night sweats

High erythrocyte sedimentation rate (ESR)

Treatment: Corticosteroids

MODALITIES: CTA

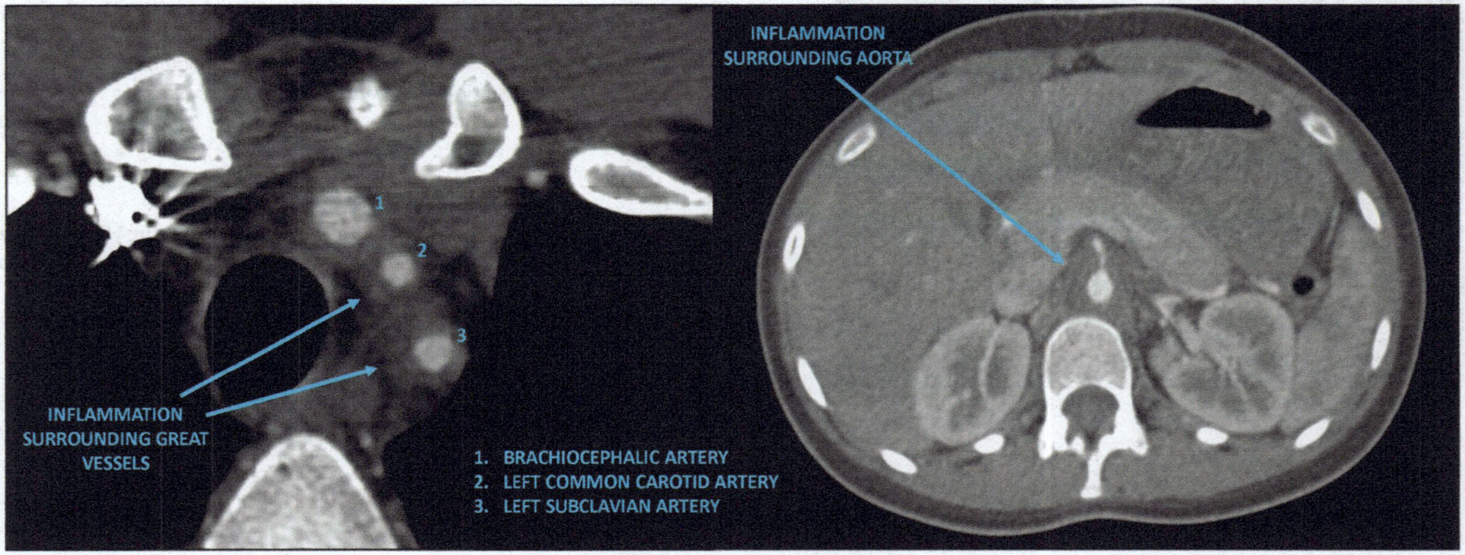

CARDIAC – VASCULAR

AORTIC OCCLUSION (LERICHE SYNDROME)

IMAGING: **Complete aortic occlusion (look to see if contrast or noncontrast exam)**

CTA: **Direct anatomical visualization of the location of the stenosis and occlusion**
Concomitant occlusive disease affecting visceral arteries

USMLE POINTS: Due to chronic peripheral artery disease of aortic bifurcation

Presentation:
- **Claudication of buttocks and hips**
- Exertional pain in early disease, rest pain in severe disease
- **Erectile dysfunction in men**
- Absent/diminished femoral pulses

Treatment:
- Anti-platelet therapy
- Treatment for underlying conditions (Hypertension & hyperlipidemia)

MODALITIES: CTA

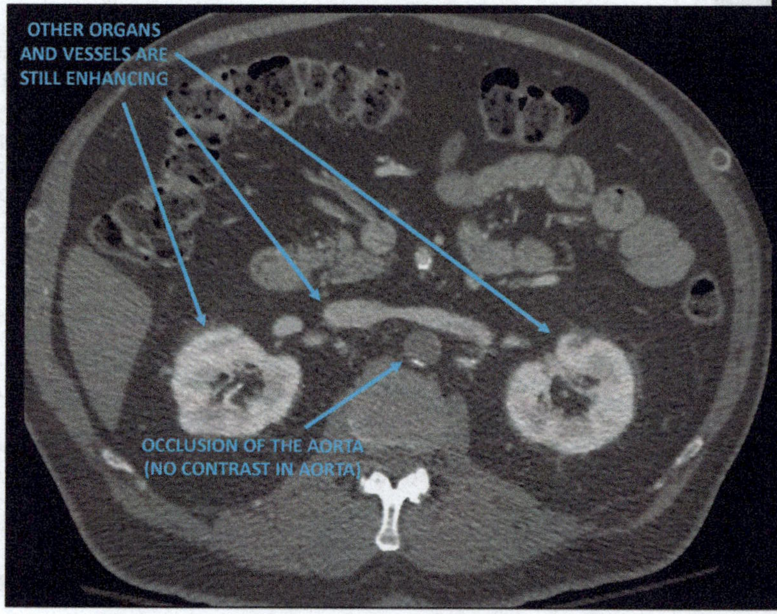

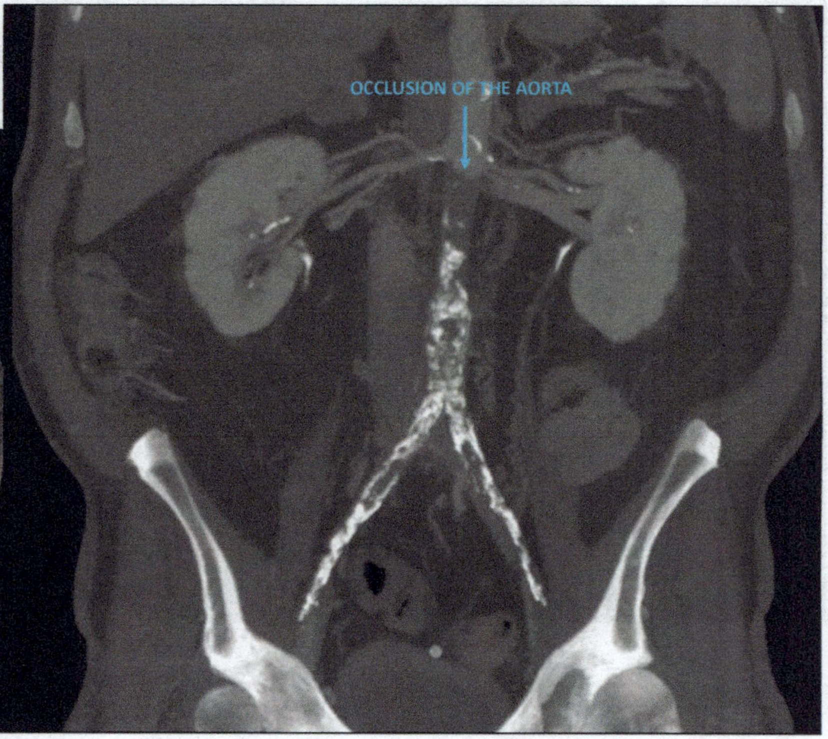

CARDIAC – VASCULAR

IMAGING: **No imaging performed**

USMLE POINTS: **Leakage of IV-administered contrast media to nearby tissues**
Common complication of contrast-enhanced CT

Presentation: Pain and tenderness
Swelling / Tightness of skin

Risk factors: Age
Emaciation
Female sex

Often no long-term consequences
Ice pack + **elevate** to reduce swelling
Rarely can **develop compartment syndrome / Skin ulceration**

MODALITIES: No imaging routinely performed
CT W – If concern for compartment syndrome

CONTRAST EXTRAVASAION

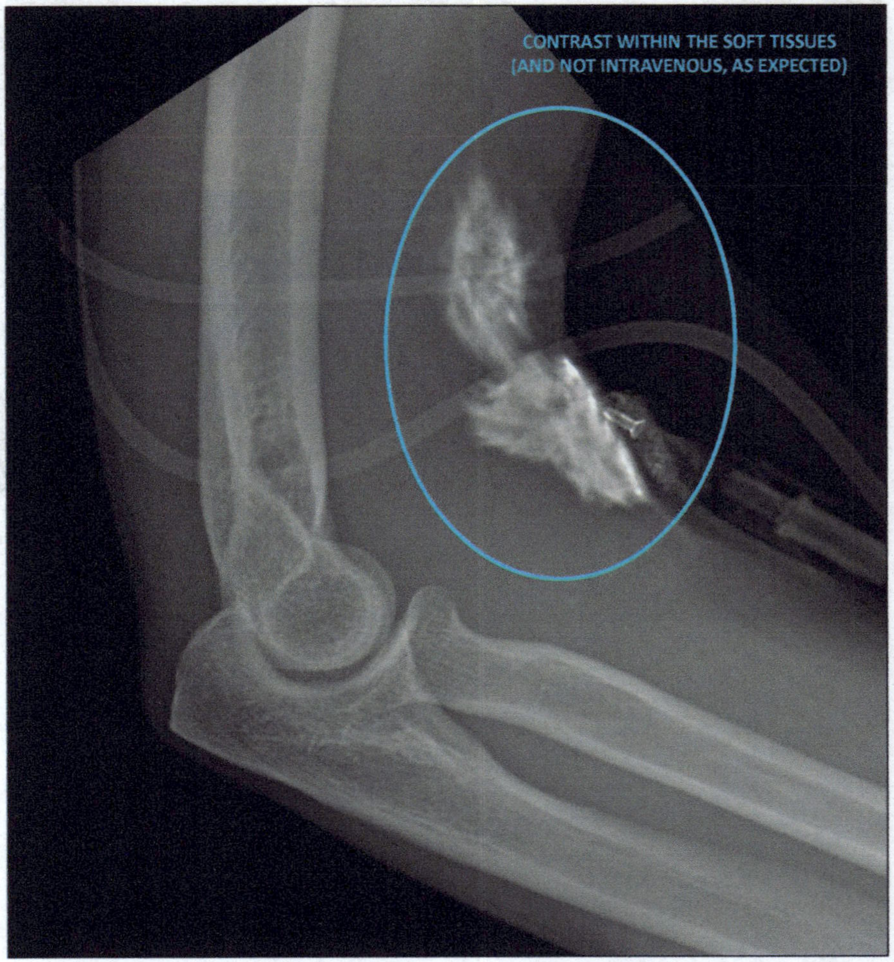

CARDIAC – VASCULAR

FIBROMUSCULAR DYSPLASIA (FMD)

IMAGING: Fusiform vascular ectasia and a **string of beads** (think of PSC of the biliary tree)

USMLE POINTS: Cause of **Renal Artery Stenosis**
Idiopathic, non-inflammatory, non-atherosclerotic **angiopathy of small and medium-sized arteries**
Proliferation of connective tissue and muscle fibers within arterial vessel walls
Most common in young women
Normal creatinine
Presentation: **Hypertension due to renal artery stenosis (female / abrupt onset)**
CNS symptoms (headache, neck pain, etc.) due to carotid and vertebral arteries
Angina, myocardial infarction due to coronary artery
Symptoms of mesenteric ischemia

MODALITIES: CTA

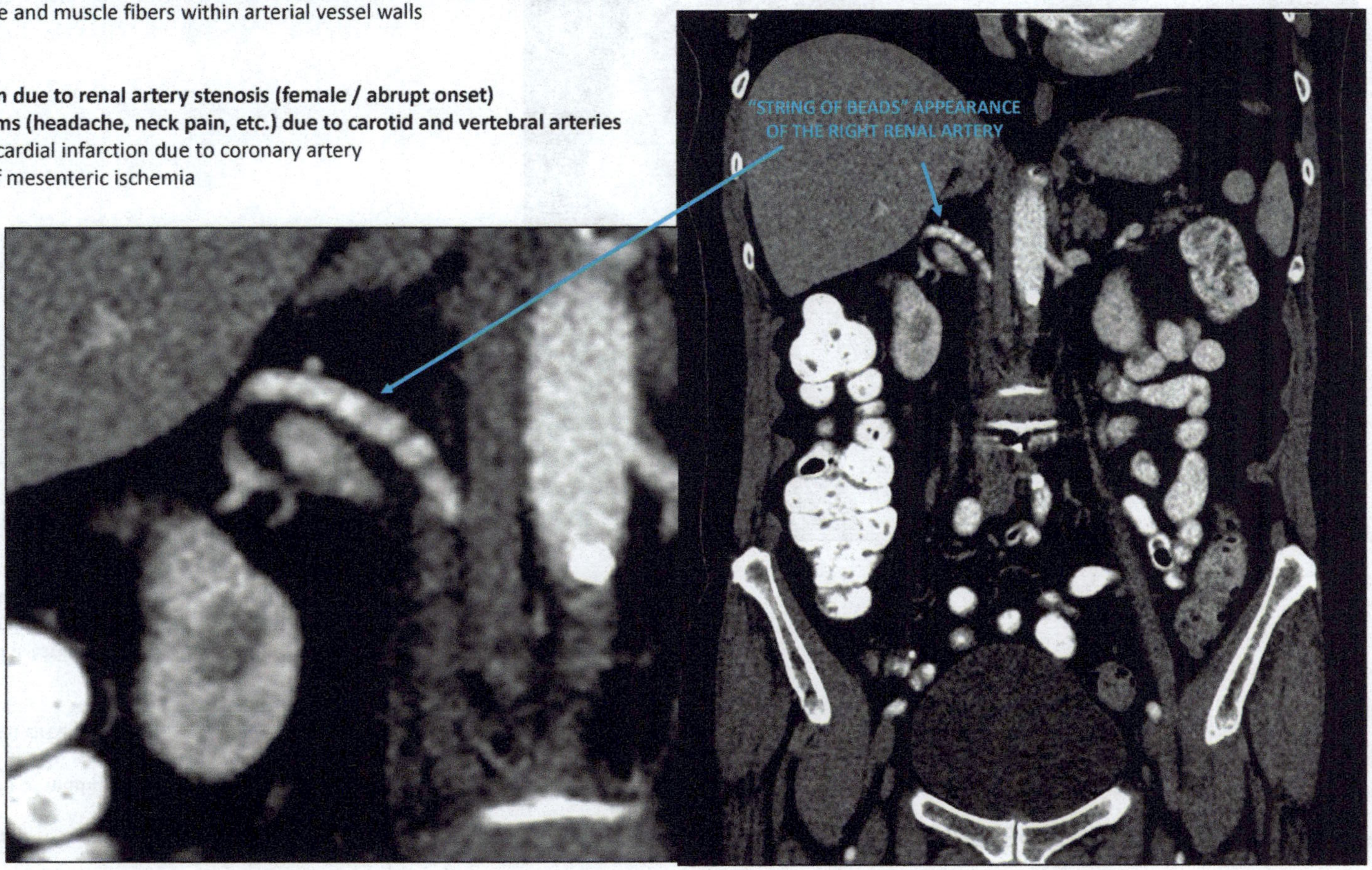

CARDIAC – VASCULAR

MONCKEBERG MEDIAL CALCIFIC SCLEROSIS

IMAGING:
Calcific deposits within the media of medium and small muscular arteries
No luminal narrowing
Calcification is typically diffuse and circumferential
Visible on plain films

USMLE POINTS:
Arteriosclerosis of medium-sized arteries
Calcification of internal elastic lamina and media of arteries that **does not obstruct blood flow**
Does not result in luminal narrowing, but does result in **stiffening → Clinically benign**
Risk factors:
- Old age
- Diabetes
- Chronic renal disease

DDX: Beurger's disease → Smokers / Corkscrew / Painful

MODALITIES: CTA

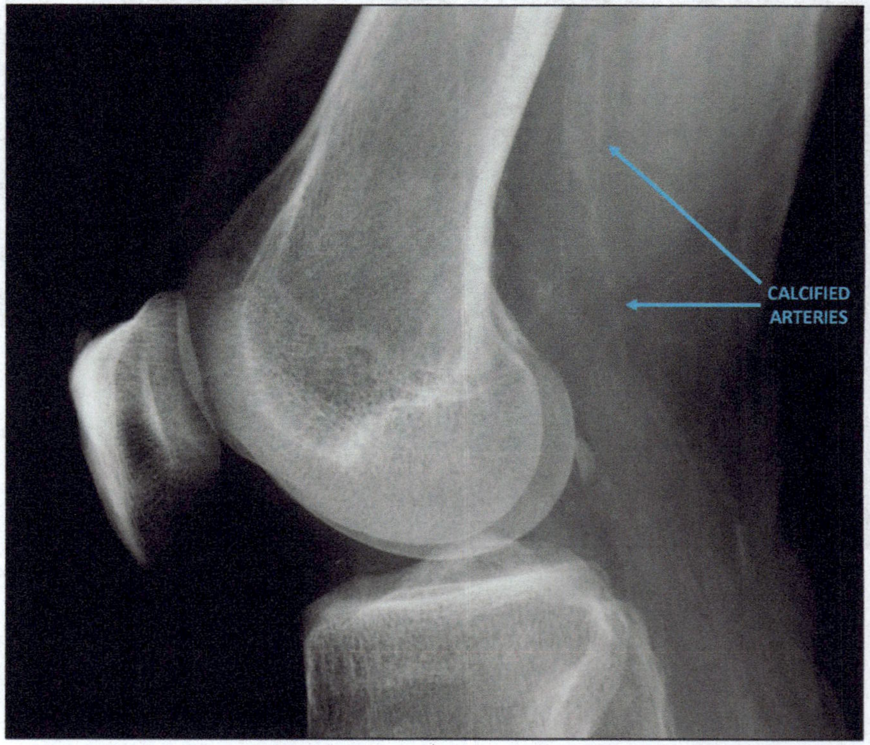

CARDIAC – VASCULAR

PERICARDIAL CALCIFICATIONS

IMAGING:

Calcification along the pericardium

Common: Right side, anterior and diaphragmatic

Uncommon: Left ventricle or cardiac apex

USMLE POINTS:

May cause **constrictive pericarditis (Kussmaul sign → increased JVD on inspiration)**

Commonly caused by **infective pericarditis**

May be asymptomatic → Heart failure

Severe cases may require pericardiectomy

Pericarditis:
- **Serous**
- **Fibrinous** **(Dressler syndrome, 1 – 3 day post MI)**
- **Hemorrhagic** **(TB)**
- **Constrictive** **(Radiation, Viral, TB)**

Friction rub

Elevated ESR / CRP

EKG: PR segment depression

Widespread ST segment elevation

MODALITIES: ECHO / CARDIAC CT / CARDIAC MRI

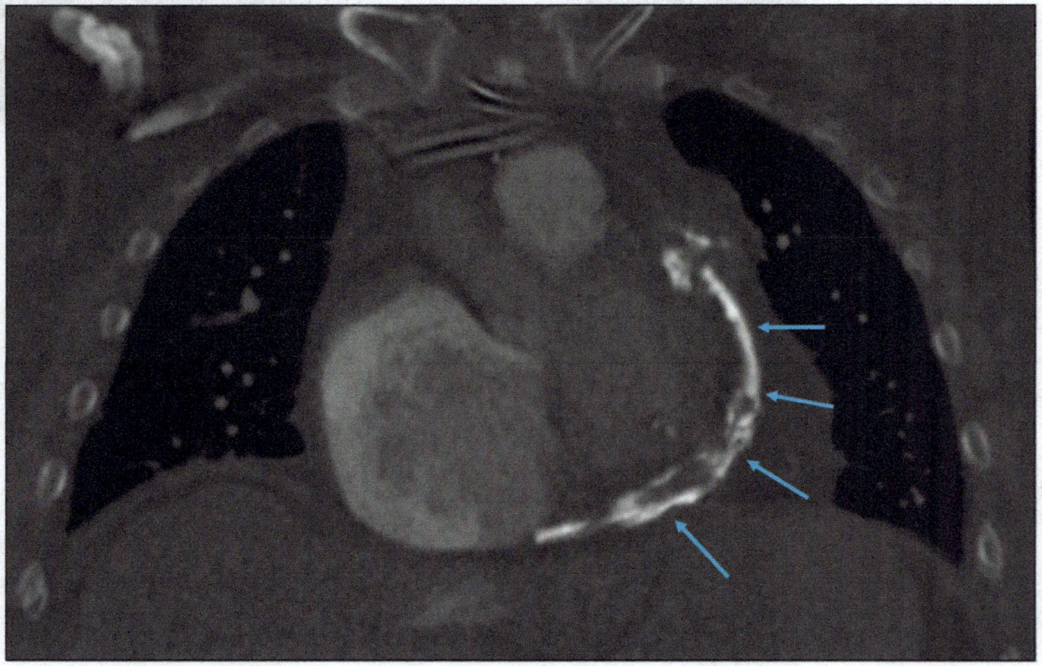

CARDIAC – VASCULAR

SUBCLAVIAN STEEL SYNDROME

IMAGING: **Flow reversal of vertebral artery ipsilateral to stenosis/occlusion of prevertebral subclavian artery**

US: Retrograde flow in the ipsilateral vertebral artery

CT: Subclavian artery stenosis or occlusion is easily identified

USMLE POINTS:

Presentation:
- Arm ischemia
- Pain
- Paresthesia
- **Vertebrobasilar insufficiency (differentiates SS syndrome vs SS phenomenon): Dizziness, Vertigo, Syncope, Ataxia, Visual changes, >15 mm Hg difference in systolic BP between arms**

Associations:
- Arteriosclerosis
- **Takayasu arteritis**
- Heart surgery
- Thoracic aortic dissection

MODALITIES: US

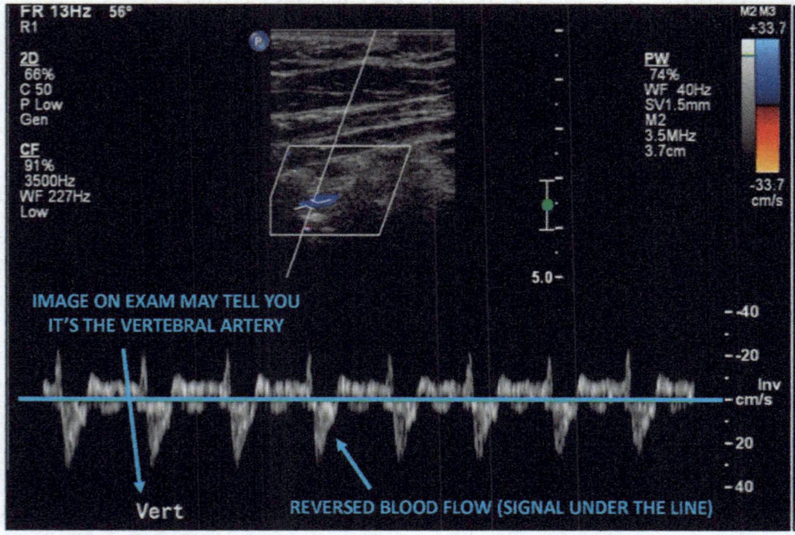

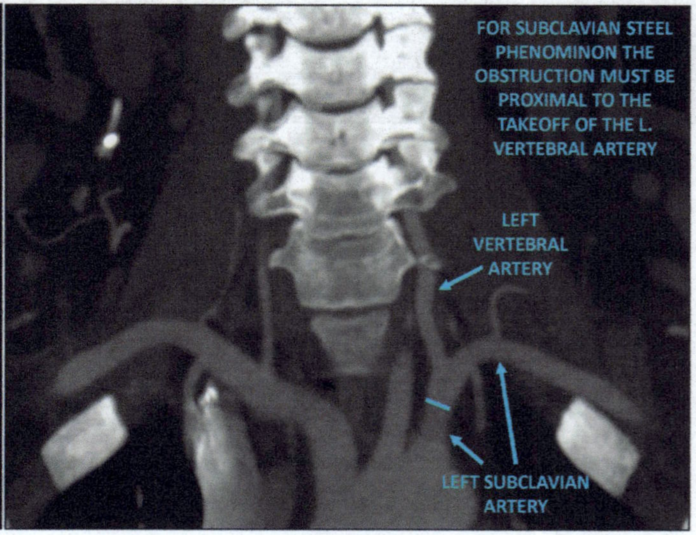

GASTROENTEROLOGY

GASTROINTESTINAL

ACHALASIA

IMAGING:
"Bird-beak" sign
Dilation of the esophagus

USMLE POINTS:
Dysphagia to both solids and liquids
Risk factor for SCC
Pseudoachalasia due to malignancy

Degeneration of inhibitory neurons (releasing NO and VIP) in **myenteric (Auerbach) plexus of esophageal** wall → Uncoordinated esophageal contraction → Dilation of esophagus

Decreased nitric oxide secretion implicated in increased lower esophageal sphincter (LES) tone

Types: 1° achalasia is idiopathic
2° achalasia commonly results from **Chagas disease – T. Cruzi**

MODALITIES:
Esophageal manometry (gold standard) → Increased LES pressure
FLX

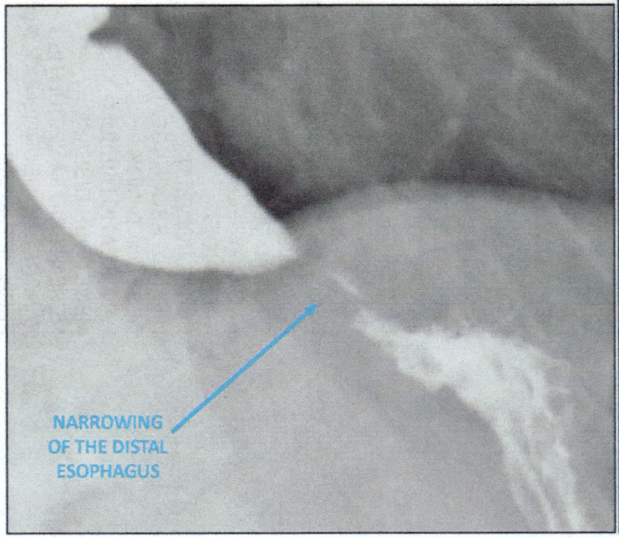

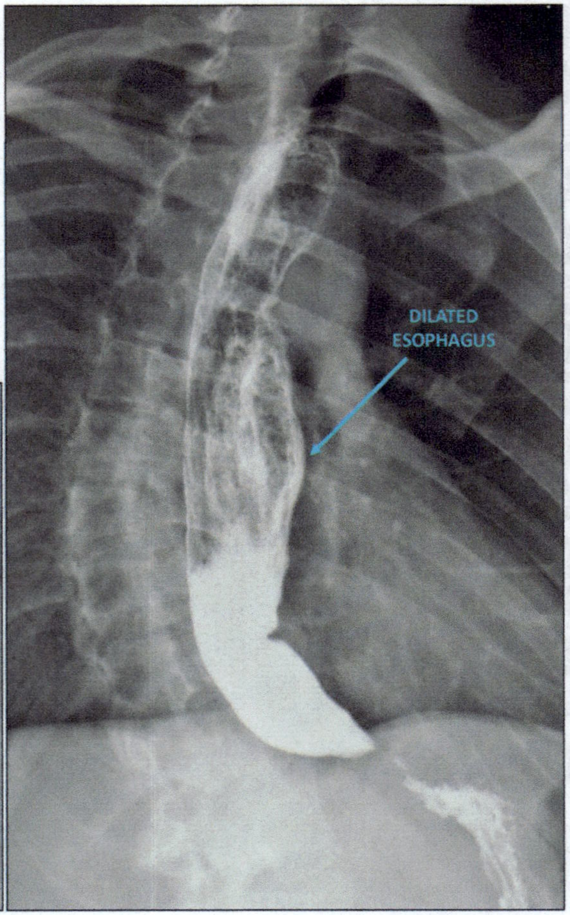

GASTROINTESTINAL

MONONUCLEOSIS

IMAGING: Enlargement of the spleen > 13 cm
Generalized lymphadenopathy
Clinical history important

USMLE POINTS: "Kissing" Disease
Avoid contact sports (susceptible to rupture)
Epstein-Barr virus (EBV) and Human herpesvirus-4 (HHV-4)
Binds to B-cells via CD21
immunocompromised patients are at risk of reactivation

Presentation:
Fatigue
Pharyngitis
Maculopapular rash
Cervical lymphadenopathy
Splenomegaly

Labs:
Positive monospot test
Increase in atypical lymphocytes

Hemolytic anemia can be treated with Rituximab

MODALITIES: US

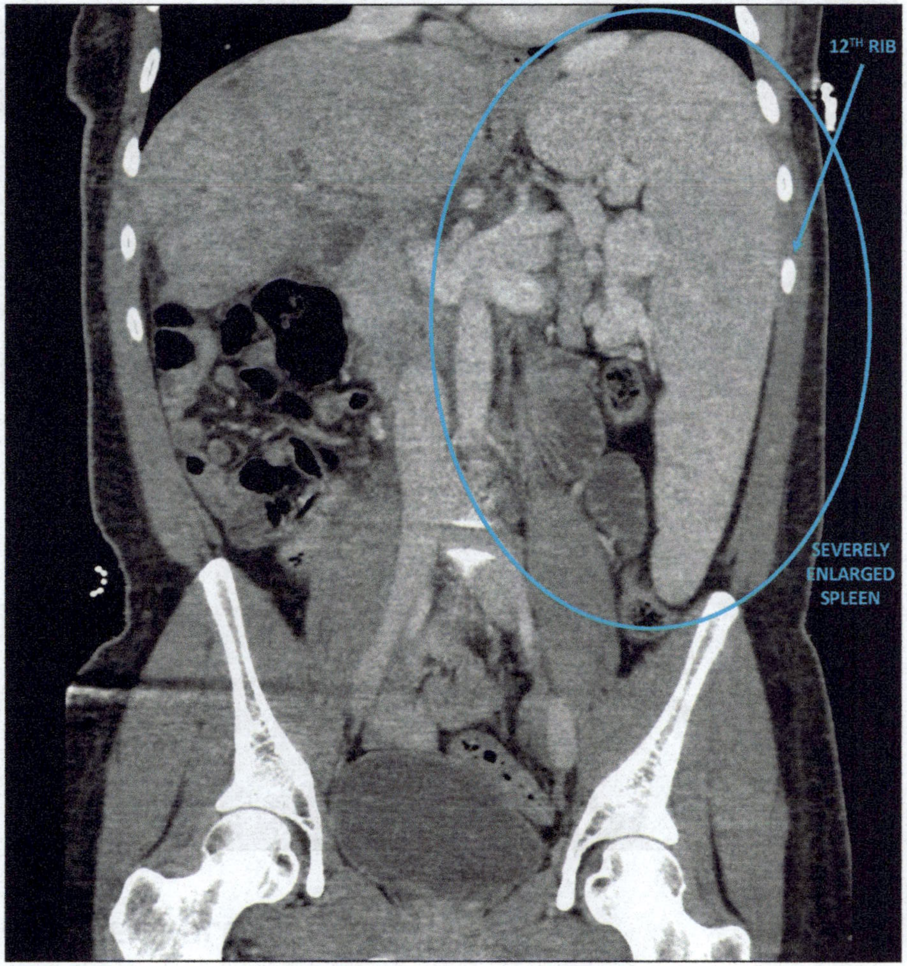

GASTROINTESTINAL

ACUTE CHOLECYSTITIS

IMAGING:
Cholelithiasis / Sludge
Gallbladder wall thickening
Pericholecystic fluid

USMLE POINTS:
Murphy sign: Inspiratory arrest upon right upper quadrant palpation due to pain
Radiation of pain to right shoulder due to irritation of phrenic nerve
Increased cholesterol and/or bilirubin, decreased bile salts, and gallbladder stasis
Acalculous cholecystitis (critically ill) → Gallbladder stasis, hypoperfusion, or infection
Emphysematous cholecystitis → Diabetics

F's: Fat, Female, Fertile, Forty, Flatulent?

EEEK: **E. coli, Enterobacter, Enterococcus, Klebsiella**

MODALITIES: US → CT W → HIDA

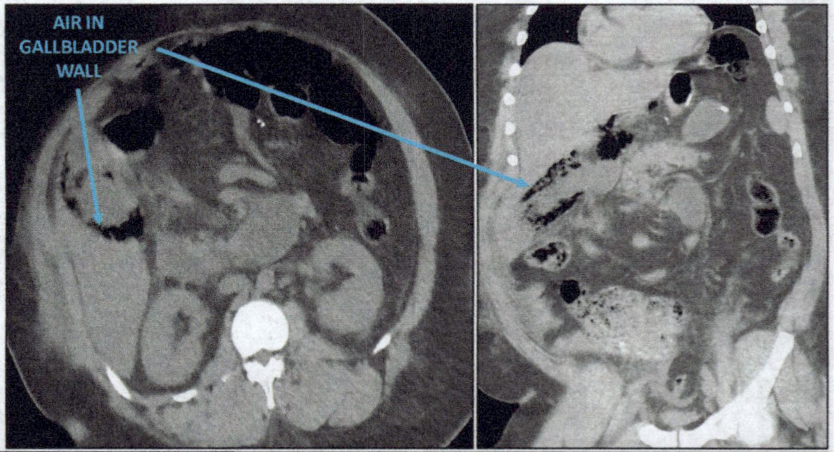

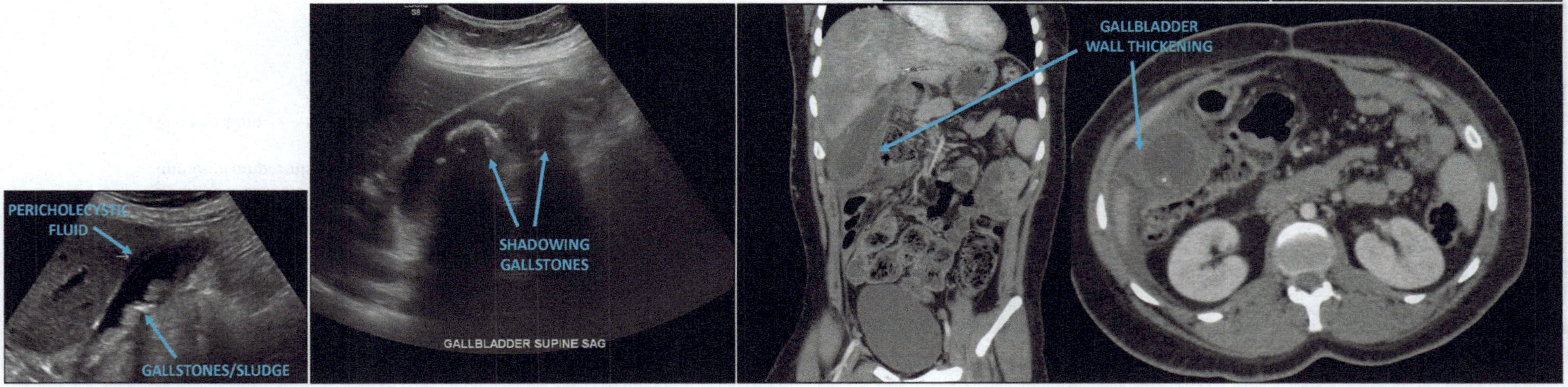

GASTROINTESTINAL

ACUTE CHOLECYSTITIS

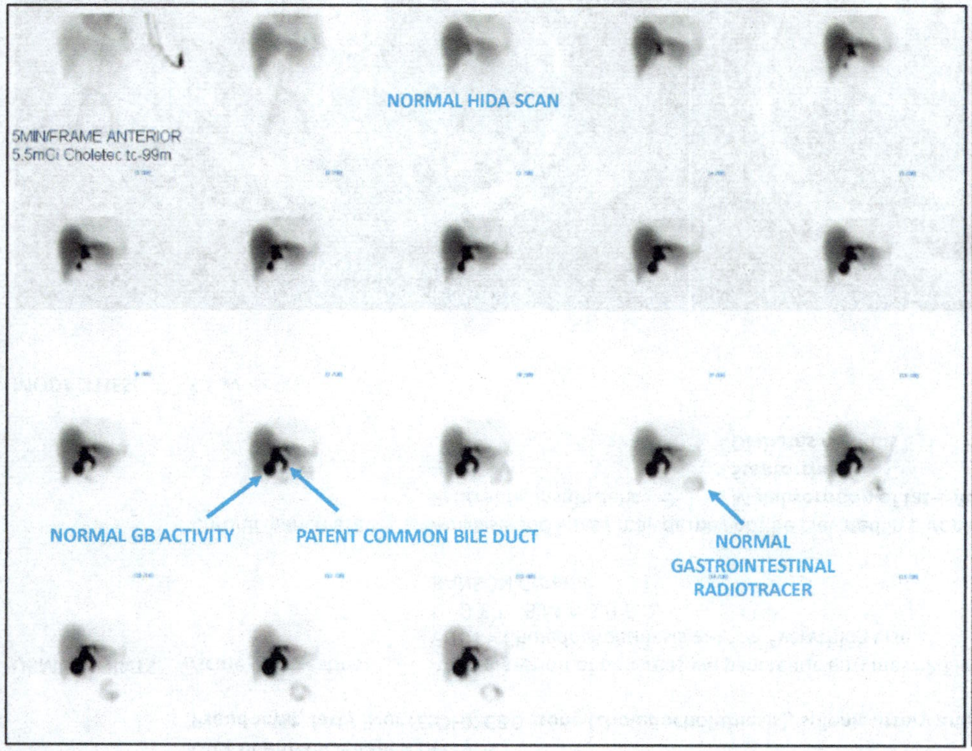

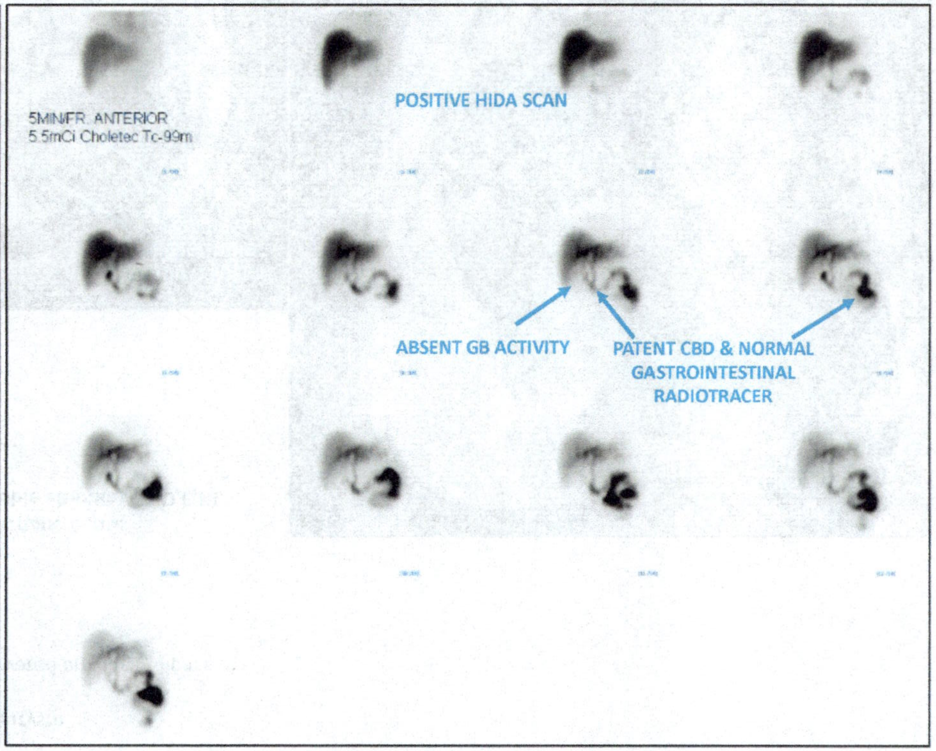

GASTROINTESTINAL

PANCREATITIS

IMAGING:

Fluid/edema surrounding the pancreas
Lack of enhancement = necrosis
Pseudocyst, fatty liver (EtOH), CBD stone (choledocholithiasis), splenic artery aneurysm

USMLE POINTS:

Acute pancreatitis:
Auto-digestion of pancreas via pancreatic enzymes → Elevated amylase / lipase
EtOH > Choledocholithiasis >>>>>> Everything else
I. **G.E.T.** S.M.A.S.H.E.D.
RANSON Criteria

Chronic pancreatitis:
Amylase and lipase may or may not be elevated in chronic pancreatitis
Pancreatic insufficiency → **Malabsorption of fat-soluble vitamins (A,D,E,K),**
Steatorrhea
Diabetes mellitus

MODALITIES: CT W → US

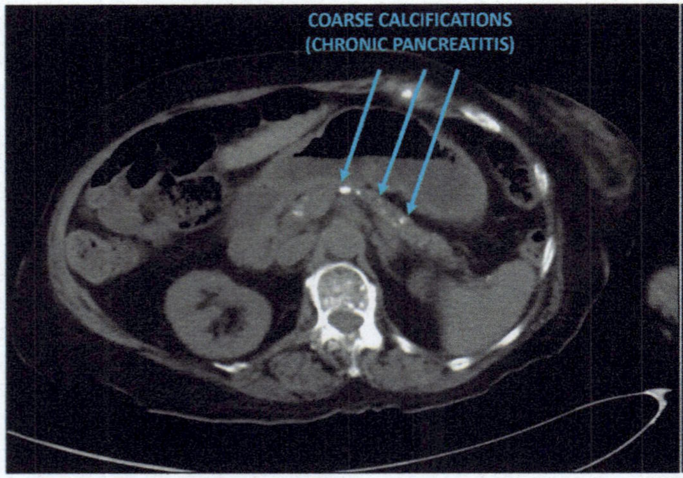

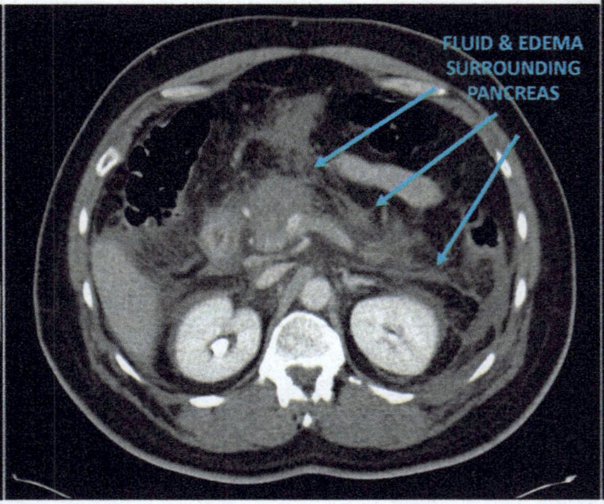

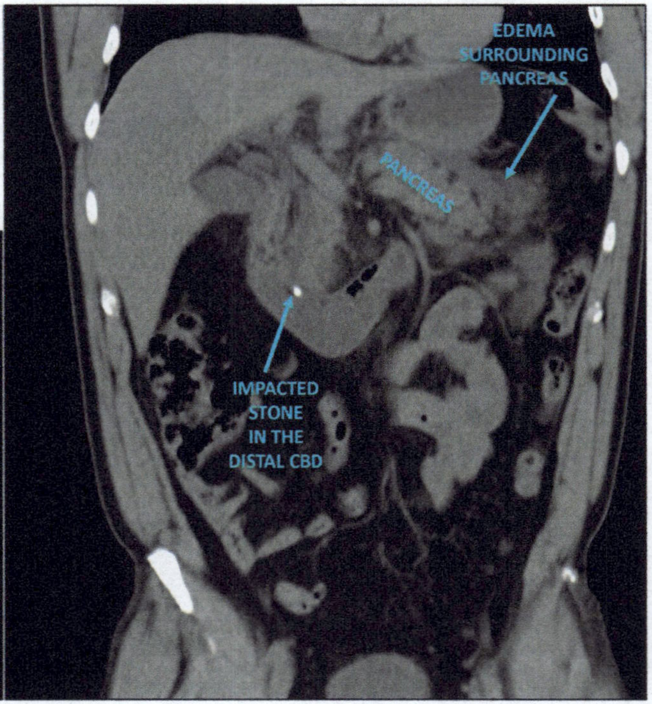

GASTROINTESTINAL

CROHN DISEASE

IMAGING:
"String-sign" sign
Colonic inflammation → Classically of the **terminal ileum**
Fistula, strictures, abscess, enterocutaneous fistula
Non-contiguous involvement (skip lesions)

USMLE POINTS:
Can occur anywhere in GI tract, though usually localized in ileum and colon
C-ANCA+, Noncaseating granulomas
Complications:
- Malnutrition due to malabsorption
- Colorectal cancer
- **Fistulas**, which can result in recurrent UTI infections
- Lower digestive tract bleeding that results in diarrhea (may or may not be bright red)
- **Calcium oxalate stones**
- **Erythema nodosum**

MODALITIES: CT W / FLX

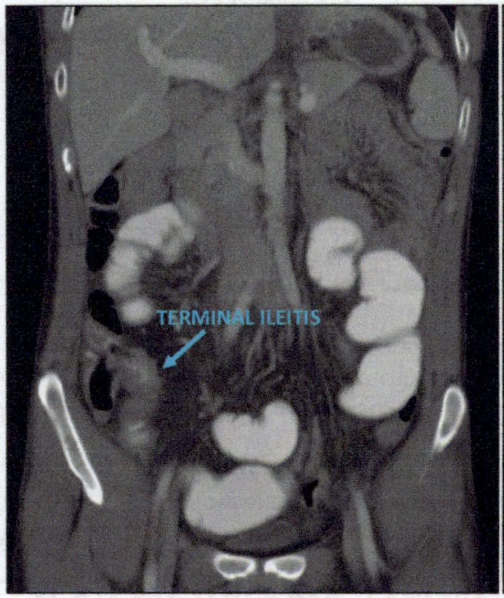

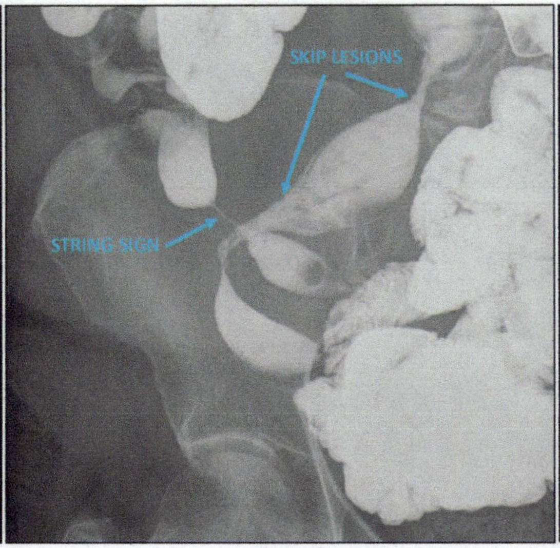

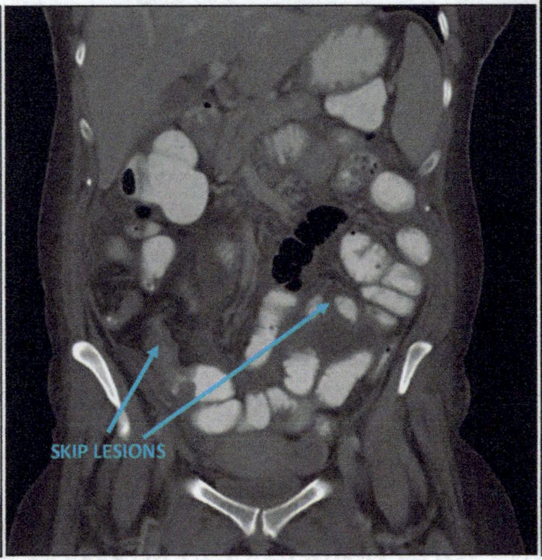

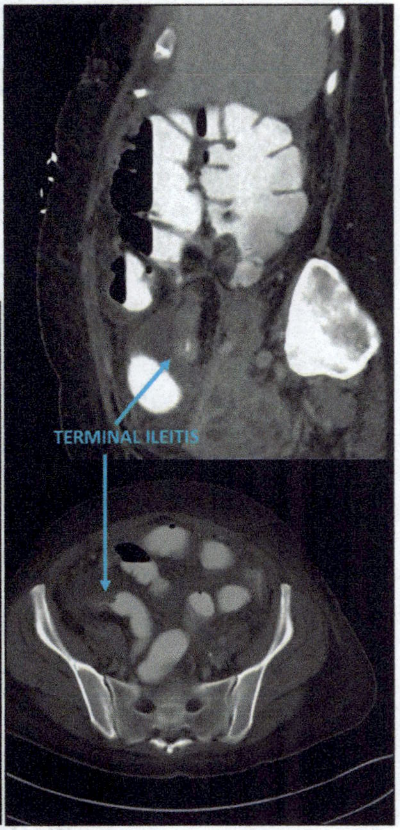

PRIMARY SCLEROSING CHOLANGITIS

IMAGING: **Strictures/beading of the intrahepatic biliary ducts**
Concentric "onion skin" bile duct fibrosis
Progressive liver disease (intrahepatic ducts)

USMLE POINTS: Middle-aged males with **ulcerative colitis (2/3 of patients)**
Increased risk for cholangiocarcinoma and gallbladder cancer
Presentation: **Pruritis, jaundice**

Labs: **Increased alkaline phosphatase (ALP) and ↑ GGT**
Increased bilirubin
ALT and AST may be normal
pANCA

Treatment: **Ursodeocycholic acid (pruritis)**
Liver transplant

MODALITIES: **ERCP (gold standard)**
Cholangiogram

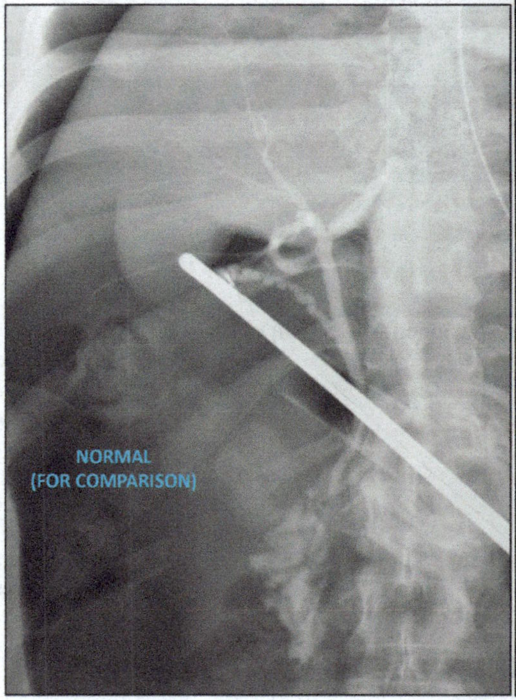

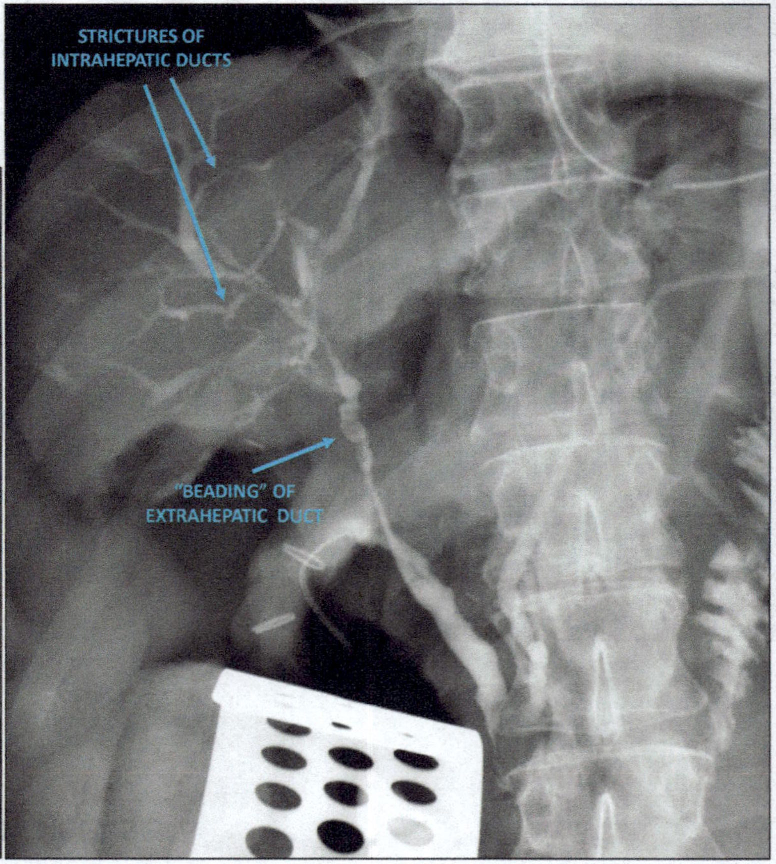

GASTROINTESTINAL

CIRRHOSIS

IMAGING: Surface/parenchymal nodularity
Portal hypertension: **Ascites (SBP)**
Splenomegaly
Paraesophageal varices
Recanalization of the umbilical vein
Portal colopathy/enteropathy

USMLE POINTS: Diffuse bridging fibrosis (via stellate cells) and regenerative nodules disrupt normal hepatic architecture
Increased risk for hepatocellular carcinoma
Prognosis: MELD score
AST:ALT > 2
Etiologies: **Alcohol, nonalcoholic steatohepatitis, Wilson disease, Hemachromatosis**
Chronic viral hepatitis (HBV / HCV)
Biliary disease (biliary atresia in children)

MODALITIES: US → CT W / MRI WWO

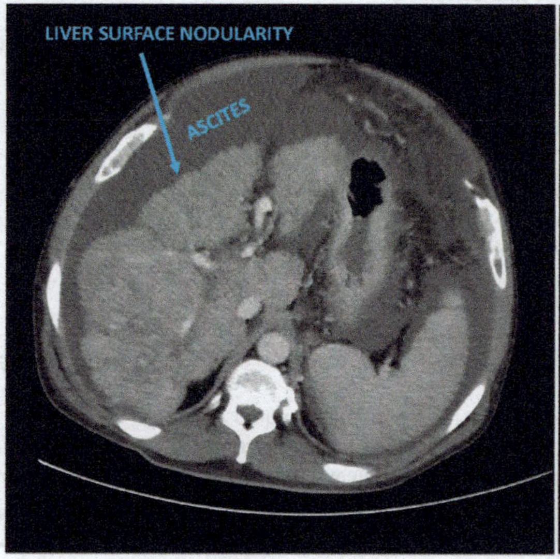

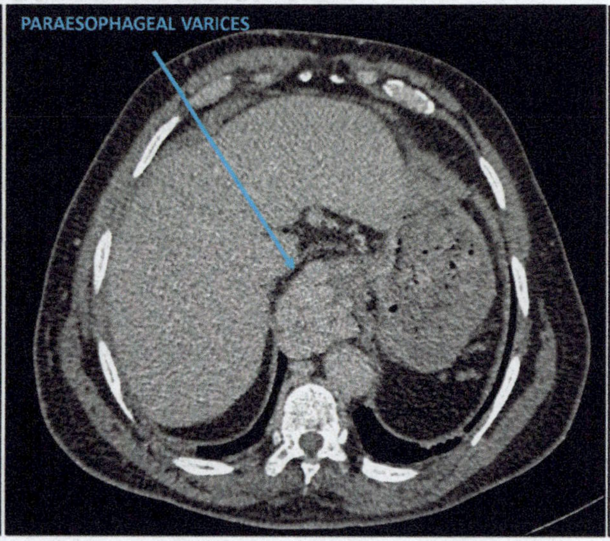

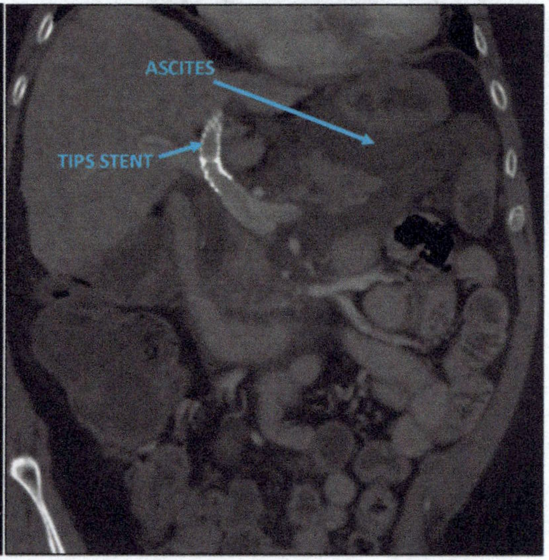

GASTROINTESTINAL

COLITIS

IMAGING:

Circumferential wall thickening + Pericolonic induration/fat stranding
Look for **abscess or free air**
DDx: Colon cancer

USMLE POINTS:

Location and history will help with etiology: **Ischemic vs. IBD (UC / Chron's) vs. Infectious (C. dificile)**
Presentation: Tenderness, loss of appetite, mucus and/or blood in stool
Complications: Perforation / Fecal peritonitis

C. dificile colitis: **Pseudomembranous colitis and diarrhea**
Diffuse thickening of the colon (pancolitis) → Almost always involves the rectum
Shaggy mucosal outline → **"Accordion" configuration**
Clindamycin, Ampicillin, Fluoroquinolones
Toxin A: Enterotoxin → Binds to the intestinal brush border
Toxin B: Cytotoxin → Depolymerizes actin → Disrupting the cytoskeleton
PO Vancomycin

MODALITIES: CT W

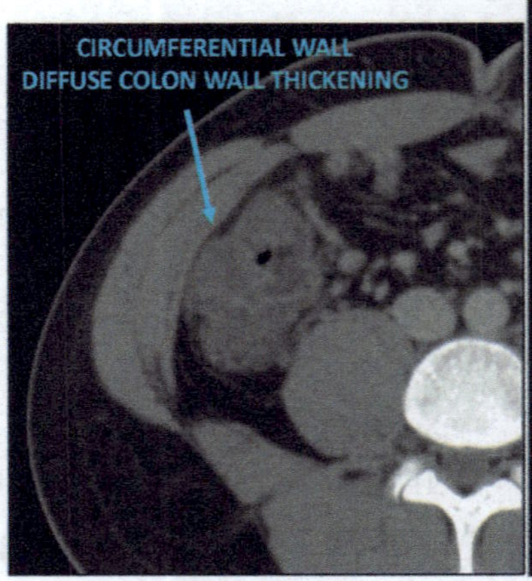

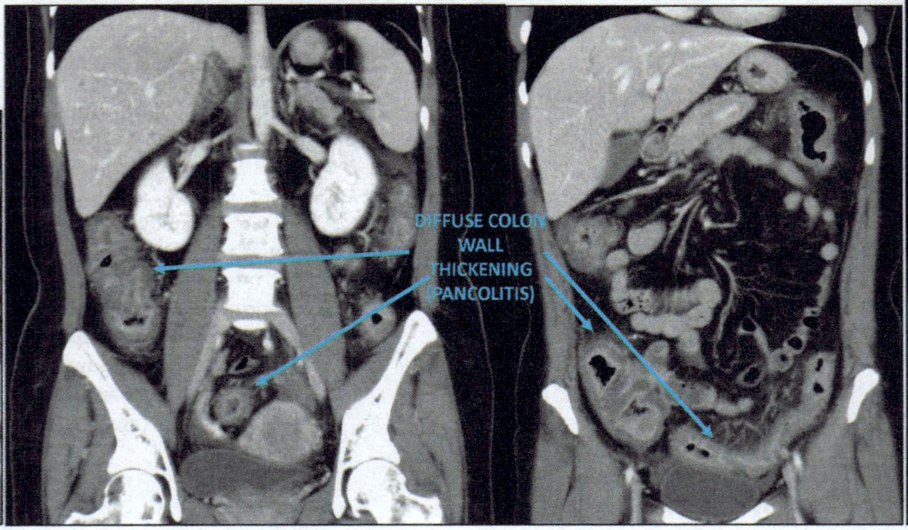

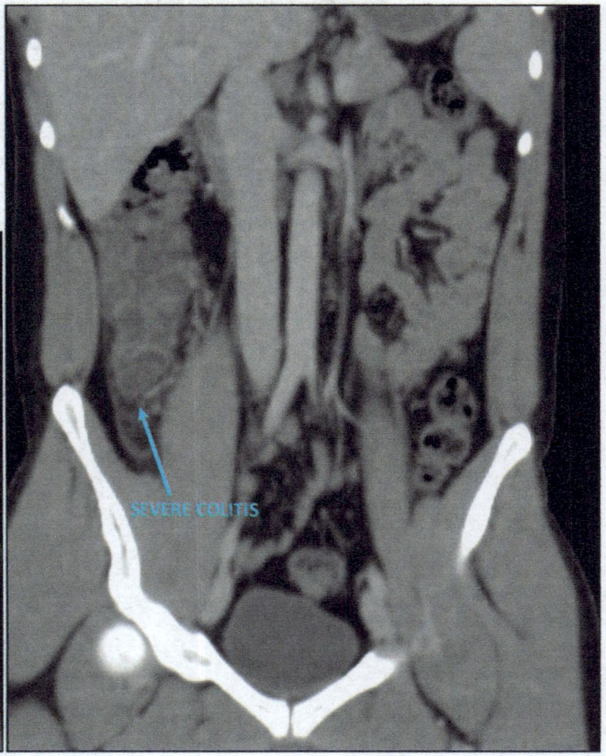

COLITIS

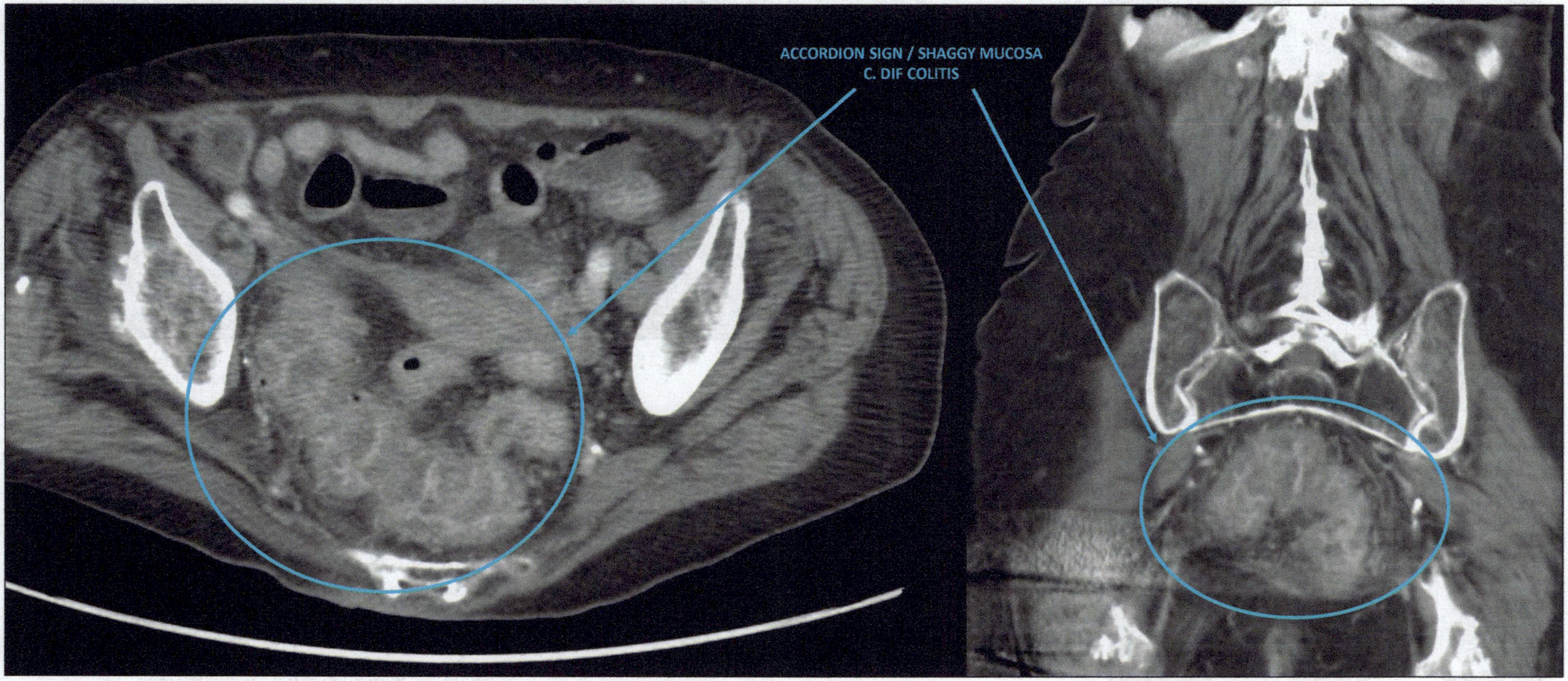

GASTROINTESTINAL

COLON CANCER

IMAGING: "Apple-core" sign
Short segment colonic narrowing (vs. colitis)

USMLE POINTS: **Rectal bleeding, unexplained iron deficiency anemia, Age** > 50 years old

Associations: Carnivorous diet, iron deficiency anemia in males, and postmenopausal females
Lynch syndrome, UC / Chron's disease, Streptococcus gallolyticus

Chromosomal instability: APC/B-catenin mutation, KRAS mutation, p53 mutation
Microsatellite instability pathway

Screening:

Average risk:	**First screen at 50 with colonoscopy**
First-degree relative w/ colon cancer:	**First screen at 40 with colonoscopy**

MODALITIES: Colonoscopy (gold standard)
CT W + PO

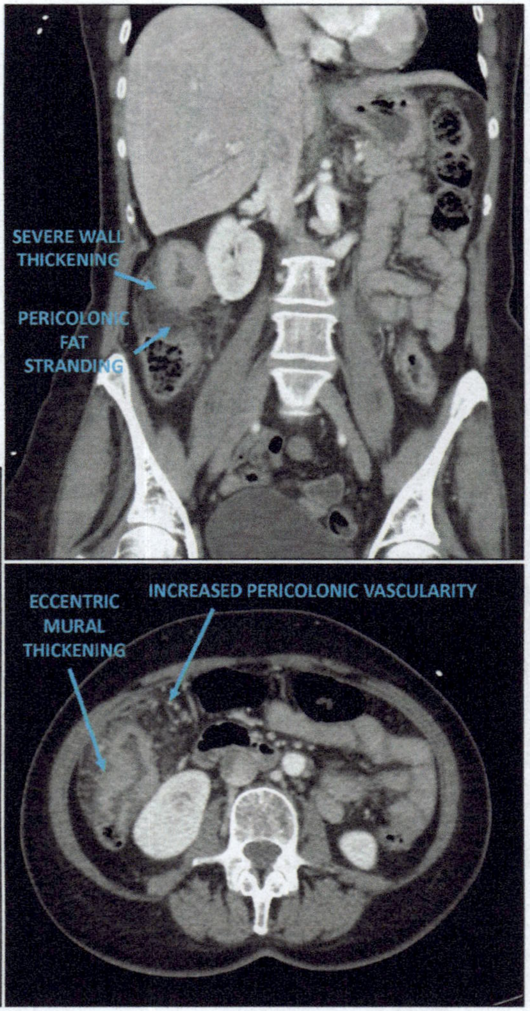

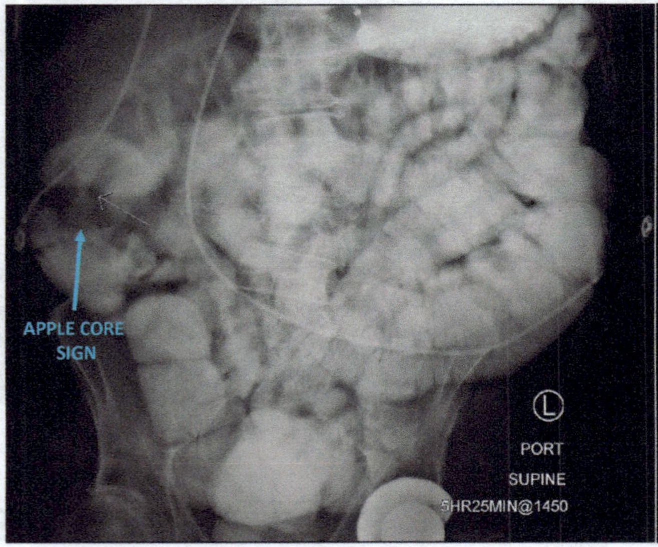

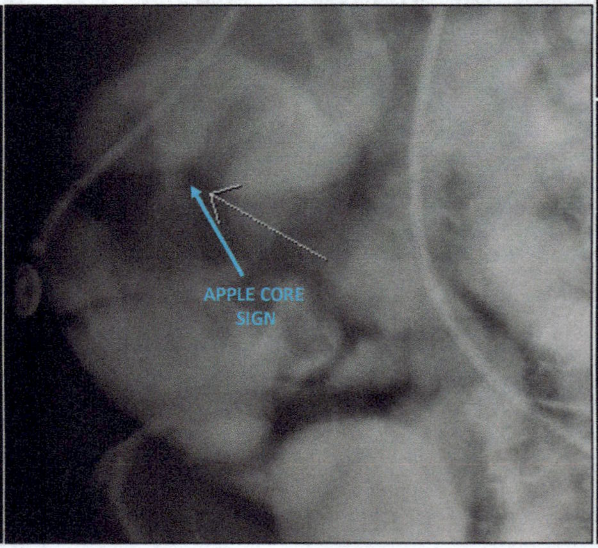

GASTROINTESTINAL

DIVERTICULITIS

IMAGING:
Focal peri-diverticular inflammation
Look for perforation or abscess
Most commonly sigmoid colon

USMLE POINTS:
Erosion of the diverticular wall from increased intraluminal pressure / inspissated food particles within diverticula
LLQ pain + Fever + Leukocytosis
May require surgery if perforated / abscess (draining considered if > 3 cm)
Complications: Abscess
Perforation
Fistula

MODALITIES: CT W

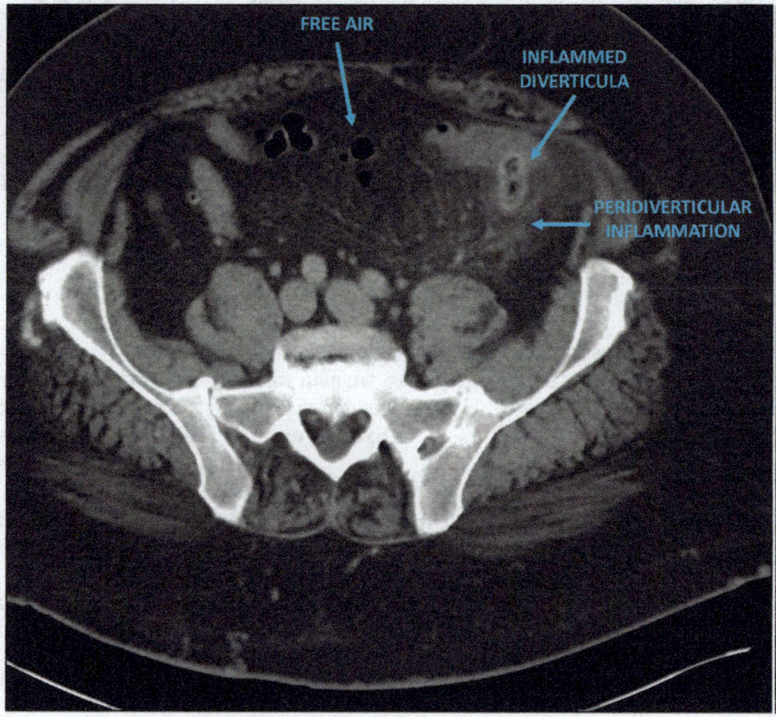

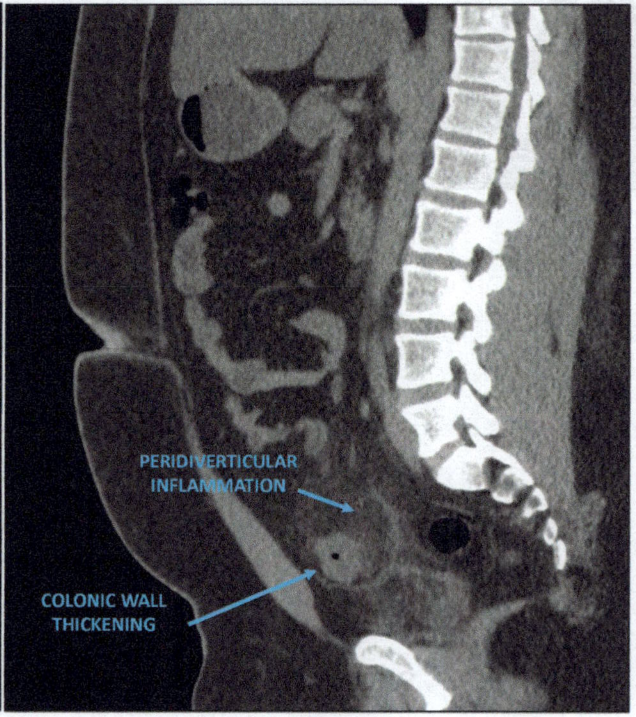

HEPATIC STEATOSIS & HEMACHROMATOSIS

IMAGING:
Hepatic steatosis: Diffusely **decreased attenuation** (hypodense) Beware of fatty sparing
Hemachromatosis: Diffusely **increased attenuation** (hyperdense)

USMLE POINTS:
Hepatis steatosis: Macrovesicular fatty change (intrahepatic fat of at least 5% of liver weight)
Results from **alcohol abuse** – possibly reversible with cessation

Hemachromatosis: **Increased intestinal absorption of iron**
Commonly presents after age 40 when iron >20 g
Iron loss via menstruation slows progression in females
Presentation: Cirrhosis, Diabetes mellitus, Skin pigmentation
Treatment: **Repeated phlebotomy, iron chelation with deferasirox, deferoxamine, deferiprone**

MODALITIES: US / CT WO

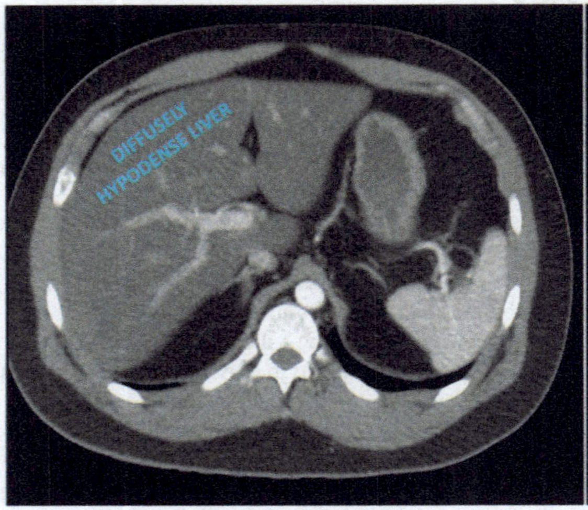

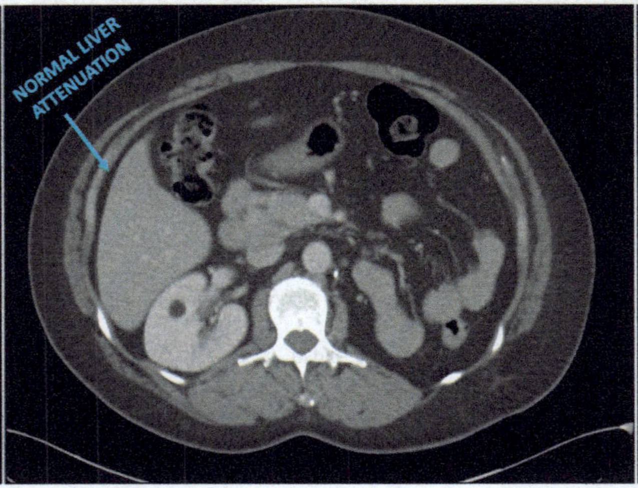

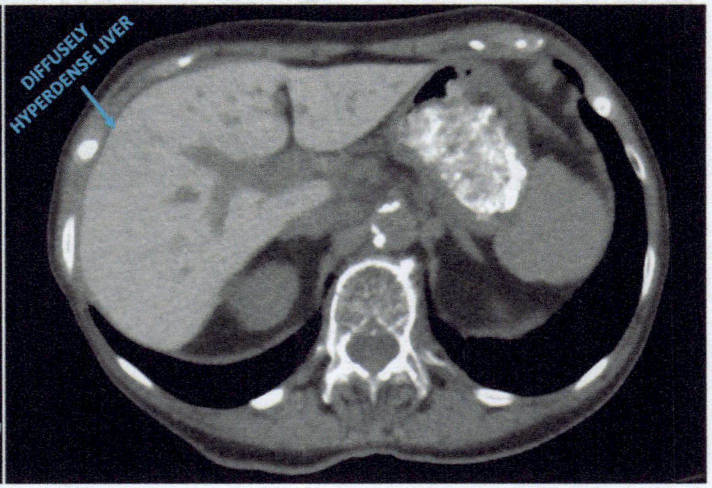

GASTROINTESTINAL

PNEUMOPERITONEUM (FREE AIR)

IMAGING:
- XR: **Curvilinear lucency under the diaphragm**
- CT: **Look anterior to liver**

USMLE POINTS:
- Make sure patient is not post-op
- Etiologies: **Diverticulitis, SBO, Volvulus**; **Intestinal perforation/enteritis**; **Pneumatosis intestinalis/coli**
- Treatment: Emergent surgery

MODALITIES: XR → CT W

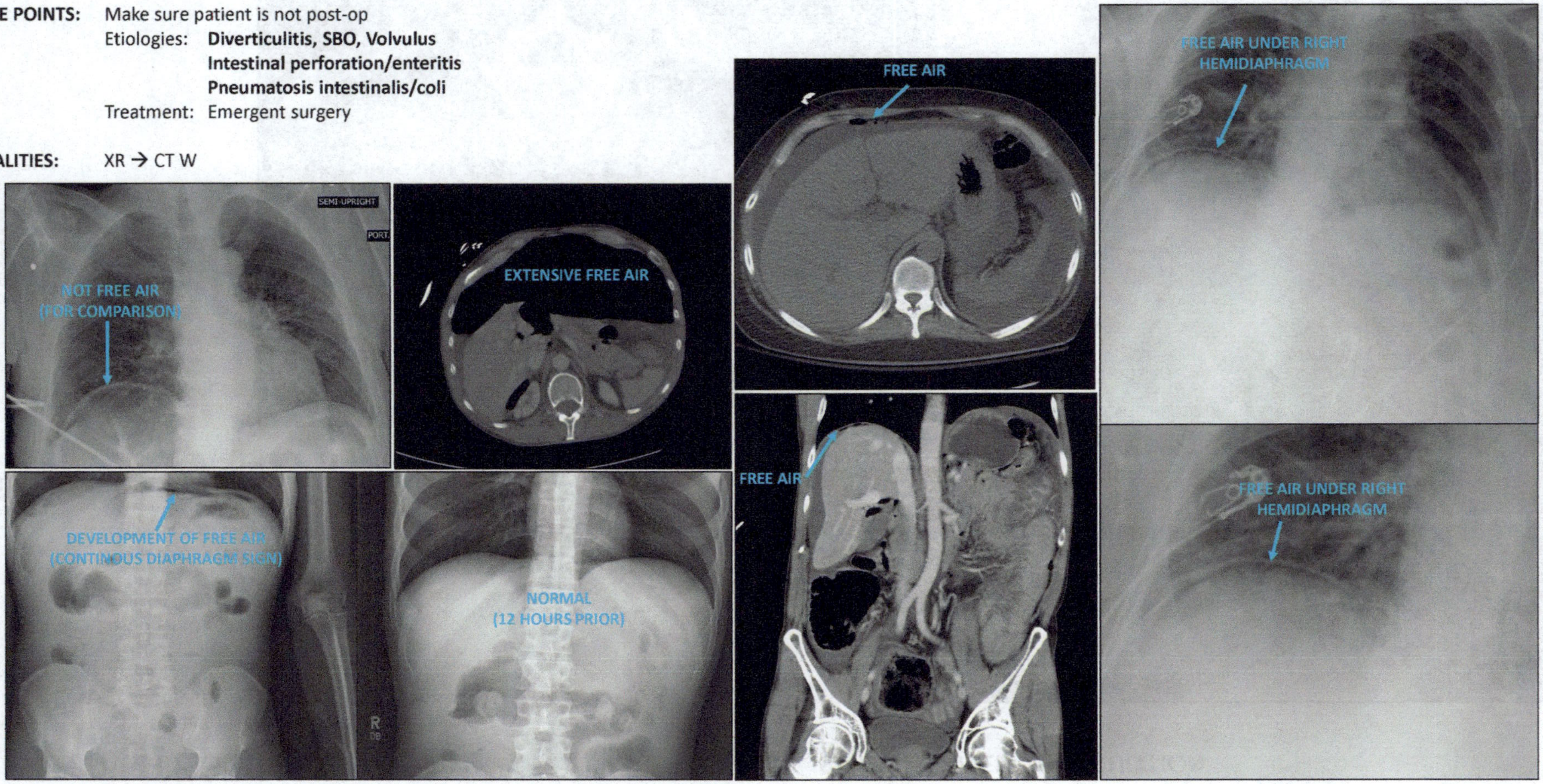

GASTROINTESTINAL

SMALL BOWEL OBSTRUCTION

IMAGING:
XR: **Dilated small bowel with air fluid levels**
CT: **Diffusely dilated loops of small bowel**
Look for free air

USMLE POINTS:
Post-operative adhesions, Hernias, Cancer
Can lead to perforation / fecal peritonitis

Partial SBO may resolve (NG Tube)
Complete SBO often require surgery

MODALITIES:
XR → CT W + PO
FLX: Small bowel follow-through with water-soluble contrast

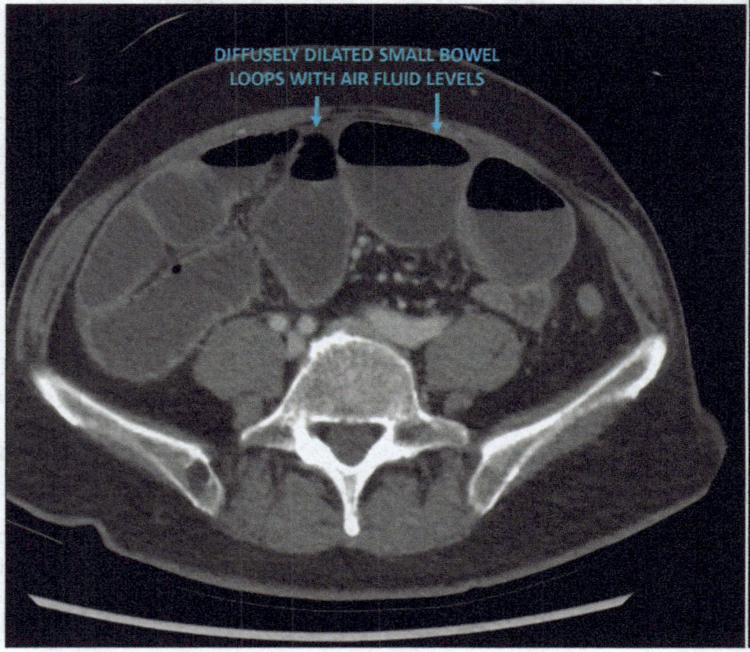

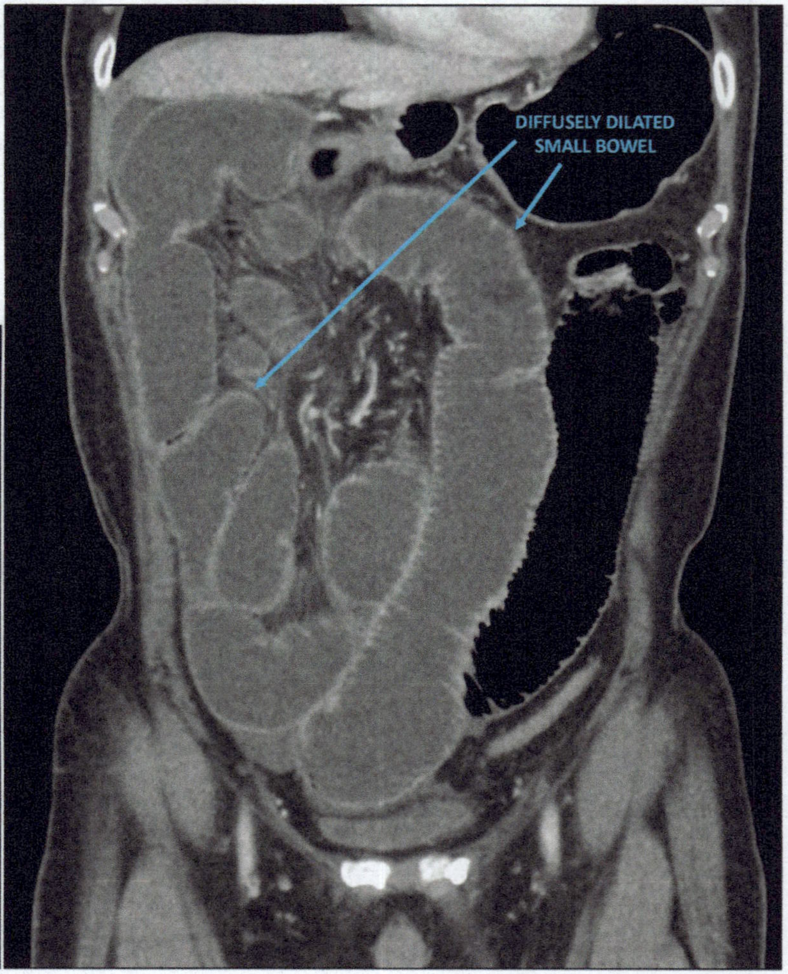

SMALL BOWEL OBSTRUCTION

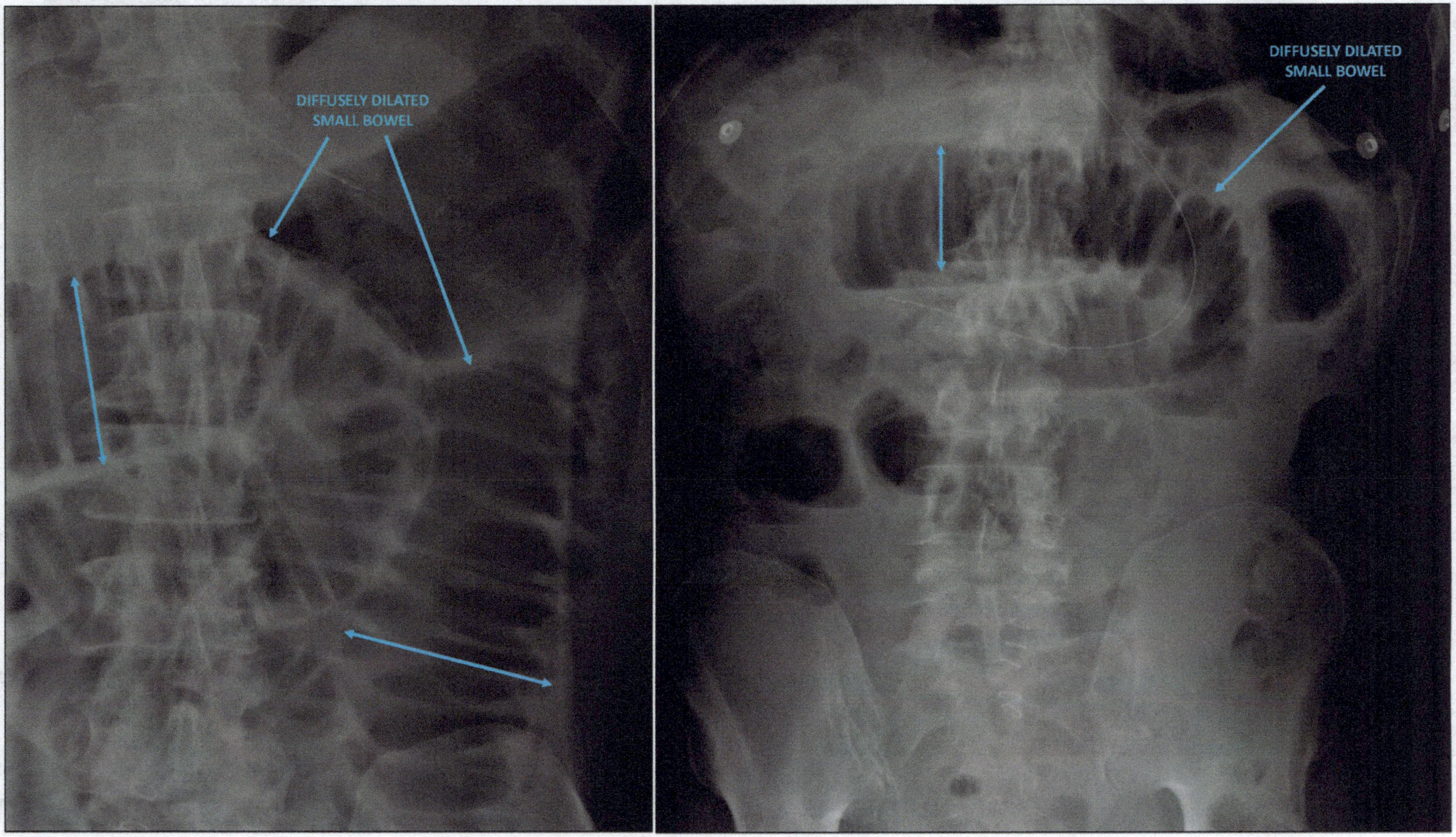

GASTROINTESTINAL

SPLENIC TRAUMA

IMAGING:
- **Laceration (linear low attenuation) within the spleen**
- **Contrast blush → IR/vascular surgery**
- Look for **rib fractures**

USMLE POINTS:
- Blunt or penetrating trauma or secondary to medical intervention
- Spleen is most frequently injured internal organ due to **blunt trauma**
- **Splenomegaly / Mononucleosis**
- Presentation: LUQ pain, left shoulder tip pain
- Treatment: **Splenic artery embolization if unstable**

MODALITIES:
- **FAST** US
- CT W / CTA

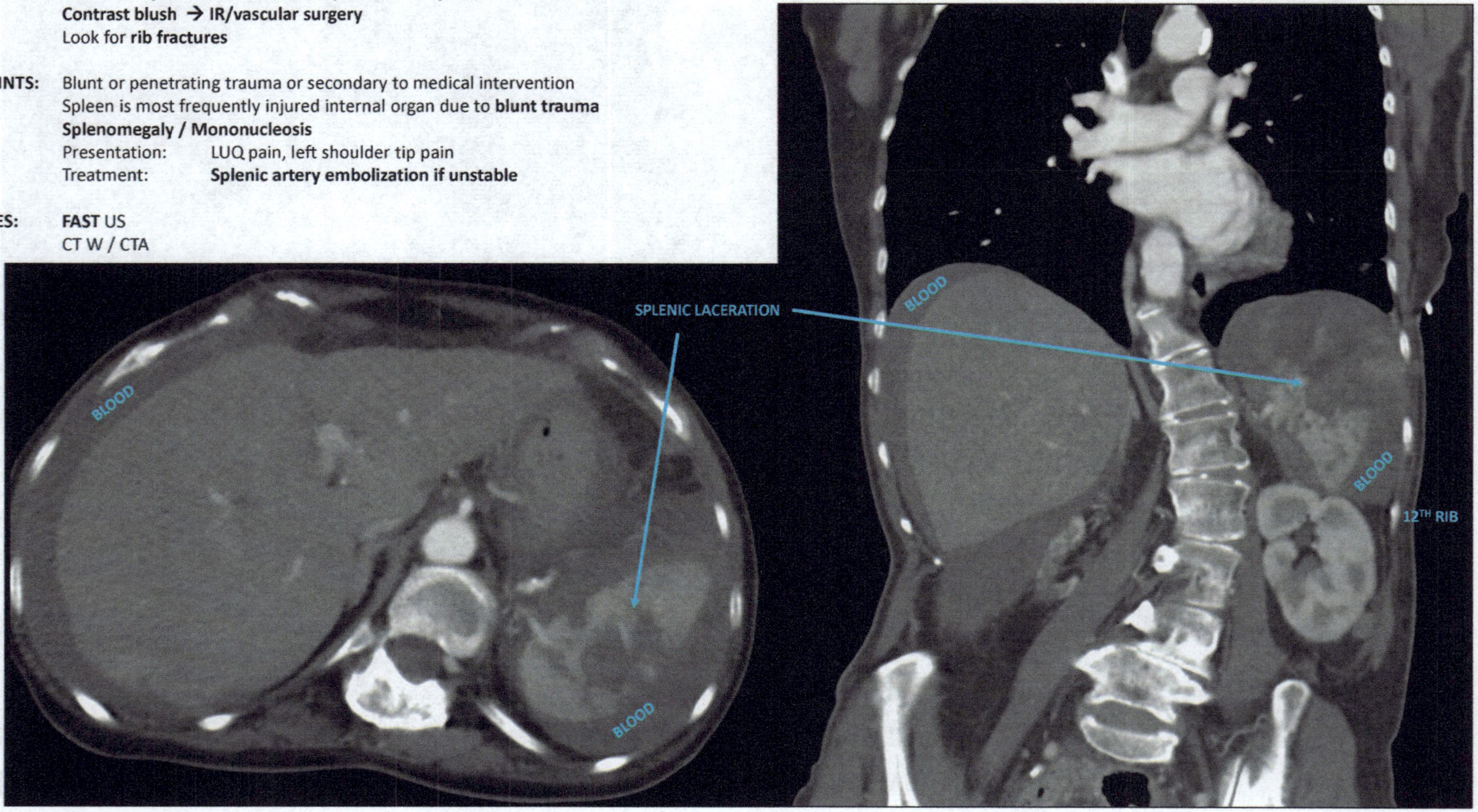

GASTROINTESTINAL

ANGIOMYOLIPOMA (TUBEROUS SCLEROSIS)

IMAGING: Extensive Angiomyolipomas: **Macroscopic fat containing** lesion (hamartoma)
TS associated findings: **AML, LAM, SEGA, Cortical tubers**

USMLE POINTS: Diagnostic of Tuberous Sclerosis (multisystem hamartomas)
Tumor suppressor genes TSC1 and TSC2 (Autosomal dominant)
Triad: **"Zits, Fits, Nitwits" → Facial angiofibroma, Epileptic seizures, MR**

MODALITIES: CT WO

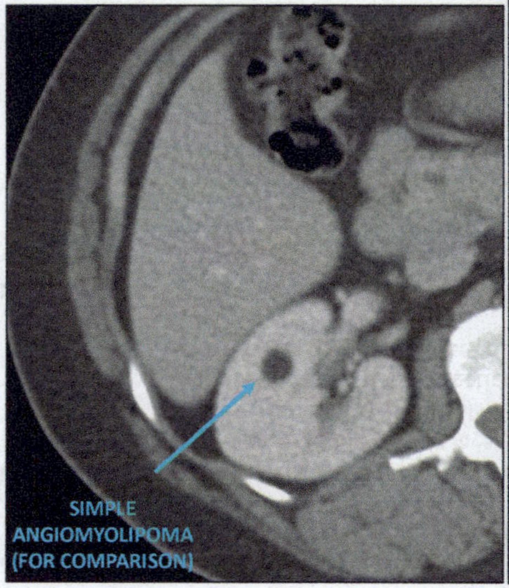

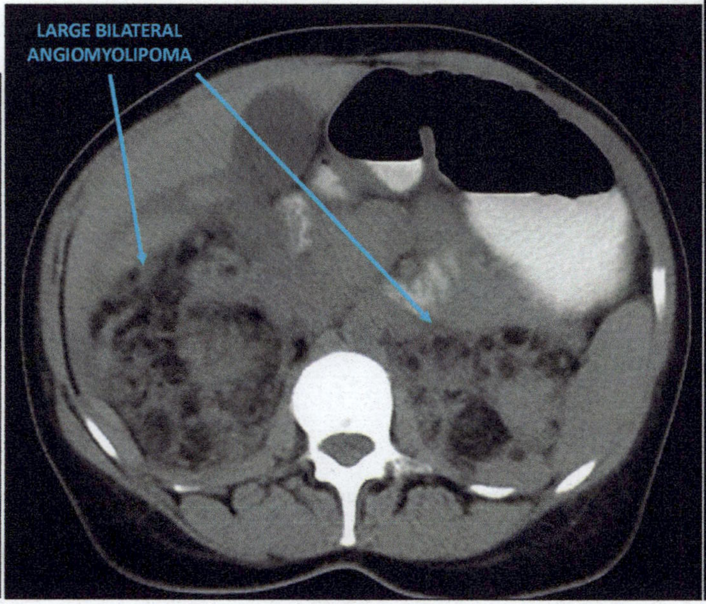

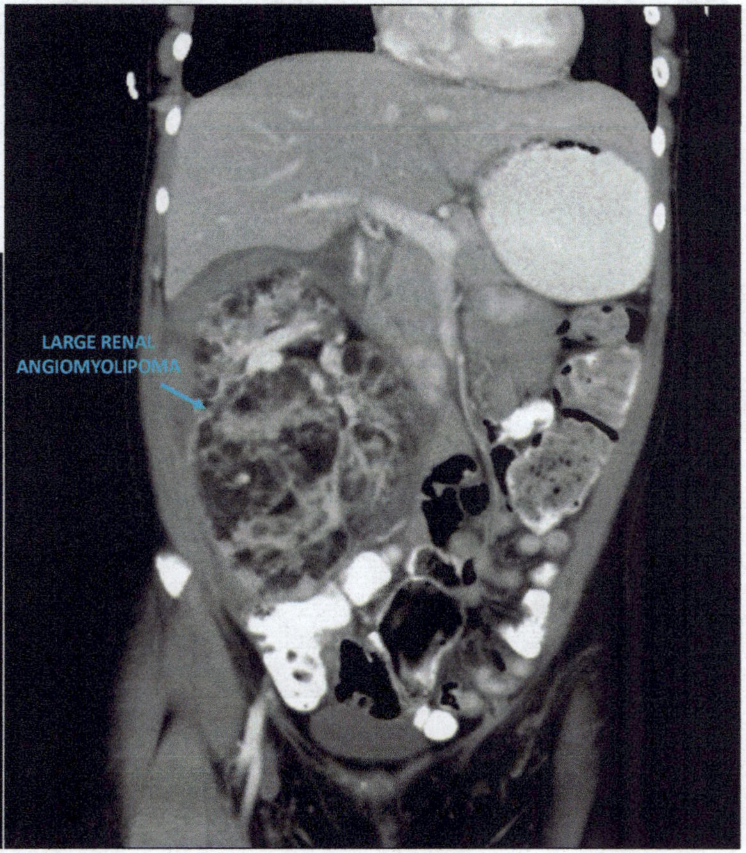

GASTROINTESTINAL

ZENKER DIVERTICULUM

IMAGING: **Posterior outpouching of the hypopharynx**
Proximal to the upper esophageal sphincter

USMLE POINTS: **"False" diverticulum → Herniation of mucosal tissue due to failure of esophageal muscles in contracting**
Weakness in the muscle layer called the Killian dehiscence
Presentation: **Halitosis**
Obstruction
Aspiration

MODALITIES: FLX

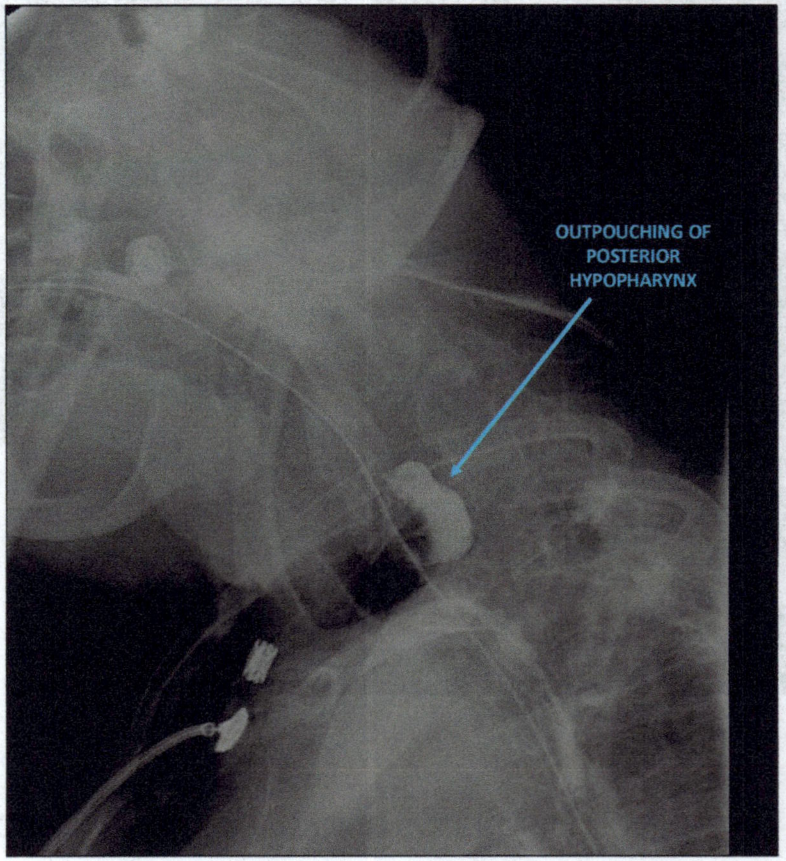

GASTROINTESTINAL

BOERHAAVE SYNDROME

IMAGING:
FLX: **Extraluminal contrast**
CT: **Extraluminal air**

USMLE POINTS:
Will have history of **retching / vomiting (EtOH)**
Longitudinal, transmural rupture due to violent retching **(distal esophagus)**
Sudden increase in intraesophageal pressure + negative intrathoracic pressure
Chemical mediastinitis
High morbidity and mortality
Chet wall crepitus
DDx: Mallory-Weiss syndrome (non-transmural, associated with hematemesis)

MODALITIES: FLX → CT WO

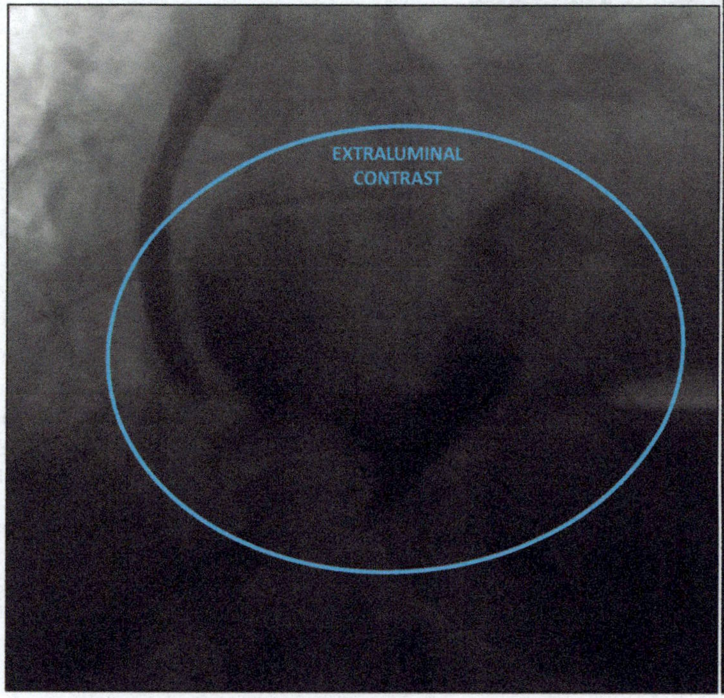

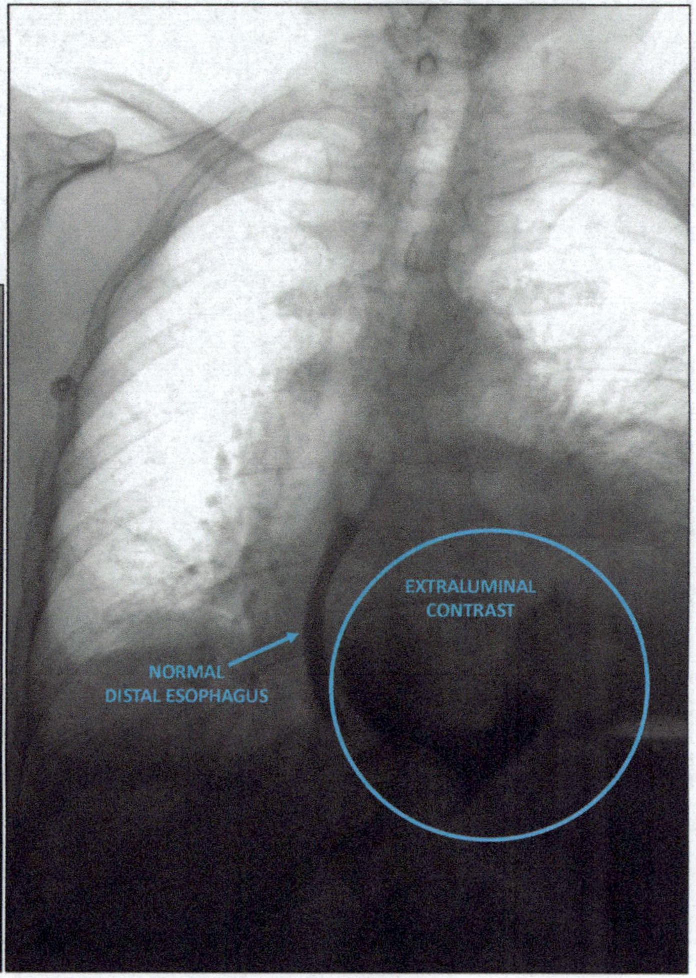

GASTROINTESTINAL

CHOLEDOCHOLITHIASIS

IMAGING: **Filling defects within the common bile duct**
May be shown on XR, US, MRCP, ERCP

USMLE POINTS: **Look for symptoms of pancreatitis / cholangitis**

Elevated labs:
- **Increased alkaline phosphatase**
- Increased GGT
- **Increased total and direct bilirubin**

MODALITIES:

High risk:	**ERCP**
Intermediate risk:	MRCP / EUS
Low risk	US

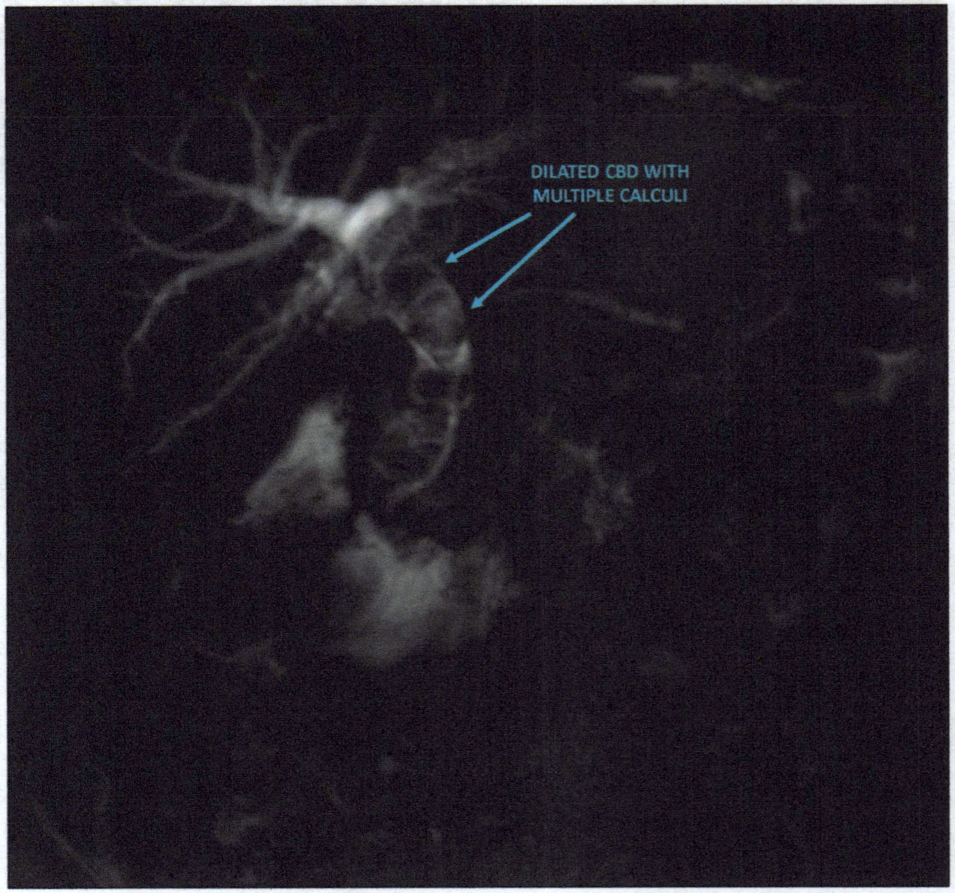

GASTROINTESTINAL

ISCHEMIC COLITIS

IMAGING: **Colitis (wall thickening & pericolonic stranding) at splenic flexure**

Watershed blood supply:

Splenic flexures	→	Junction of SMA / IMA
Rectosigmoid	→	Junction of IMA / Superior rectal artery

Ischemic small bowel: **Air within bowel wall + PV**

USMLE POINTS: Location of colitis helps differentiate
Pain worse after eating (chronic mesenteric ischemia)

MODALITIES: CT W

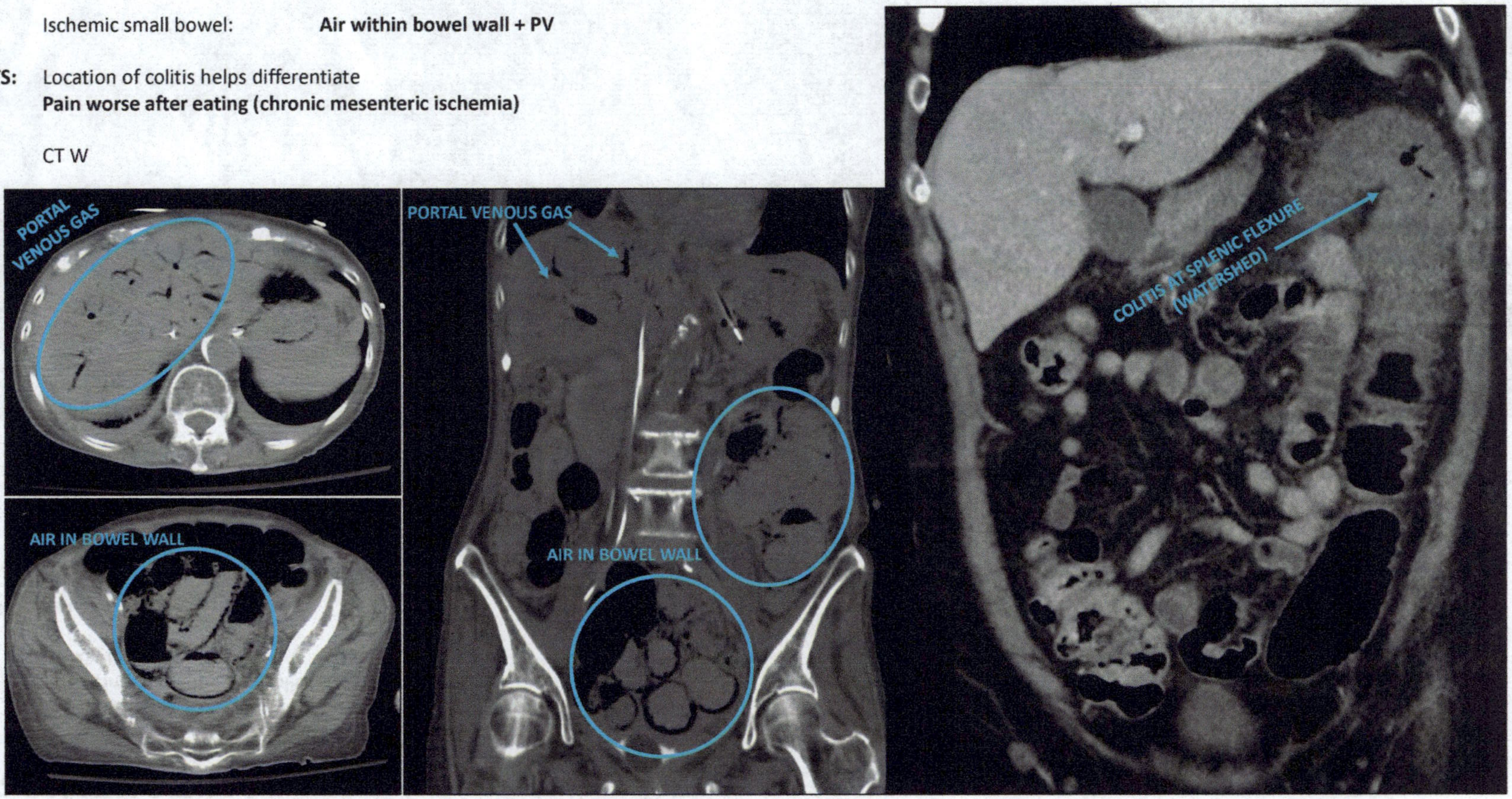

GASTROINTESTINAL

ULCERATIVE COLITIS

IMAGING:

Colitis starting at rectum → Sigmoid → Descending → Transverse → Ascending
Loss of haustra → "Lead-pipe" appearance
Narrowing of the luminal caliber, and pseudopolyps
No skip lesions

USMLE POINTS:

Recurring inflammation.
Limited to the mucosal layer of the colon

Presentation:	Bloody diarrhea
Association:	**Primary sclerosing cholangitis, Uveitis**
Treatment:	Infliximab, **Colectomy**, 6-mercaptopurine

MODALITIES: CT W + PO

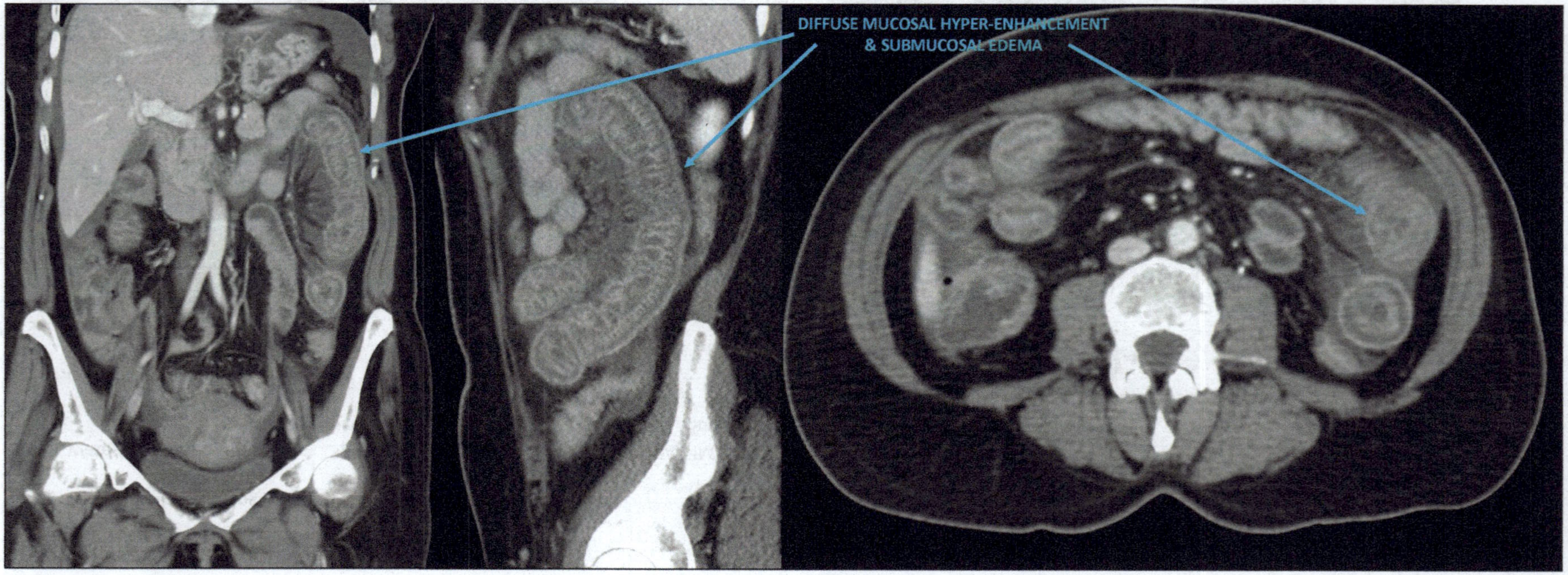

GASTROINTESTINAL

GASTRIC ULCER

IMAGING:
Pocket of barium filling the ulcer crater
Edematous collar of swollen mucosa

USMLE POINTS:
H. pylori infection in 70% of cases
NSAIDS also common
Greater pain after eating because of increased H+ secretion

Zollinger-Ellison syndrome
Zollinger Ellison syndrome: Post-bulbar / **Multiple ulcers**
Gastrin-secreting tumor (Gastrinoma – Pancreatic neuroendocrine tumor) of duodenum of pancreas
May cause ulceration of duodenum or jejunum as a result of increased H+ secretion
Positive secretin stimulation test: Increased gastrin levels even after administration of secretin

MODALITIES: FLX / ENDOSCOPY

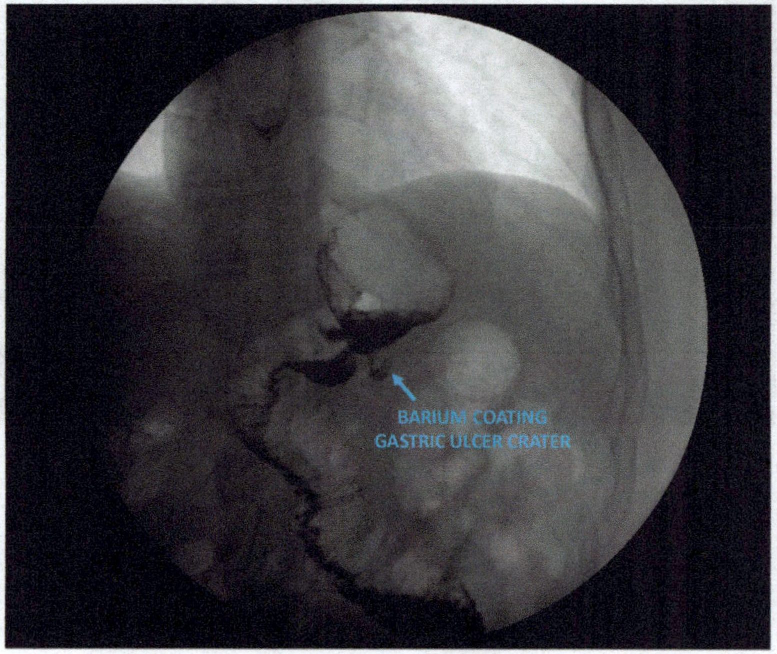

GASTROINTESTINAL

IMAGING: **Hepatic mass with underlying cirrhosis**
Washout mechanics beyond scope of USMLE / COMPLEX

USMLE POINTS: **Most common malignant primary liver tumor in adults**
HBV and other causes of cirrhosis
Increased **AFP**
Presentation: Anorexia
Jaundice
Hepatomegaly
Abdominal pain

Paraneoplastic: **Hypoglycemia**
Erythrocytosis
Hypercalcemia

DDx Adenoma: **OCP**
Anabolic steroids
Glycogen storage disease

MODALITIES: CT WWO / MRI WWO

HEPATOCELLULAR CARCINOMA

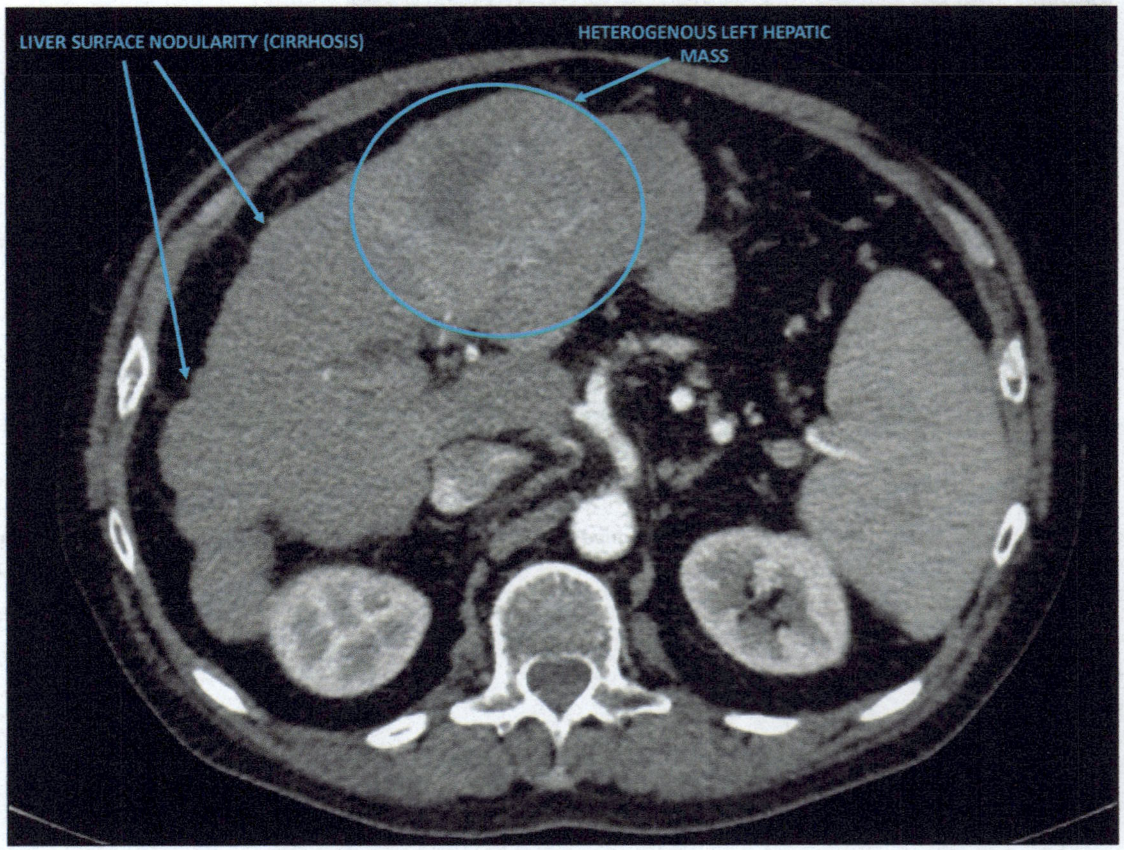

GASTROINTESTINAL

PORTAL VEIN THROMBOSIS / BUDD CHIARI SYNDROME

IMAGING:

PV Thrombosis: **Filling defect within portal vein**

Budd Chiari : **Hepatic vein thrombosis**
Mottled liver (nutmeg liver)

USMLE POINTS:

Portal vein thrombosis: Most commonly from **cirrhosis**
Look for history of **hypercoagulable state, pancreatitis**, or cholangitis
Cause of portal hypertension
Treatment → Thrombolysis + Anticoagulation

Budd Chiari Sx: **Hepatic venous outflow tract obstruction**
Congestive liver disease
Absence of jugular vein distension
Associated with **Hypercoagulable states and Polycythemia vera**

MODALITIES: CT W

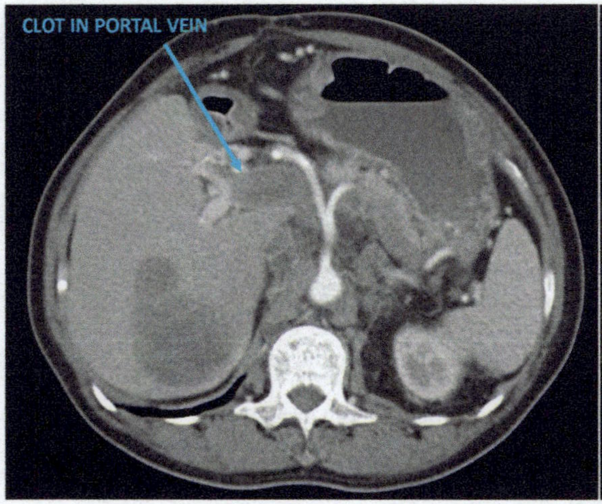

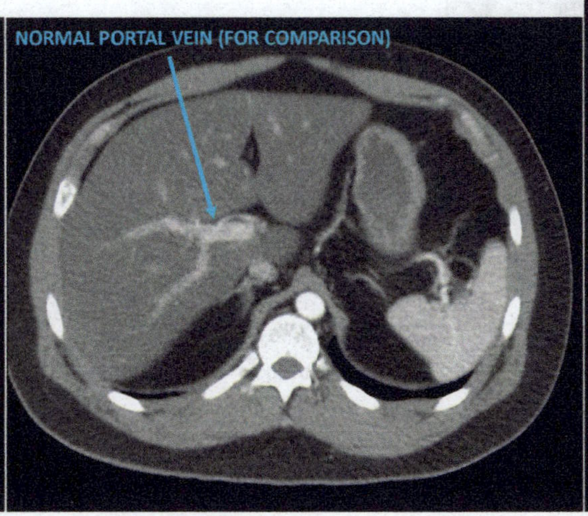

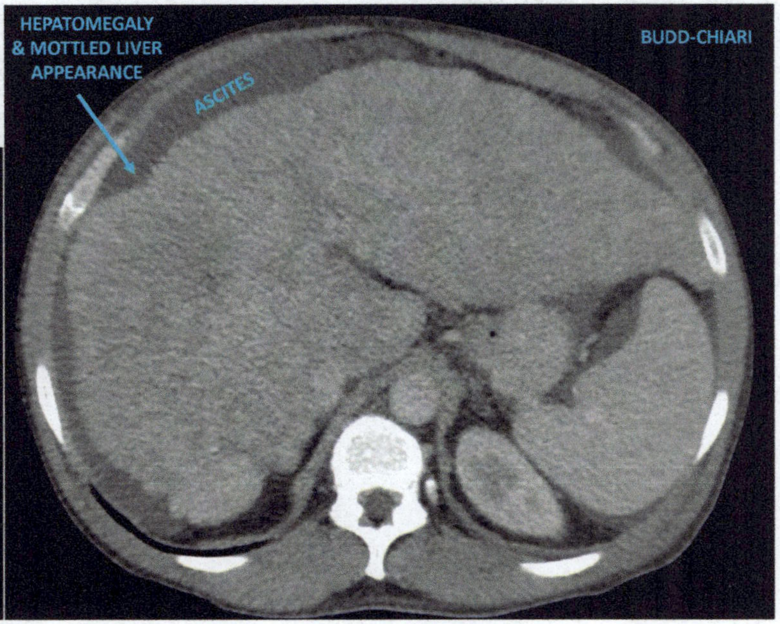

GASTROINTESTINAL

RETROPERITONEAL HEMATOMA

IMAGING: **Hemorrhage (dense fluid) within the retroperitoneum**

USMLE POINTS: **History of femoral artery line, renal trauma, renal intervention, or blunt trauma**

Retroperitoneal organs:
- **Suprarenal glands (adrenal glands)**
- **Aorta and IVC**
- **Duodenum (2nd-4th)**
- **Pancreas**
- **Ureters**
- **Colon**
- **Kidneys**
- **Esophagus**
- **Rectum**

Treatment:
- Fluid resuscitation
- Transfusion
- Anticoagulation
- Embolization

MODALITIES: CTA

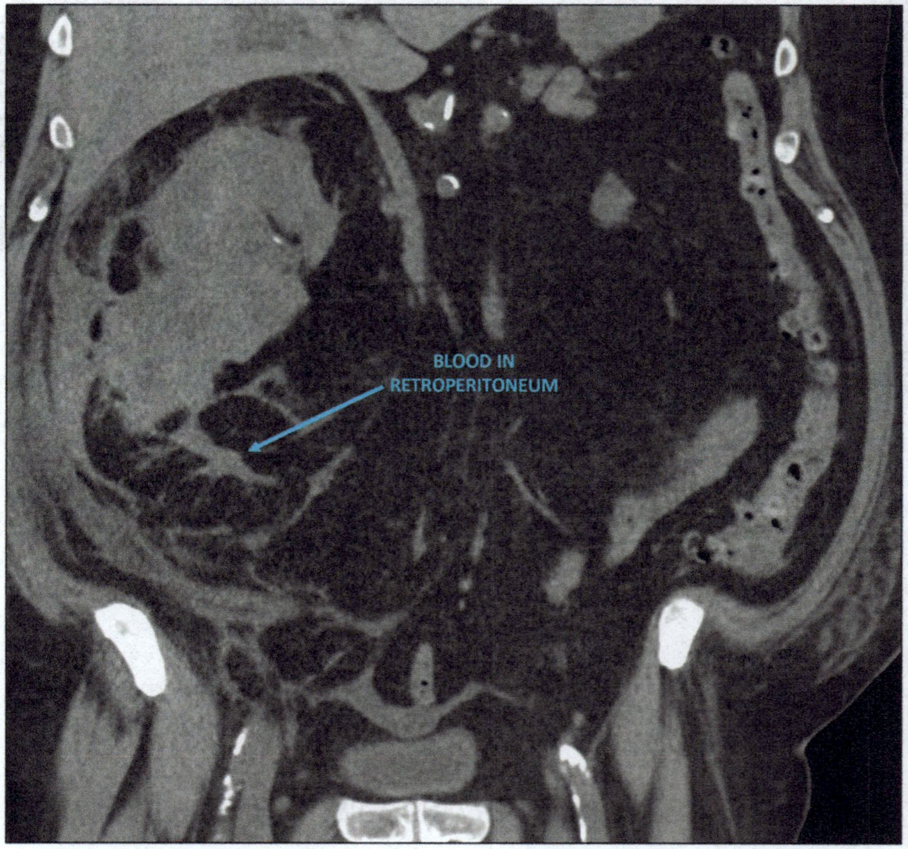

GASTROINTESTINAL

RETROPERITONEAL HEMATOMA

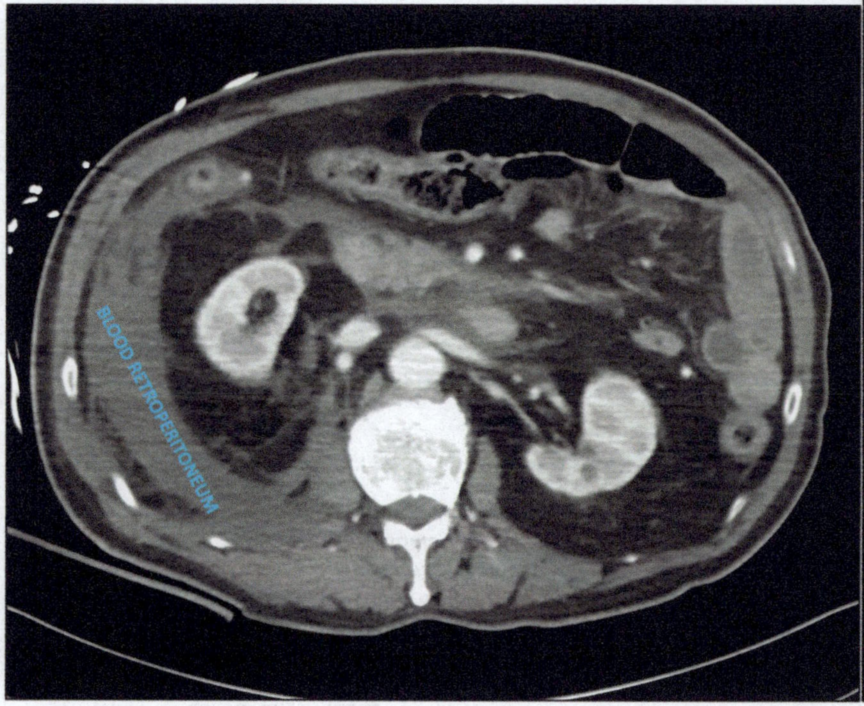

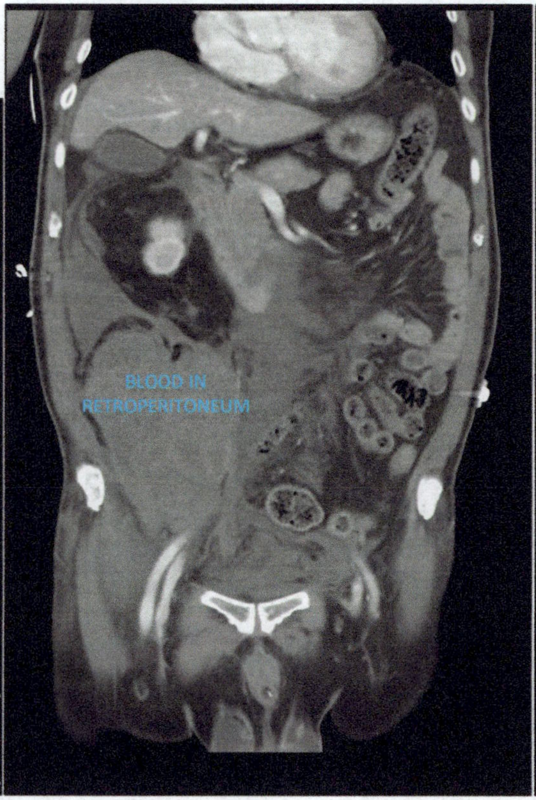

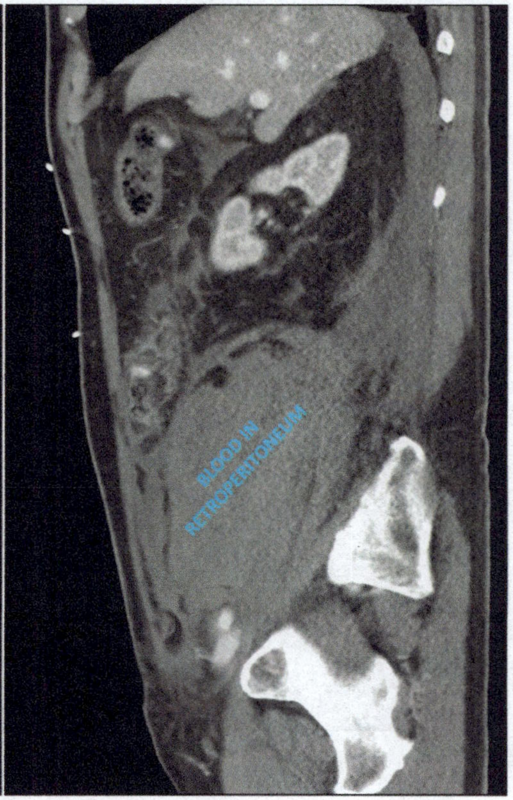

GASTROINTESTINAL

TOXIC MEGACOLON

IMAGING: **Dilation of colon > 6 cm**
Loss of haustrations
Look for free air

USMLE POINTS: Complication of colitis → Loss of neurogenic tone → Dilation → Rupture
May result as severe **complication of ulcerative colitis**
Treatment: **Steroids and other immunosuppressants**
Antibiotics
Surgery

MODALITIES: XR → CT W

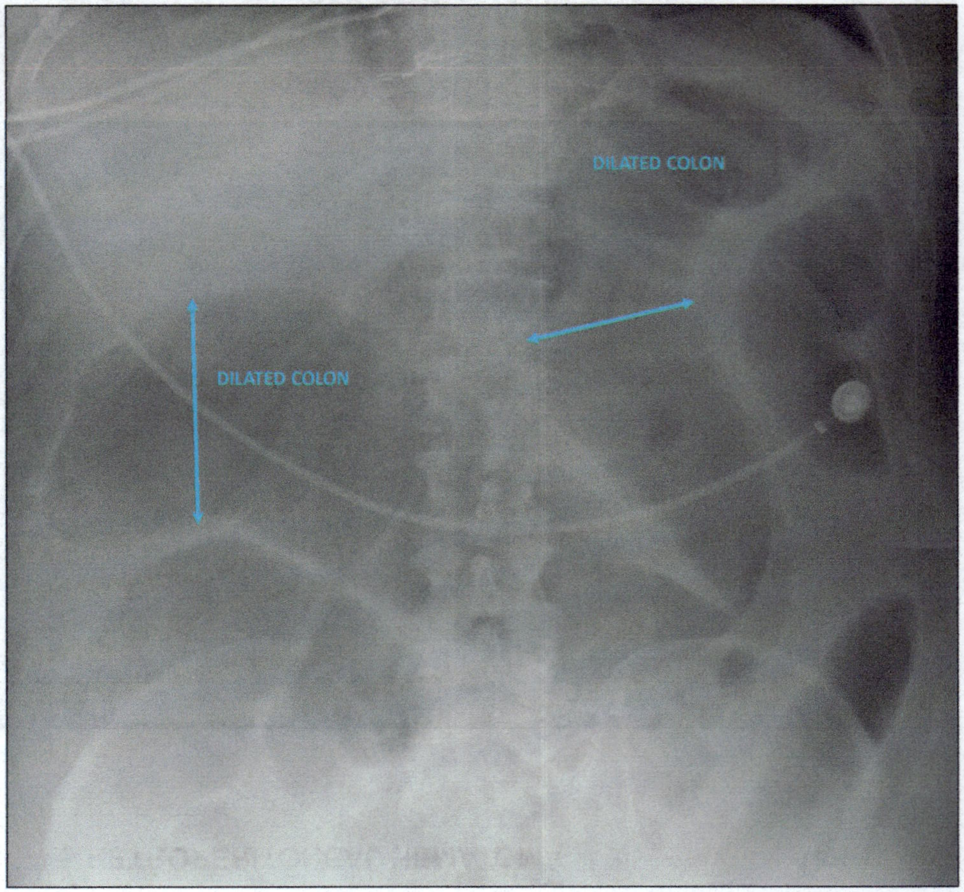

GASTROINTESTINAL

APPENDICITIS

IMAGING:

Dilated appendix > 6 mm
Appendix wall thickening + Peri-appendiceal fat stranding
Look for appendicolith, abscess, free air

USMLE POINTS:

Obstruction by fecalith/appendicolith (in adults) or lymphoid hyperplasia (in children)
Ultrasound first in children (no radiation / can be done bedside)
Initially, diffuse periumbilical pain (T10) → **McBurney's point**
Pain my decrease if ruptures
Rovsing sign, Psoas sign, Obturator sign
Appendectomy should be performed within 12 hours

MODALITIES: **US (pediatric)** → CT W + PO

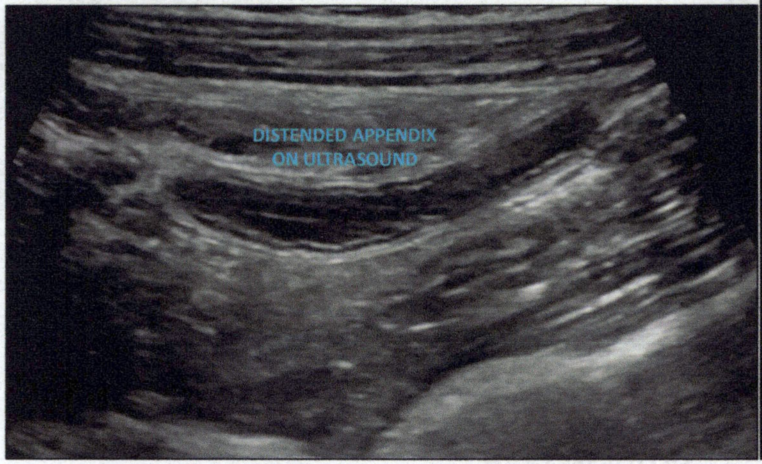

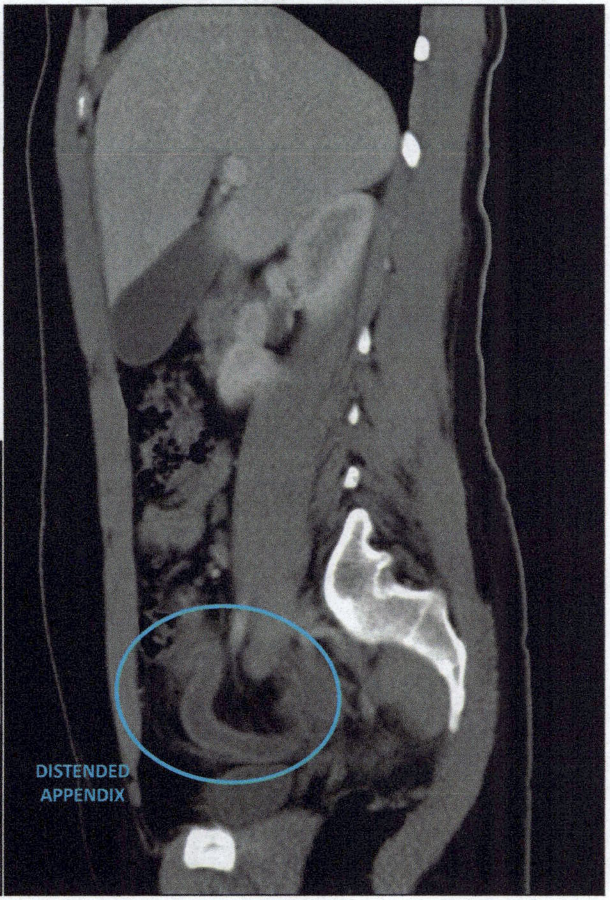

APPENDICITIS

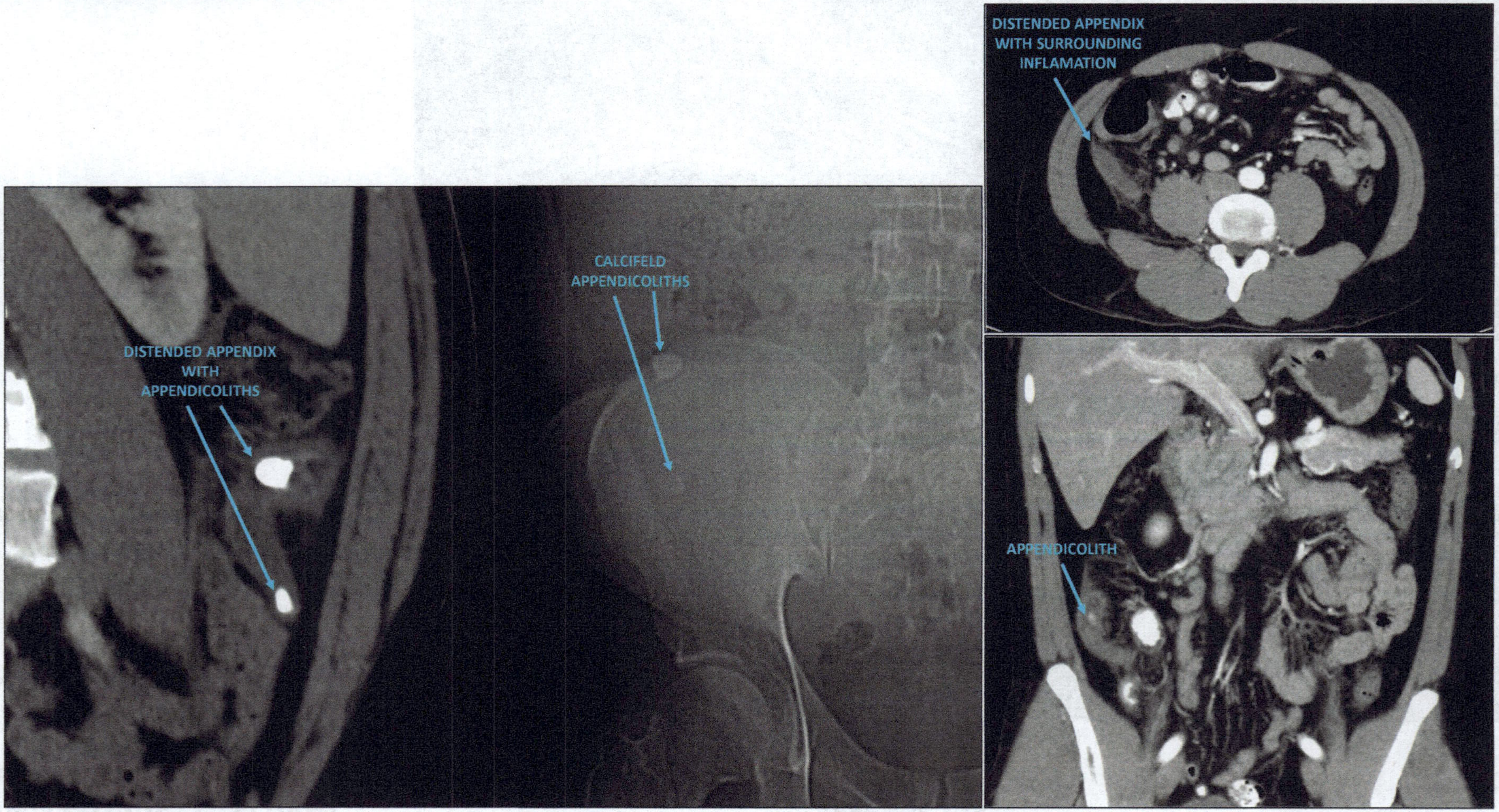

GASTROINTESTINAL

PANCREATIC LACERATION

IMAGING: **Linear low attenuation with surrounding dense fluid (hemorrhage)**
Abnormal enhancement of the pancreas

USMLE POINTS: History of **trauma**
Can be a life-threatening injury following blunt abdominal trauma
Complications:
- Pancreatitis
- Pseudocyst
- Vascular injury

MODALITIES: CT W

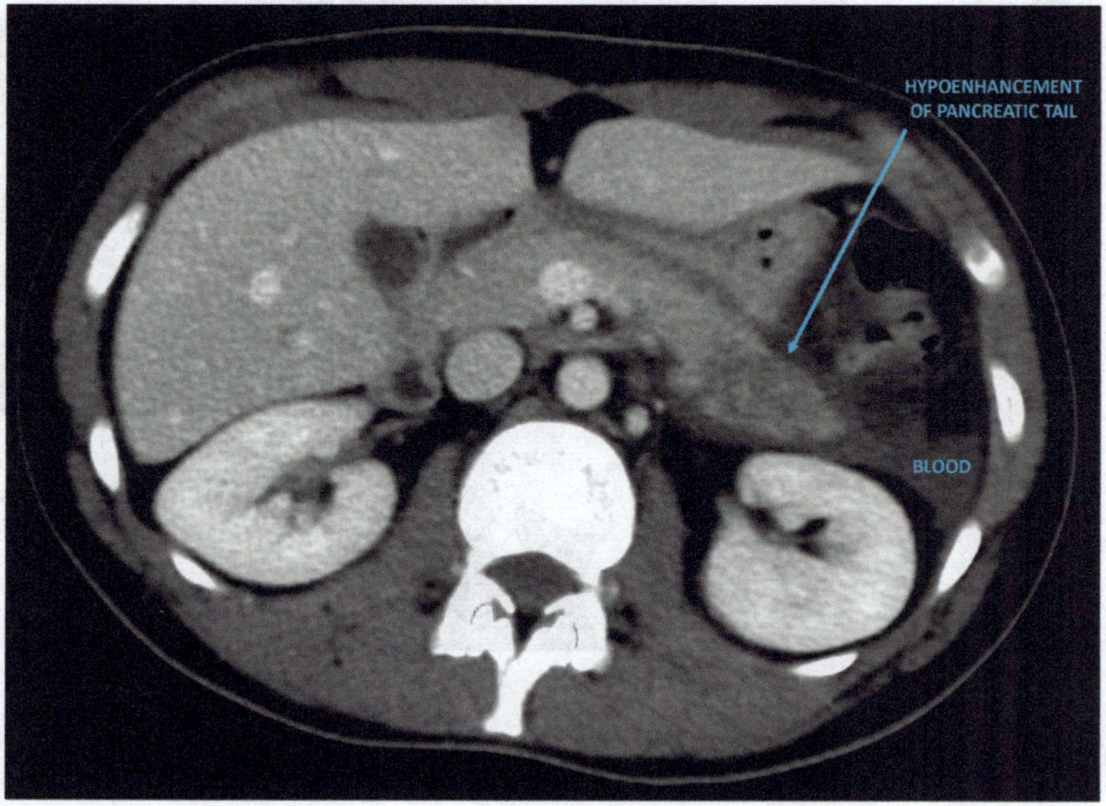

GASTROINTESTINAL

SITUS INVERSUS

IMAGING:

Heart of right side
Liver on left side
Spleen on right side (polysplenia)
Aorta / IVC Inversion

USMLE POINTS: Inverted position of chest and abdominal organs

Associations: Dextrocardia

Kartagener syndrome: Dynein arm defect in cilia → Impaired migration & orientation during development

MODALITIES: CT W

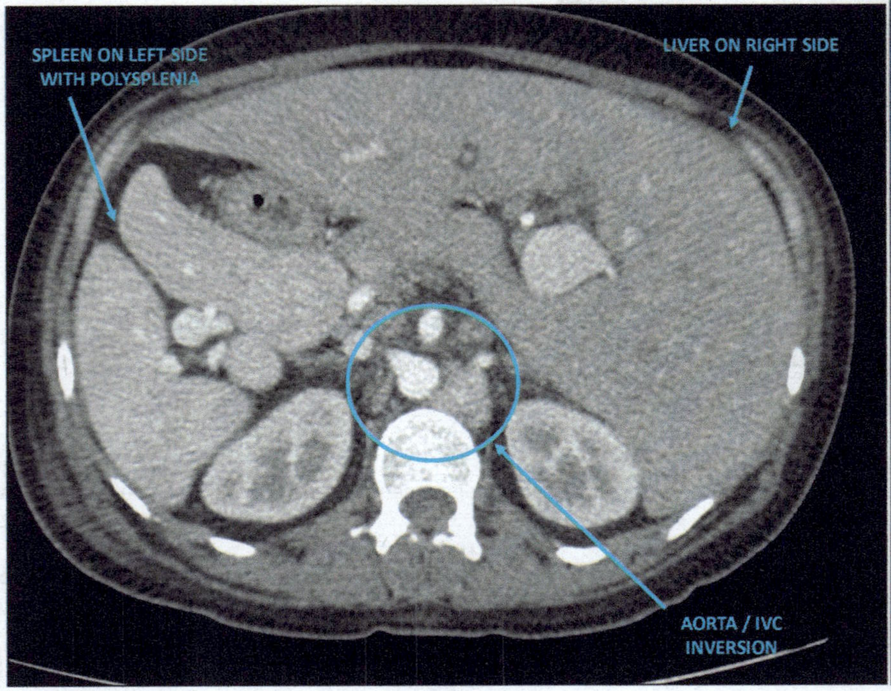

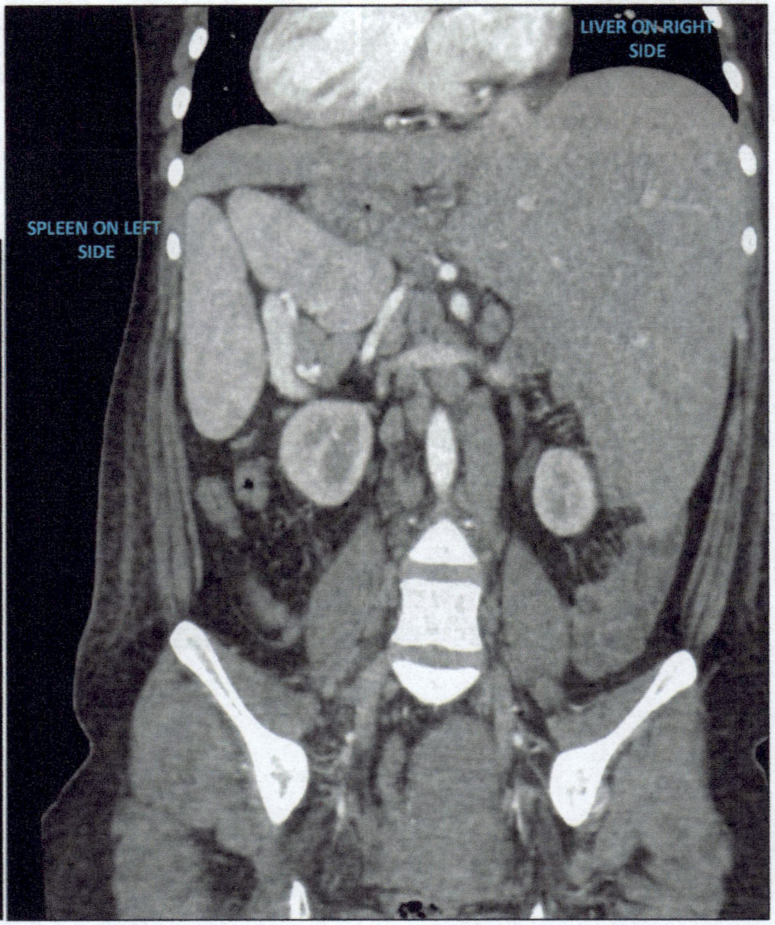

GASTROINTESTINAL

HIATAL HERNIA

IMAGING: **Retrocardiac lucency with air-fluid level**

USMLE POINTS:

Sliding: Gastroesophageal junction displaced upward as gastric cardia slides into hiatus
Associated with GERD

Paraesophageal: Gastric fundus protrudes into thorax
GE junction remaining below the diaphragm

Treatment: Weight loss, lifestyle, PPI, H2RA
Nissen fundoplication (severe symptoms, large size, risk of strangulation)

MODALITIES: FLX

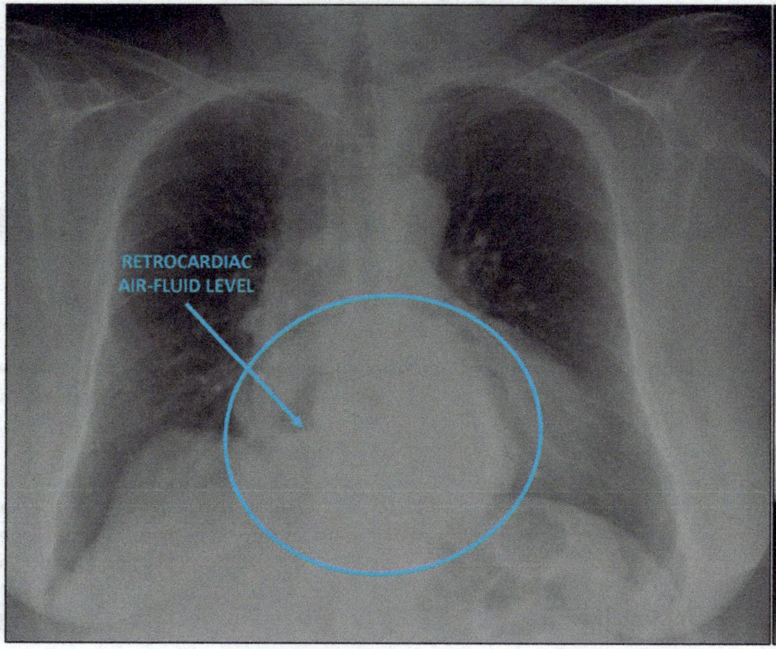

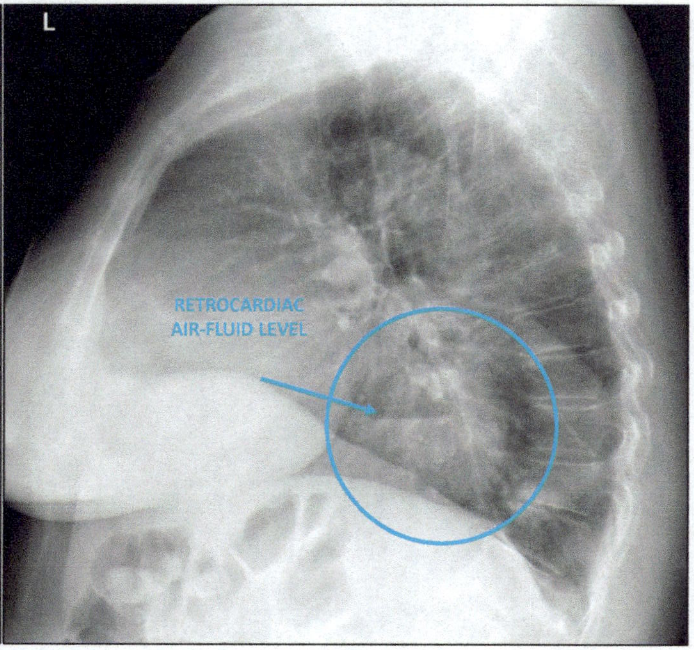

GASTROINTESTINAL

HEPATIC METASTASES

IMAGING:

Multiple hepatic masses (hypodense on CT)
If there is concomitant hepatic steatosis, the lesions may be iso or hyperattenuating
Hyper-enhancing metastases:
- Renal cell carcinoma
- Thyroid carcinoma
- **Neuroendocrine** tumors

USMLE POINTS:

Most commonly: **Gastrointestinal (portal circulation) or pancreas**
Presentation: Loss of appetite, lethargy, jaundice, abdominal distention from ascites/hepatomegaly

MODALITIES:

CT W / MRI WWO

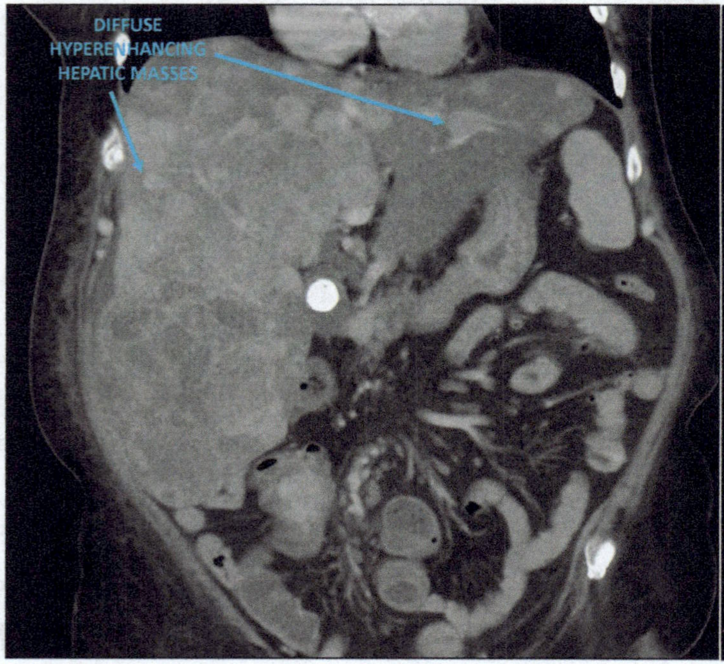

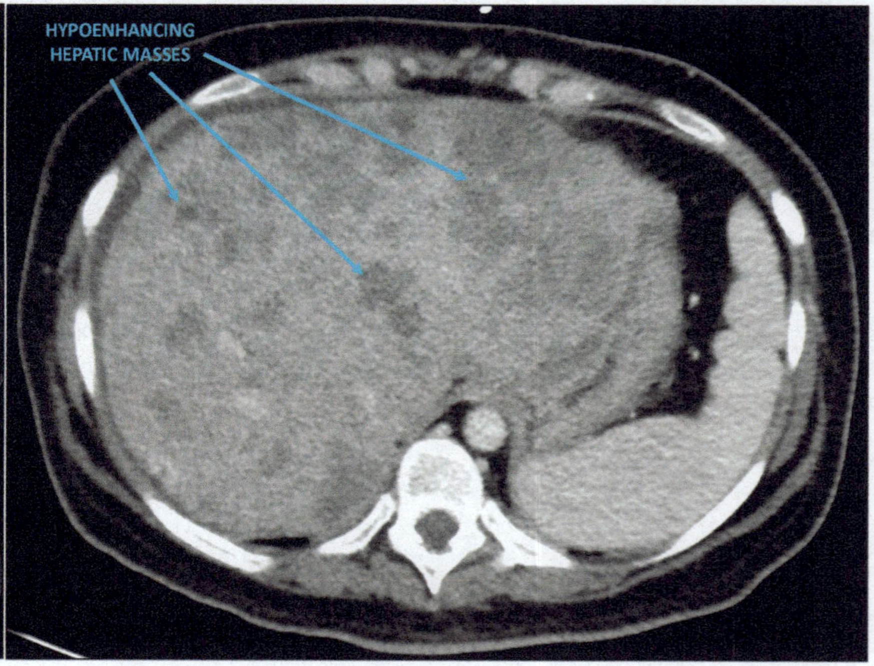

GASTROINTESTINAL

PANCREATIC ADENOCARCINOMA

IMAGING: Enhance poorly compared to adjacent normal pancreatic tissue → **Hypodense**
"Double-Duct" sign may be a clue

USMLE POINTS: Very **aggressive**, commonly metastatic at presentation (arises from pancreatic ducts)
90% of pancreatic cancers are pancreatic adenocarcinoma / CA 19-9 tumor marker

Risk factors: **Tobacco, Smoking,** Chronic pancreatitis, Diabetes, Age > 50 years old

Presentation: Abdominal pain, weight loss, obstructive jaundice

Double-Duct sign: May be due to gallstones that reach Ampulla of Vater
Carcinoma of head of pancreas and ampullary tumors (cancer of Ampulla of Vater)
Cholangitis / pancreatitis

Treatment: Whipple procedure if resectable (often not resectable)

MODALITIES: CT W / MRI WWO

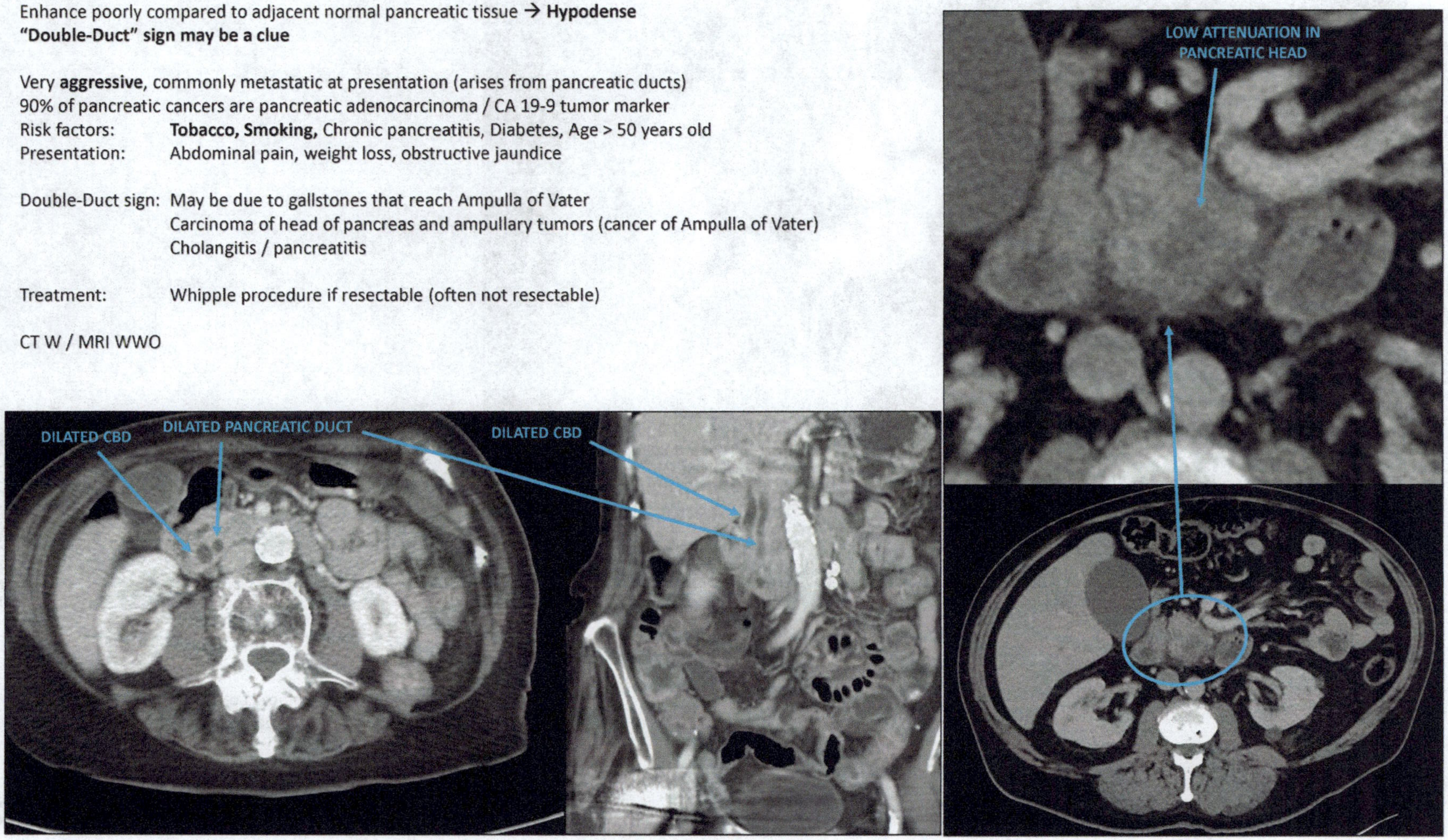

GASTROINTESTINAL

PORCELAIN GALLBLADDER

IMAGING: **Thin, peripheral gallbladder wall calcifications**

USMLE POINTS: **Needs to be surgically removed** (increased risk of gallbladder cancer)
Calcified gallbladder due to chronic cholecystitis

MODALITIES: XR → US → CT W

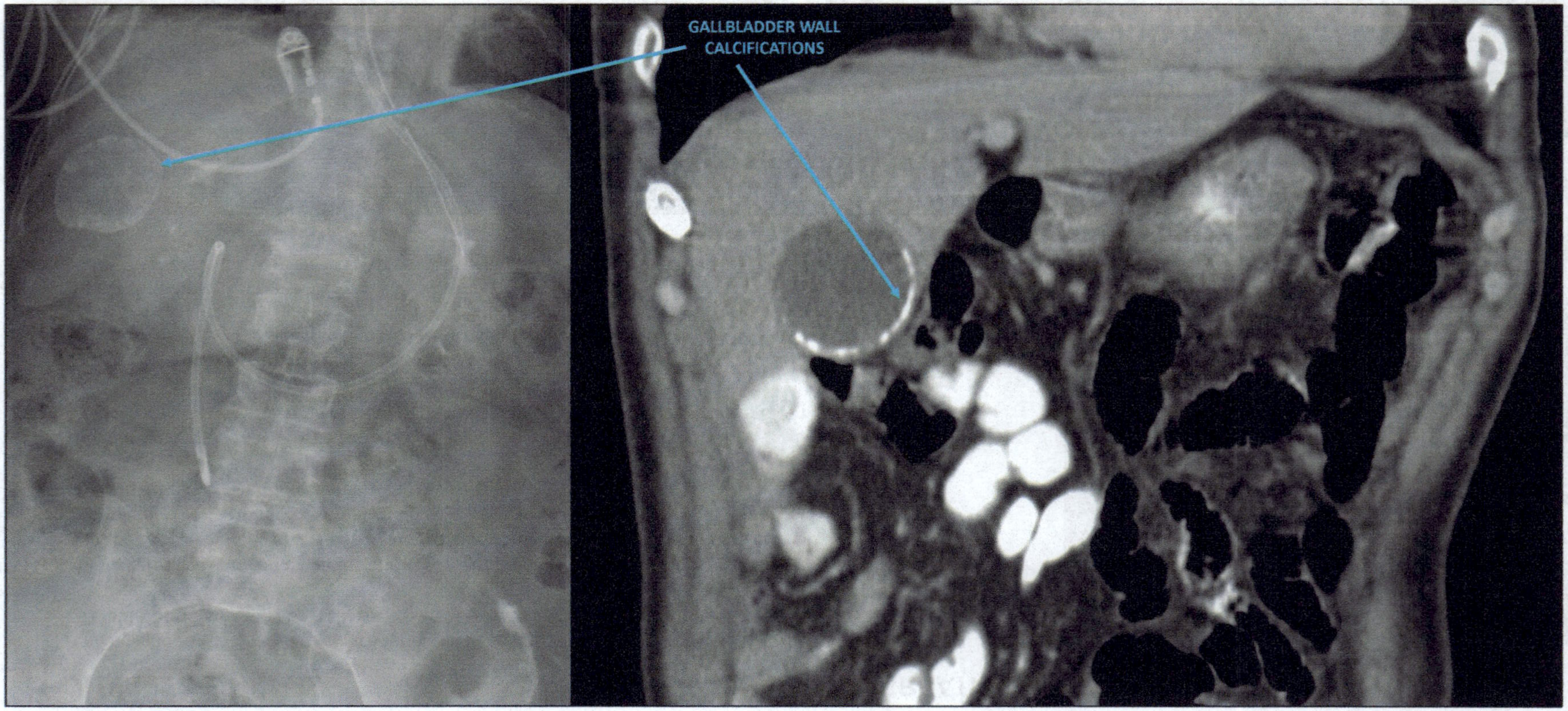

GASTROINTESTINAL

SIGMOID VOLVULUS

IMAGING: **Large bowel obstruction (dilated colon) due to the sigmoid colon twists on its mesentery**
Large gas-filled loop lacking haustra → forms a closed-loop obstruction
Whirl sign: Swirling of mesentery

USMLE POINTS: Elderly
Complications: **Bowel perforation and fecal peritonitis**
Treatment: Endoscopic detorsion
Emergency surgery

MODALITIES: CT W

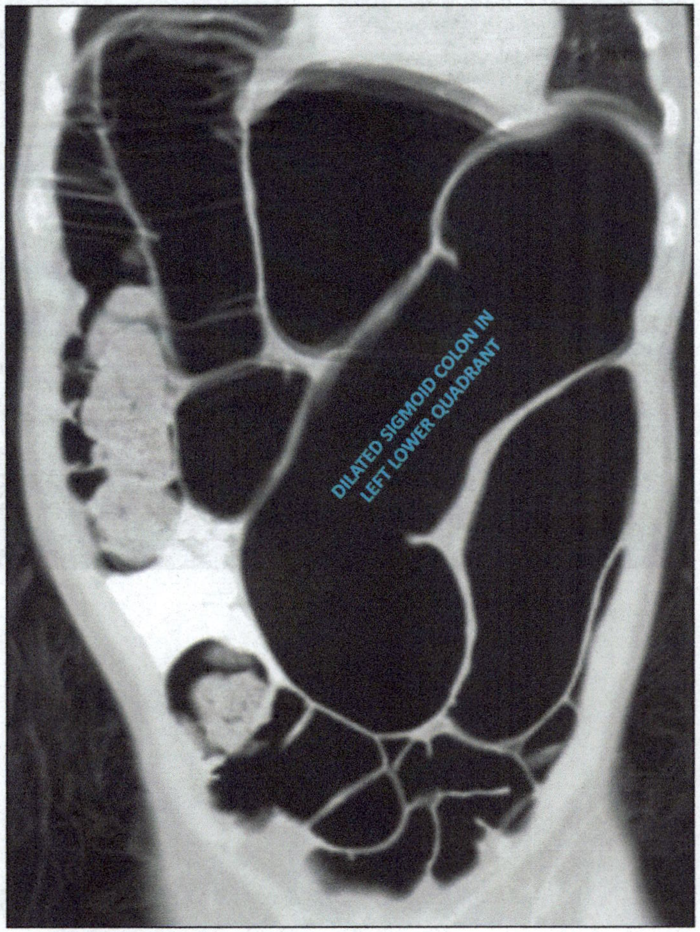

GASTROINTESTINAL

ANGIODYSPLASIA

IMAGING:

Ectatic vessels but no discrete lesion
Focal areas of contrast enhancement in the bowel wall

USMLE POINTS:

Common cause of lower gastrointestinal bleed (diverticulosis most common)
Most common vascular anomaly within the gastrointestinal tract
Most often found in right-sided colon

Associations:
- ESRD
- Von-Willebrand disease
- **Aortic stenosis**

Treatment:
- Endoscopic treatment
- Angiography / Embolization
- Surgery

MODALITIES:

CTA
Endoscopy preferred

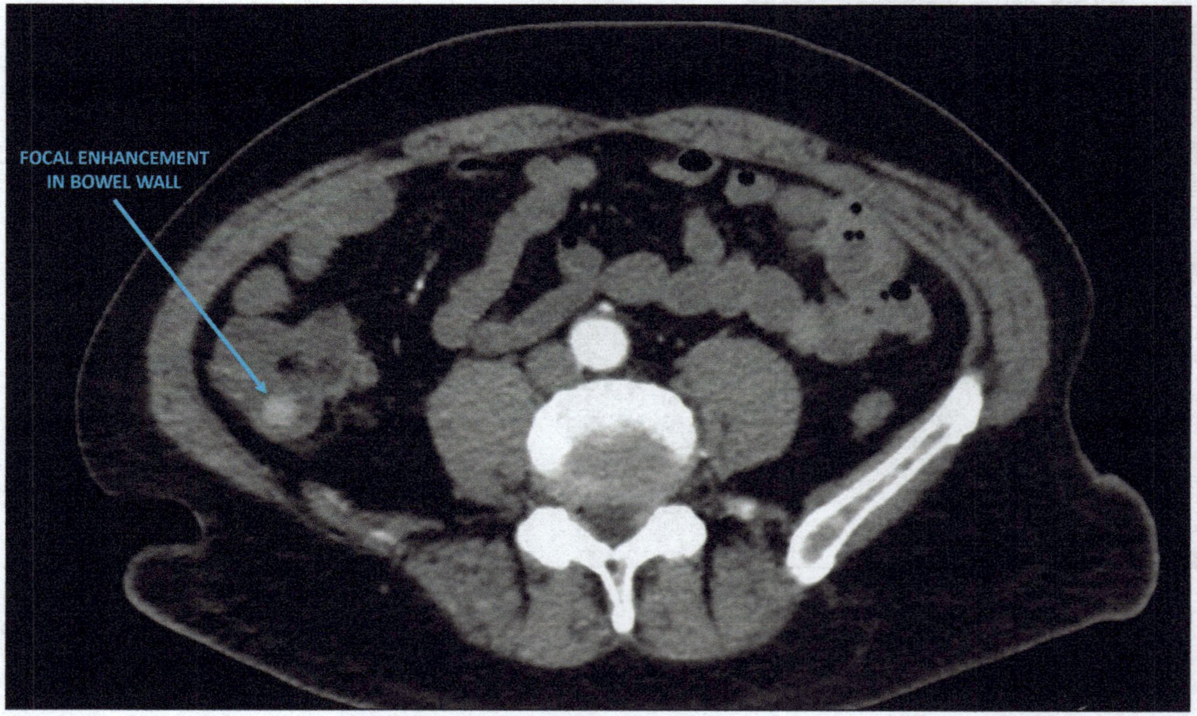

GASTROINTESTINAL

CARCINOID

IMAGING:

Calcified mesenteric mass
Tethering of adjacent mesentery secondary to desmoplastic reaction

USMLE POINTS:

Carcinoid syndrome: **Neuroendocrine cells (intestine** or lung) → Secretes 5-HT → carcinoid syndrome (systemic circulation)
Episodic flushing, diarrhea, wheezing, right-sided valvular heart disease / "TIPS"

Gastrointestinal tract is most common location (small bowel)

Associated with Pellagra (B2 deficiency)
Urinary excretion of 5-HIAA ≥ 25mg/day

Rule of thirds:
1/3 metastasize
1/3 present with 2nd malignancy
1/3 are multiple

Treatment:
Surgical resection
Somatostatin analog

MODALITIES:

CT W + PO
In-111 octreotide scan

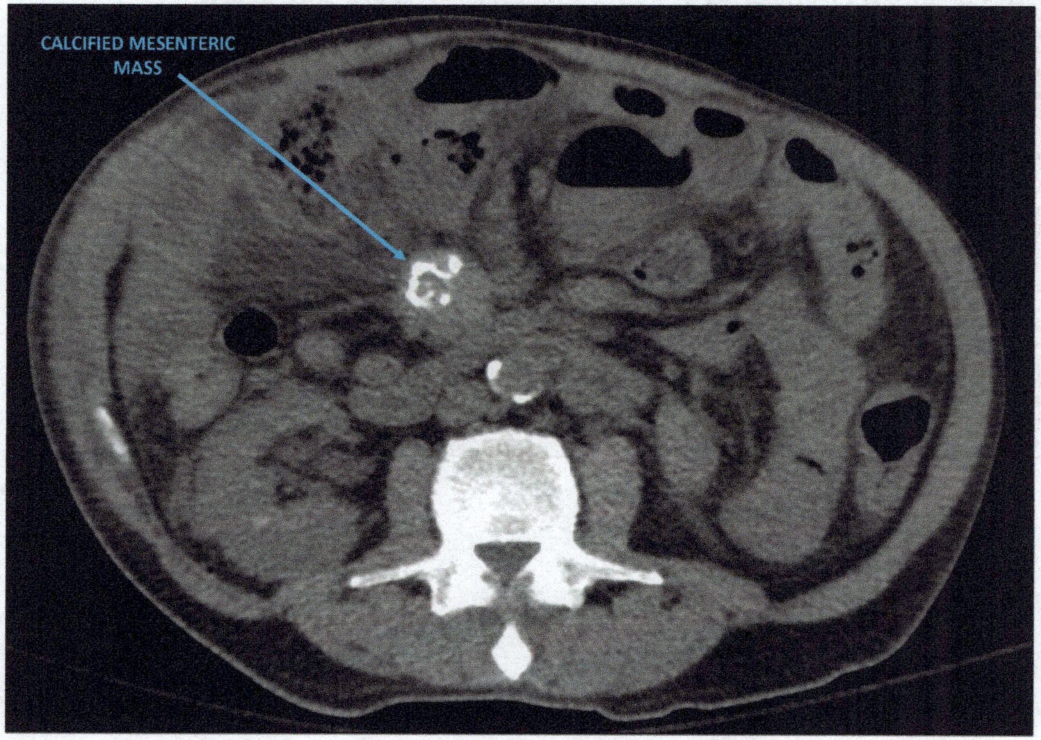

GASTROINTESTINAL

CECAL VOLVULUS

IMAGING: Torsion of the cecum around its mesentery → colonic obstruction → bowel perforation / fecal peritonitis
Look in **RLQ for severely dilated colon**
"Coffee bean" sign

USMLE POINTS: Rotation or torsion of a mobile cecum and ascending colon, commonly resulting in obstruction
Complications: **Bowel perforation and fecal peritonitis**
Presentation: Colicky abdominal pain, vomiting, abdominal distention

MODALITIES: XR → CT W

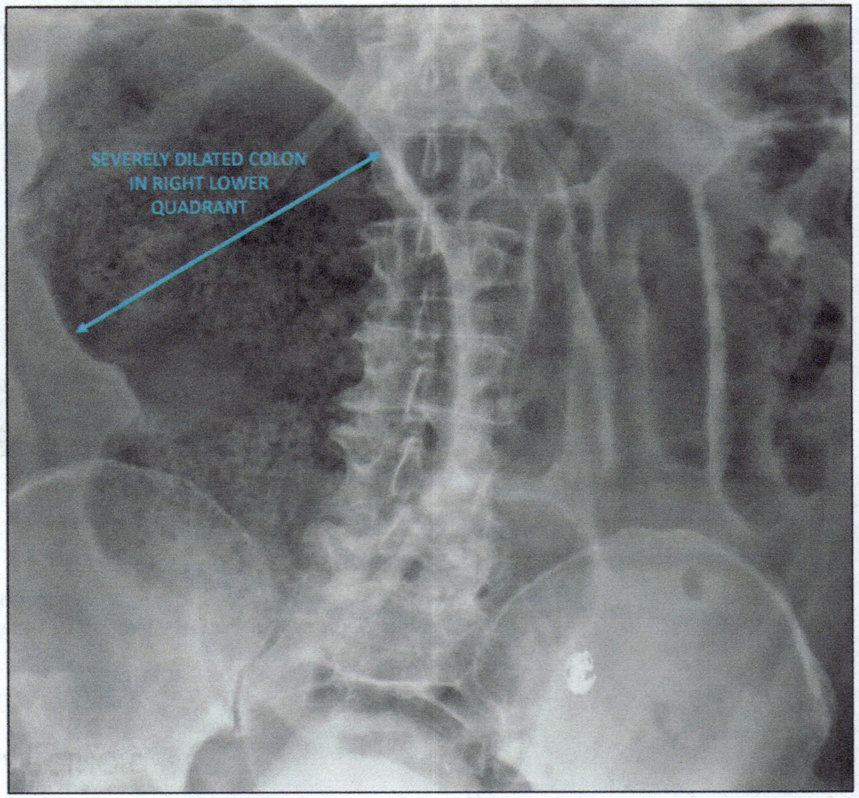

GASTROINTESTINAL

DIFFUSE ESOPHAGEAL SPASM

IMAGING: **"Cork-Screw" appearance of the esophagus**

USMLE POINTS: Normal peristalsis is interrupted by many tertiary (non-propulsive) contractions
Can be difficult to distinguish from cardiac chest pain

Diagnosis: FLX, esophageal **manometry**

Presentation: **Dysphagia or regurgitation**

Treatment: **Nitrites, CCB,** Botox, Myotomy

MODALITIES: FLX / Manometry is gold standard of testing

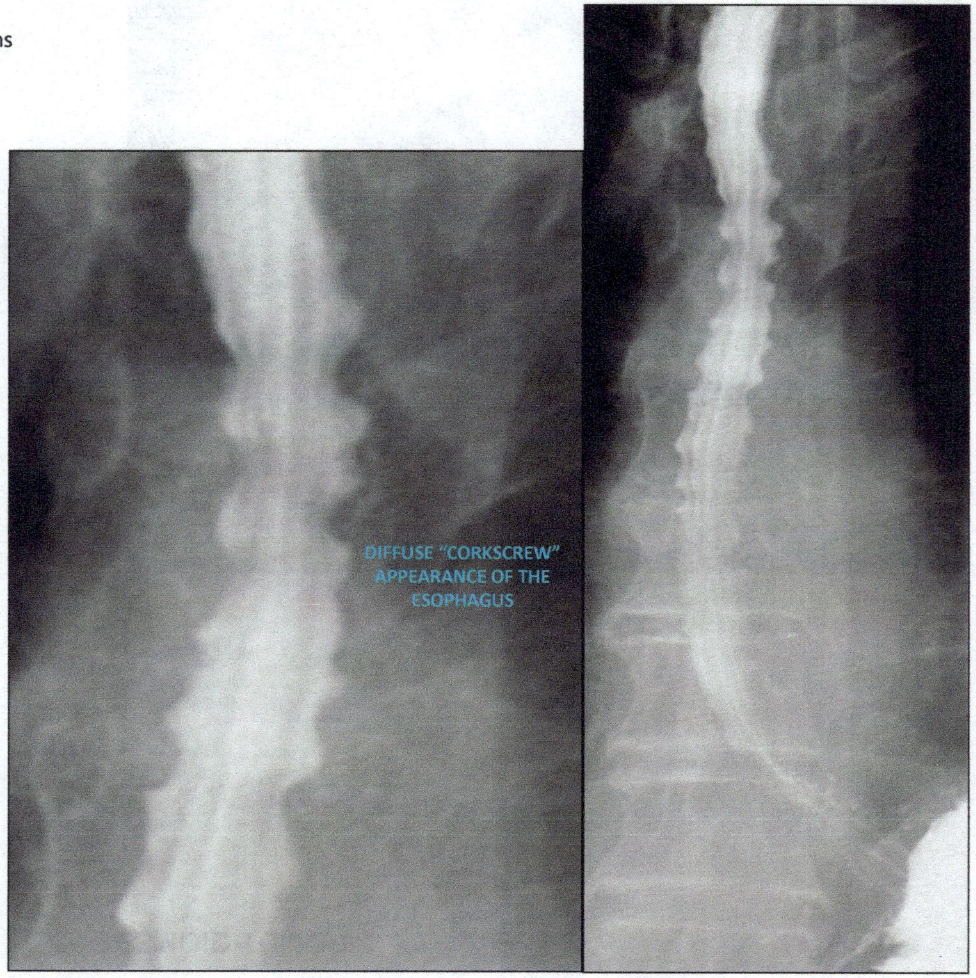

GASTROINTESTINAL

DESMOID TUMOR

IMAGING: Non-inflammatory fibroblastic tumors
Well circumscribed
Tendency for **local invasion and recurrence**

USMLE POINTS: Presentation depends on location (mass, swelling, pain, cramping)
Noncancerous growths in connective tissue → Does not metastasize

Gardner syndrome (subtype of **FAP**): Osteomas
Desmoid tumors
Congenital retinal hypertrophy
Nasal angiofibroma
Tx: Prophylactic colectomy
Routine screening for extra-colonic tumors

MODALITIES: CT W + PO

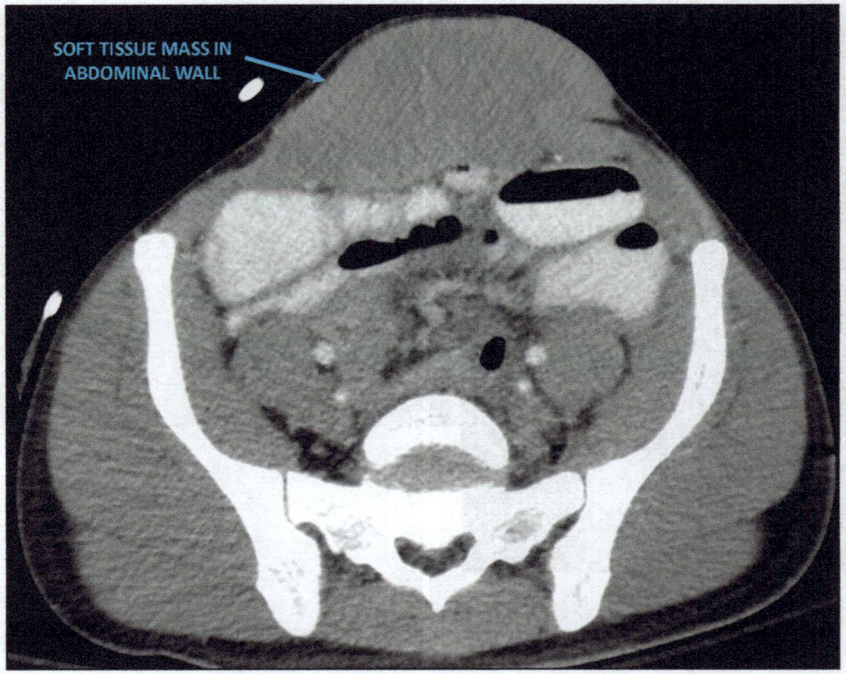

GASTROINTESTINAL

PANCREATIC DIVISUM

IMAGING: **Dorsal pancreatic duct (main pancreatic and Santorini ducts) directly entering the minor papilla**
No communication with the ventral duct (Wirsung)

USMLE POINTS: Ventral and dorsal parts of pancreas fail to fuse at around 7 weeks of development
Two separate pancreatic systems

Presentation: Chronic abdominal pain
Pancreatitis

MODALITIES: MRCP

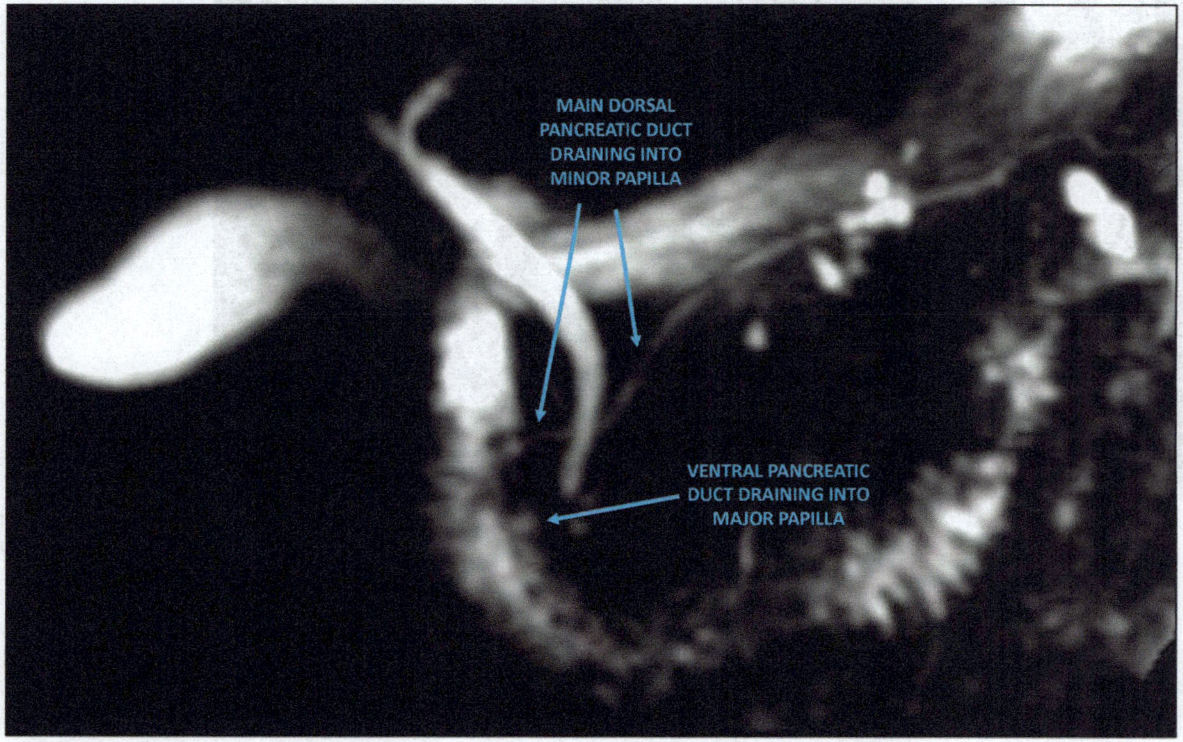

GASTROINTESTINAL

MENETRIER DISEASE

IMAGING:

Rugae along stomach wall enlarge, creating giant folds due to overgrowth of mucous cells
Antrum may be spared. Worse along the gastric body
May resemble a brain

USMLE POINTS:

Hypertrophic gastropathy from **hyperplasia of mucus-producing cells**
Protein loss in stomach due to low levels of stomach acid
Pediatric cases can be associated with CMV infections
Increased risk for adenocarcinoma

Presentation: Pain, Nausea, Vomiting, Diarrhea

Treatment: Cetuximab
Gastrectomy in severe cases

MODALITIES: FLX / CT W

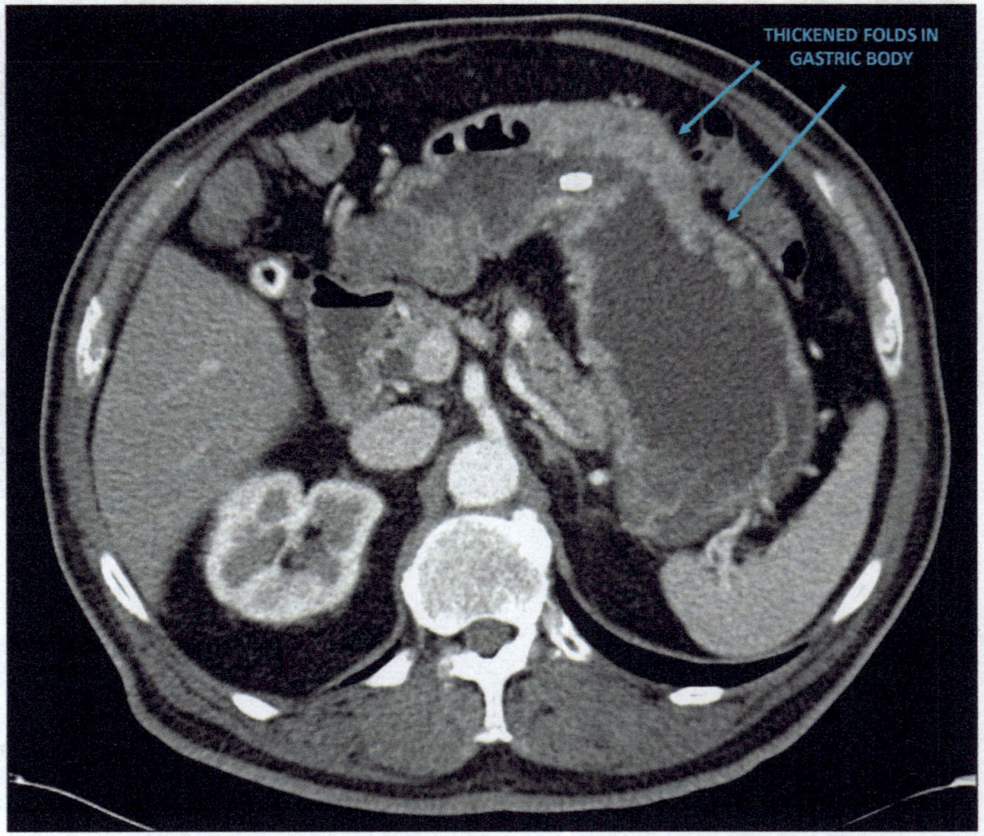

GASTROINTESTINAL

MESENTERIC PANNICULITIS

IMAGING: **Focal area of mesenteric induration**
Often with enlarged mesenteric lymph nodes

USMLE POINTS: Inflammatory disease that affects adipose tissue of mesentery of small intestine and colon
AKA Sclerosing mesenteritis
Abdominal pain
Often self limiting

MODALITIES: CT WO

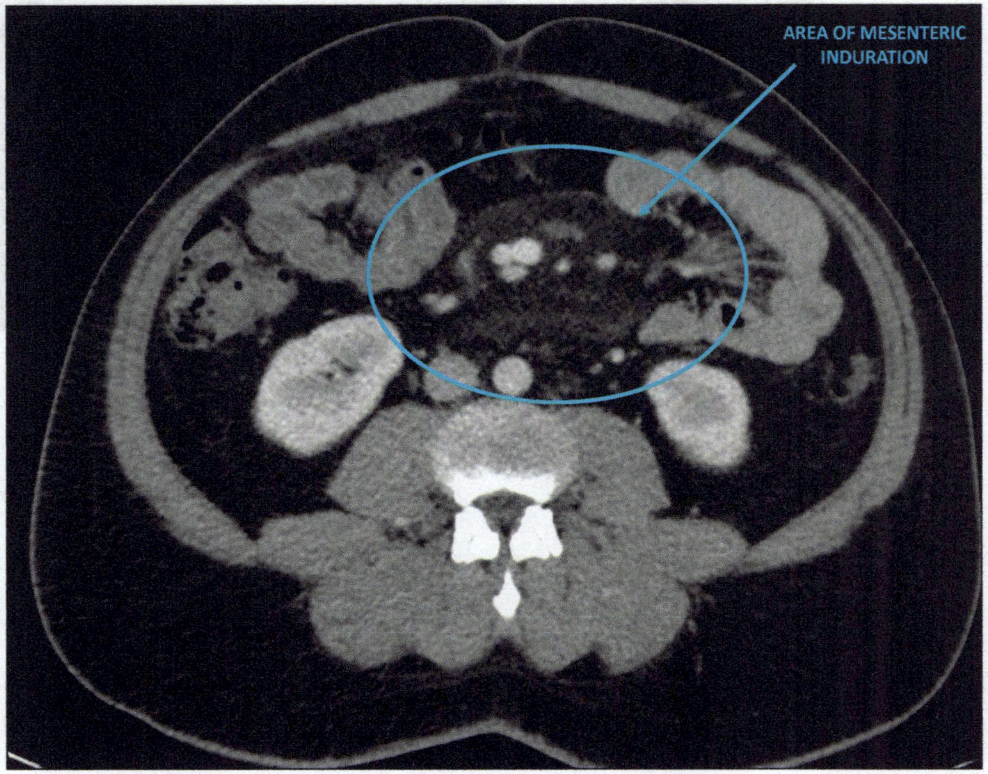

GASTROINTESTINAL

PANCREATIC NEUROENDOCRINE TUMOR

IMAGING: **Hyperdense** pancreatic lesion (vs. adenocarcinoma which is hypodense)

USMLE POINTS: Islet cells of pancreas
Autosomal dominant – MEN 1 inherited syndrome

Glucagonoma	a-islet cells	Rash, weight loss, diabetes	**Octreotide**
Insulinoma	b-islet cells	**Increased C-peptide**	Surgery
VIPoma		Facial flushing, NAG Metabolic acidosis, **WDHA Syndrome**	**Octreotide**
Gastrinoma		**Zollinger Ellison syndrome**	Surgery, PPI / H2-R antagonist
Somatostatinoma		Achlorhydria, steatorrhea	5-FU, Streptozotocin

MODALITIES: CT W / MRI WWO

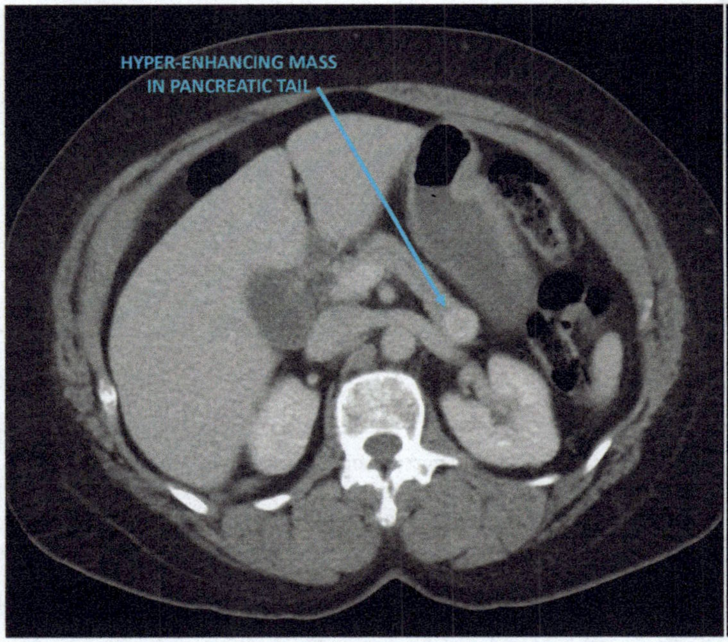

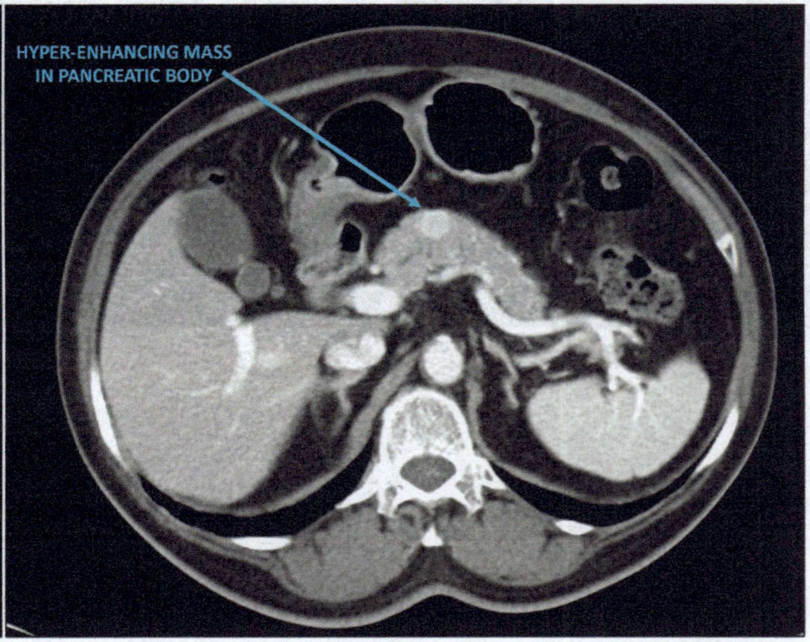

GASTROINTESTINAL

FECAL IMPACTION

IMAGING:

XR: Stool within a distended large bowel, most commonly the rectum

CT: Severe distention of the rectum with stool

Often has thickening of the rectal mucosa (stercoral colitis)

USMLE POINTS:

Inability to spontaneously evacuate solid feces

Almost always very **elderly**

Can perforate, leading to fecal peritonitis

Presentation: Constipation, **Rectal pain**, Abdominal pain

Risk factors:

- **Constipation**
- Sedentary lifestyle
- Low-fiber diet
- Opioids

MODALITIES: XR / CT WO

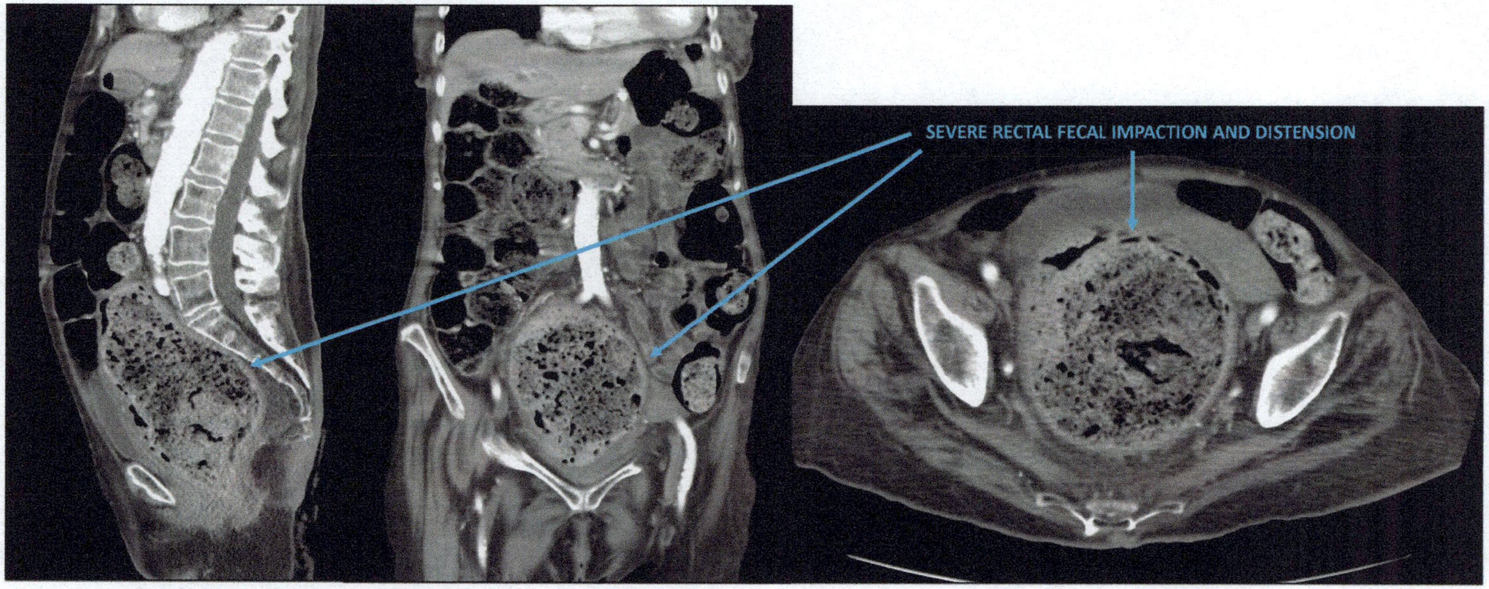

PEDIATRICS

PEDIATRICS

CHILD ABUSE – NONACCIDENTAL TRAUMA

IMAGING: Shaken baby syndrome:

- **Posterior rib fractures**
- **Retinal hemorrhages**
- **Metaphyseal corner fractures**
- **Subdural hematoma**
- **Skull fracture**
- **Scapular fractures**

Not toddler fractures

- **Commonly occur in young children (9 months – 3 years)**
- **Usually seen in tibia**
- **Often stable and nondisplaced**

USMLE POINTS:

- **Injury in non-ambulatory child**
- **Injury and history inconsistent**
- **Multiple fractures without history of osteogenesis imperfecta**
- **History of "household falls"**
- **Multiple fractures with different stages of healing**

MODALITIES: XR (SKELETAL SURVEY) / US / CT

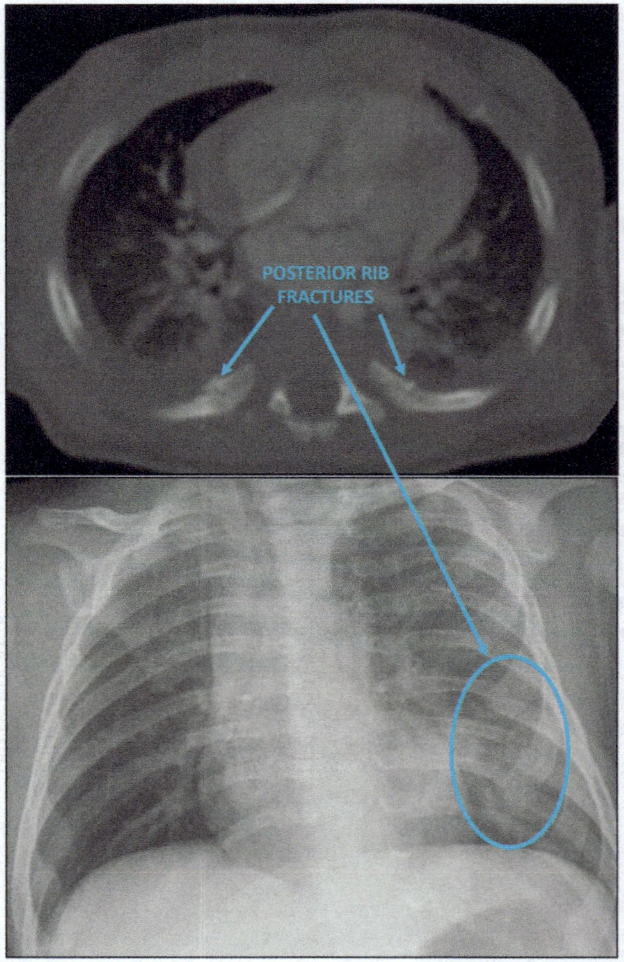

CHILD ABUSE – NONACCIDENTAL TRAUMA

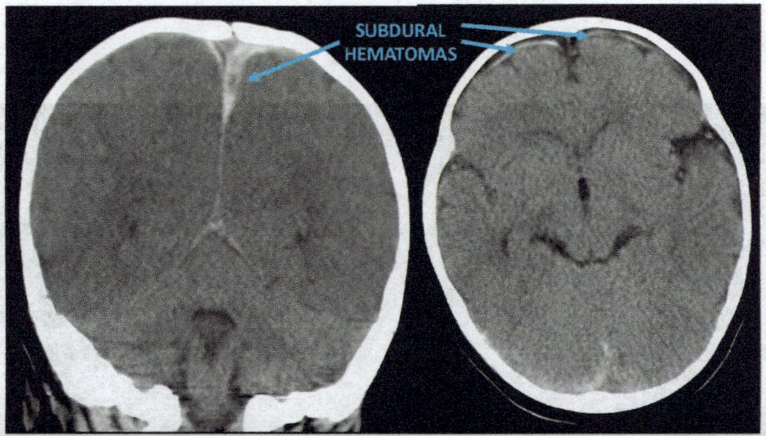

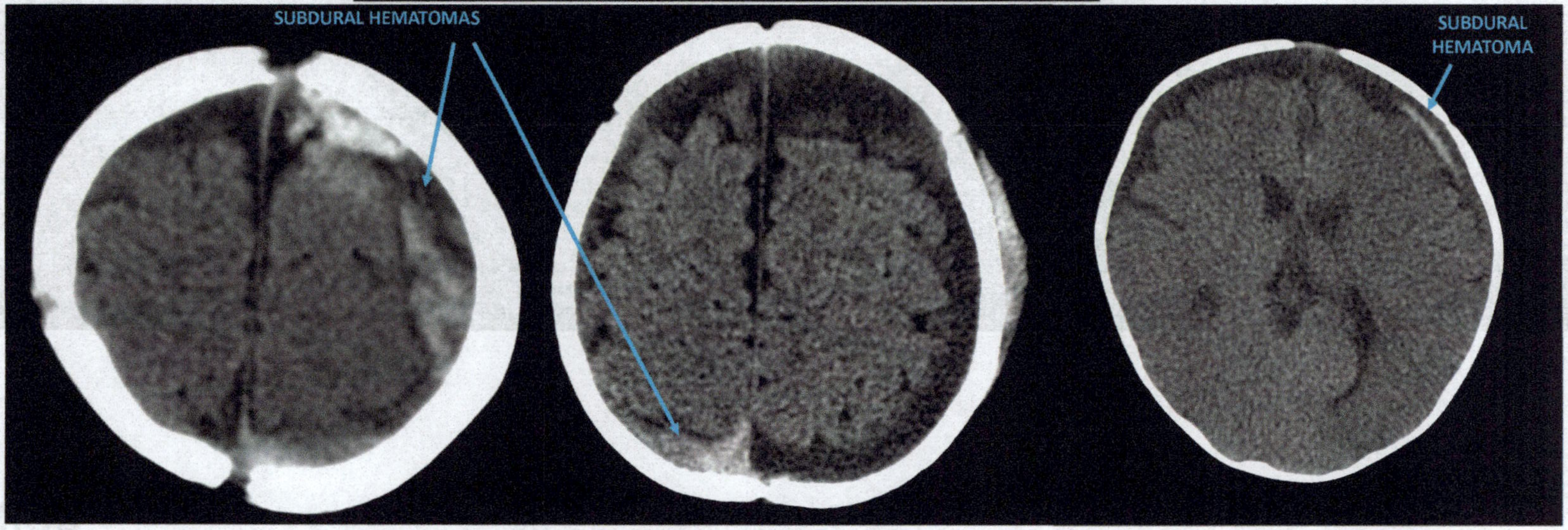

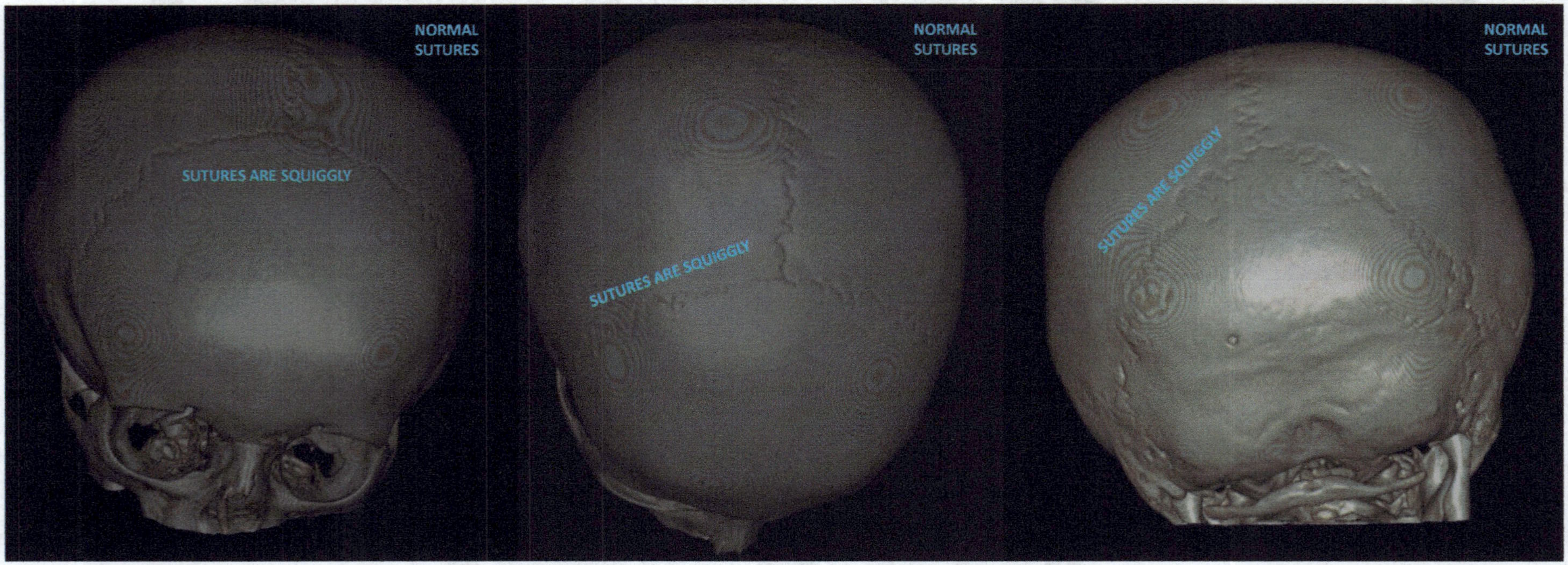
NORMAL SUTURES
SUTURES ARE SQUIGGLY
NORMAL SUTURES
SUTURES ARE SQUIGGLY
NORMAL SUTURES
SUTURES ARE SQUIGGLY

CHILD ABUSE – NONACCIDENTAL TRAUMA

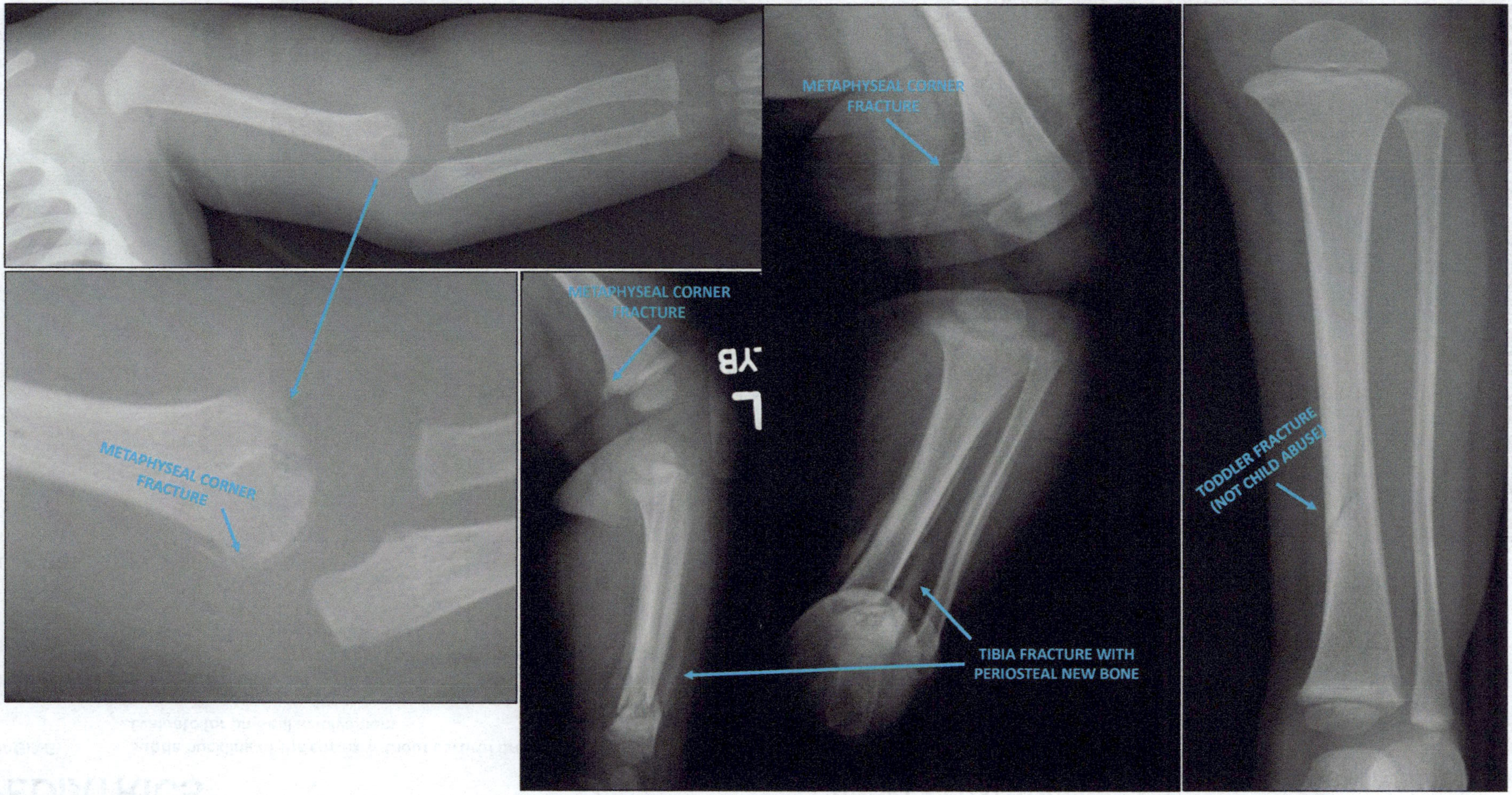

PEDIATRICS

BUCKLE FRACTURE

IMAGING:
Subtle buckling of the cortex without cortical break
Evaluate for physeal involvement

USMLE POINTS:
Pediatric fracture
Axial force applied to immature bone results the **cortex buckling on the compression (concave) side**
Tension (convex) side remains intact
Rarely operated on

MODALITIES: XR → CT

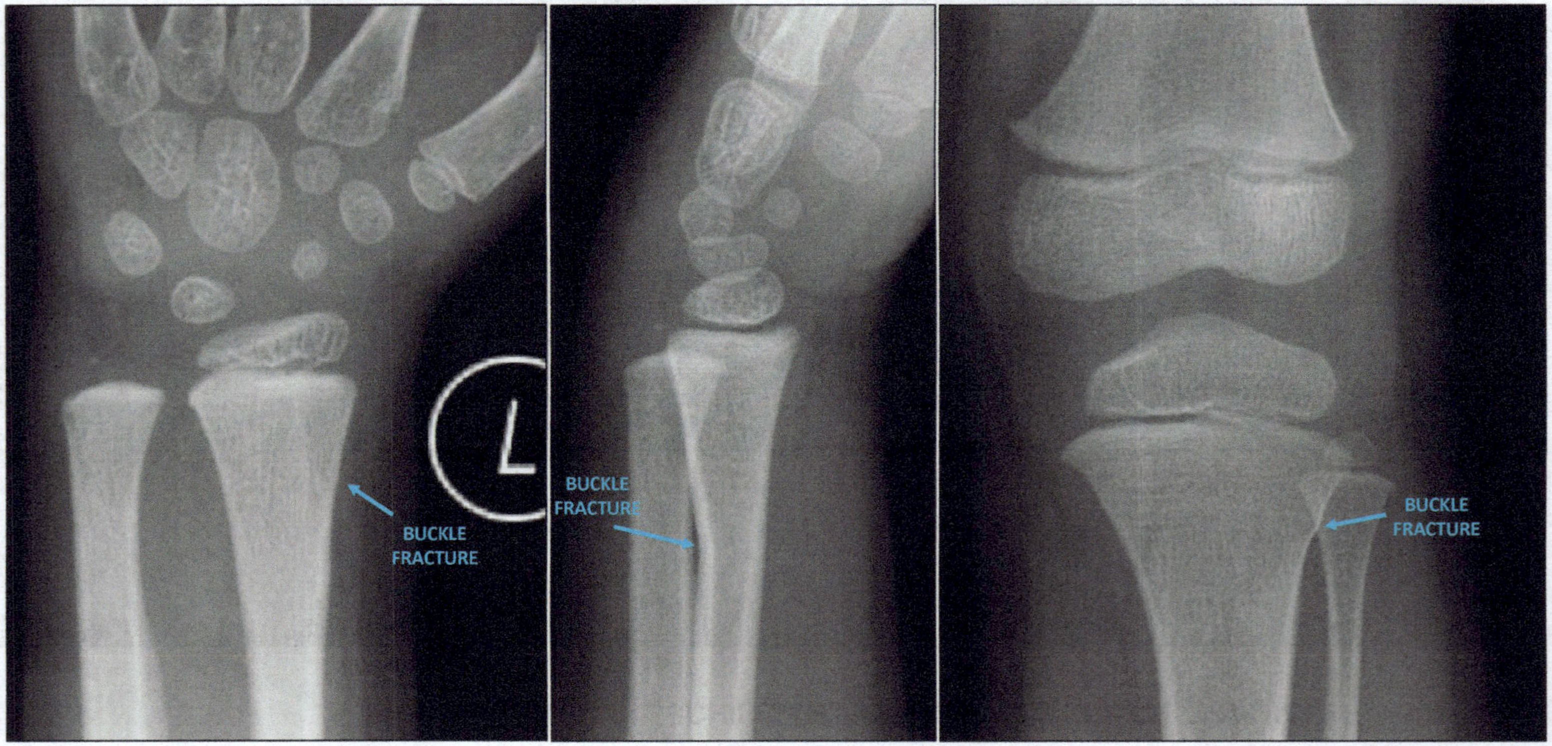

PEDIATRICS

NURSEMAID ELBOW

IMAGING: **Dislocation of the radial head**
Anterior humeral and radiocapitellar lines

USMLE POINTS: Common elbow injury in **children < 5 years old**
Results from sudden pull on arm (often from a caretaker in dangerous circumstance), when immature annular ligament slips over head of radius
Treatment: Supinate wrist + Flex elbow

MODALITIES: XR → CT

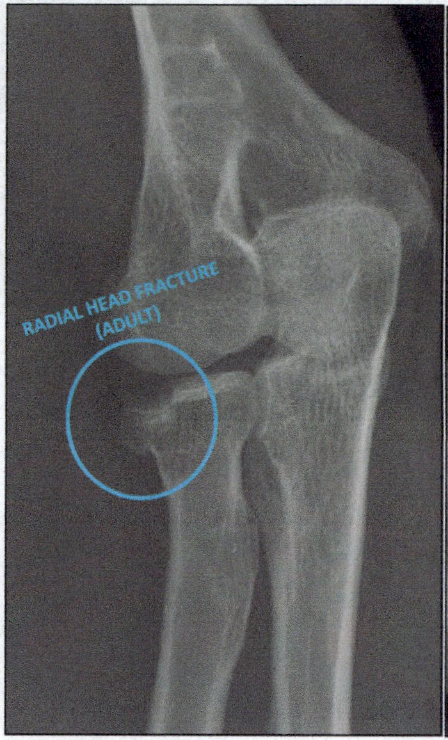

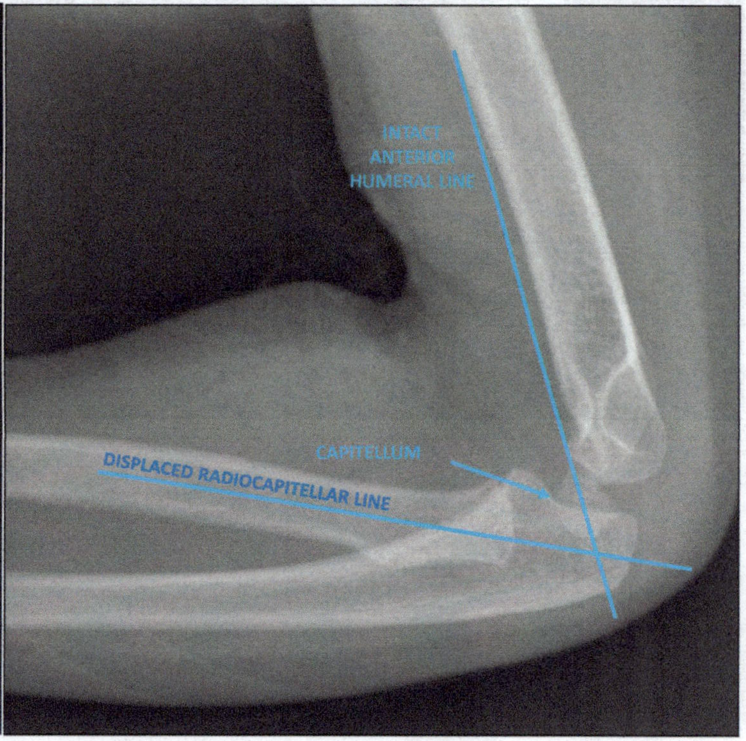

PEDIATRICS

SUPRACONDYLAR FRACTURE

IMAGING:
Anterior humeral line
Joint effusion → Positive anterior fat pad sign (sail sign)

USMLE POINTS:
Most common elbow fracture in child
May result in injury to the **median nerve** → "Pope's Blessing" when making a fist (loss flex at the PIP and DIP)
Extension type injury → Olecranon process forced against the weaker supracondylar humerus
FOOSH

MODALITIES:
XR

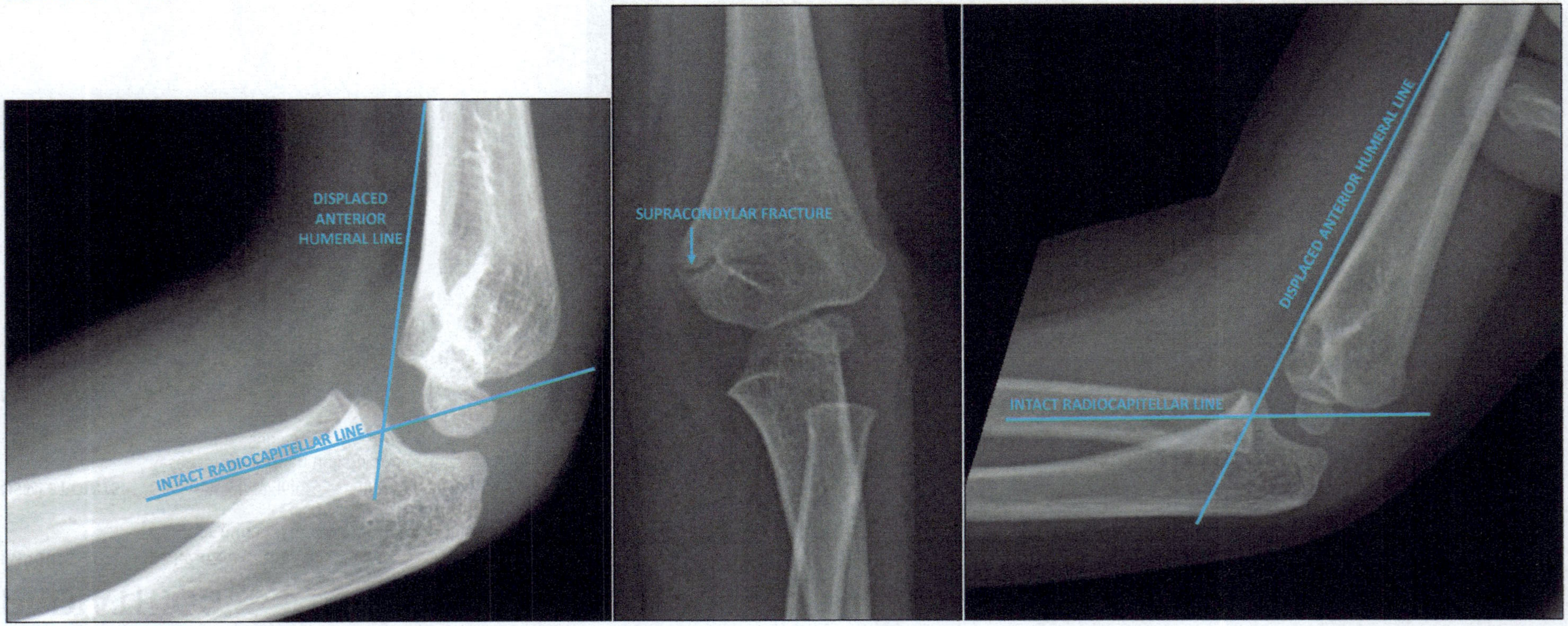

PEDIATRICS

GREENSTICK FRACTURE

IMAGING: **Incomplete fracture with cortical break of only one side**
Commonly mid-diaphyseal + Angulated

USMLE POINTS: **Usually <10 years old**
Incomplete fracture extends partway through width of bone following bending stress
Bone fails on tension side, compression side intact
Bone bent like a "green twig"

MODALITIES: **XR** → CT

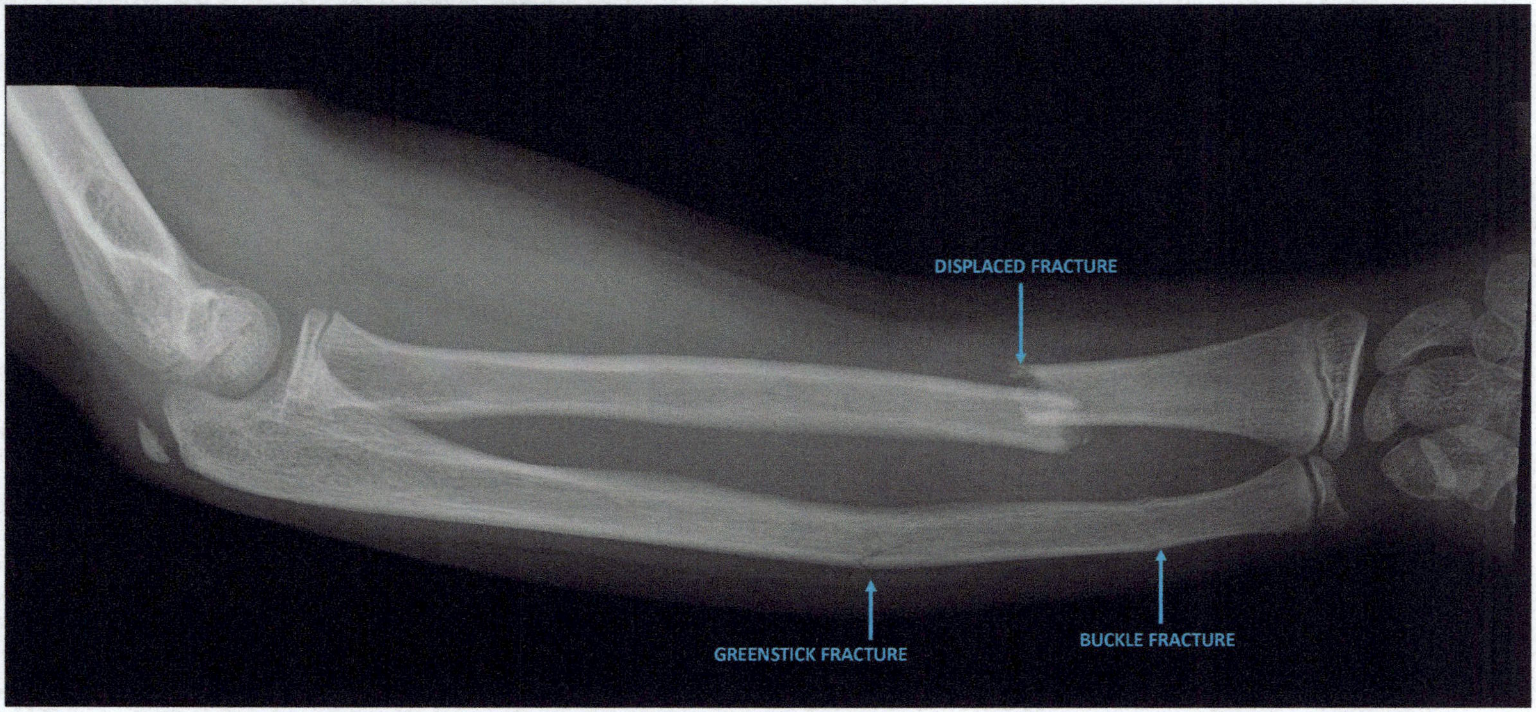

PEDIATRICS

EWING SARCOMA

IMAGING:
Aggressive, poorly marginated tumors
Permeative appearance
Codman triangle / spiculated sunburst appearance
"Onion-skin" pattern of osteolytic lesions

USMLE POINTS:
Age: **10 – 20 years old**
Diaphysis of long bones (especially femur), pelvic flat bones
PNET: Anaplastic small blue cells of neuroectodermal origin
Aggressive with early metastases
Responsive to chemotherapy
Resection is a treatment option for local disease

MODALITIES: XR → MRI WWO

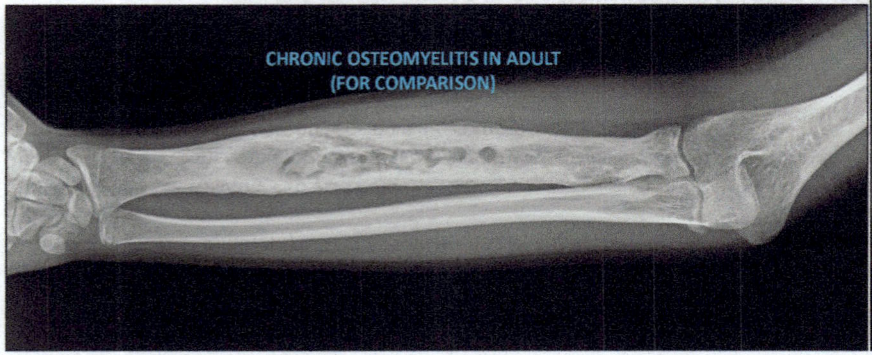

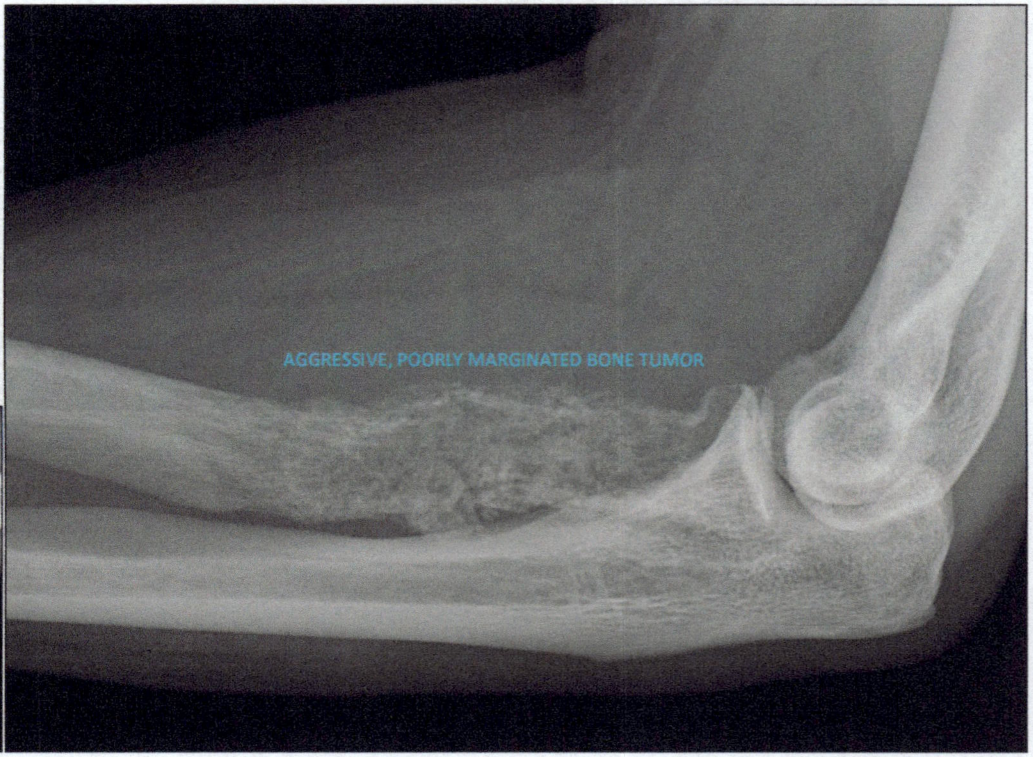

PEDIATRICS

OSTEOGENESIS IMPERFECTA

IMAGING: **Multiple fractures in baby**

USMLE POINTS: Genetic bone disorder → **COLIA1** and COLIA2
Autosomal dominant
Decreased production of normal type I collagen

Common complications:		
	Bones	Multiple fractures and bone deformities after minimal trauma
	I	Eye → **Blue sclera** (due to translucent connective tissue over choroidal veins)
	Teeth	Dental imperfections
	Ear	Conductive hearing loss due to abnormal ossicles

Confused with child abuse

MODALITIES: XR

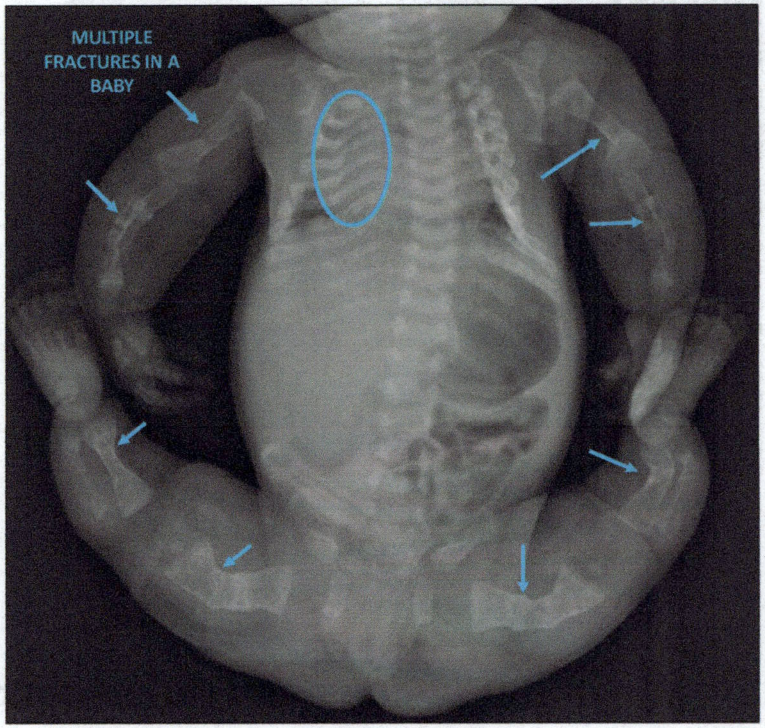

PEDIATRICS

OSGOOD-SCHLATTER DISEASE

IMAGING:
Bone fragmentation at the tibial tuberosity
Soft-tissue swelling anterior to the tibial tuberosity

USMLE POINTS:
Traction apophysitis
Overuse injury → Repetitive strain and chronic avulsion of secondary ossification center of proximal tibial tubercle
Adolescents after growth spurt
Progressive anterior knee pain
More common in boys
Treatment: **Conservative**

MODALITIES: XR → MRI WO

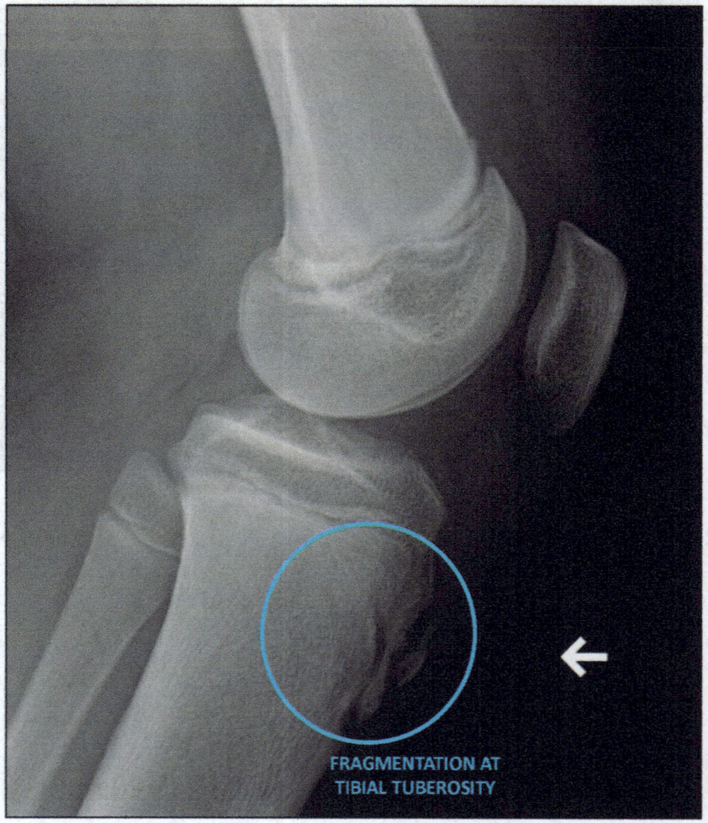

PEDIATRICS

SCFE

IMAGING:
Remember the **ice-cream cone**
Pre-slip phase: Widening of the growth plate + irregularity / blurring of the physeal edges
Line of Klein
Obtain **frog-leg lateral**

USMLE POINTS:
Age: 8 – 15 years old
Obese young adolescents with hip/knee pain and altered gait
Mechanical overload → Excessive shear force on physis
Increased axial force on femoral head results in epiphysis displaced relative to femoral neck

Treatment: **Percutaneous pinning**
Non-weightbearing while awaiting surgery

MODALITIES:
XR → MRI WO

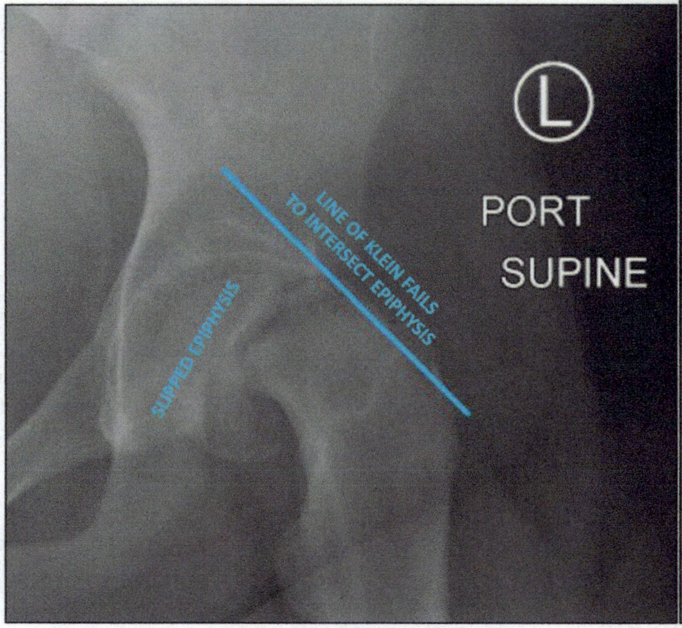

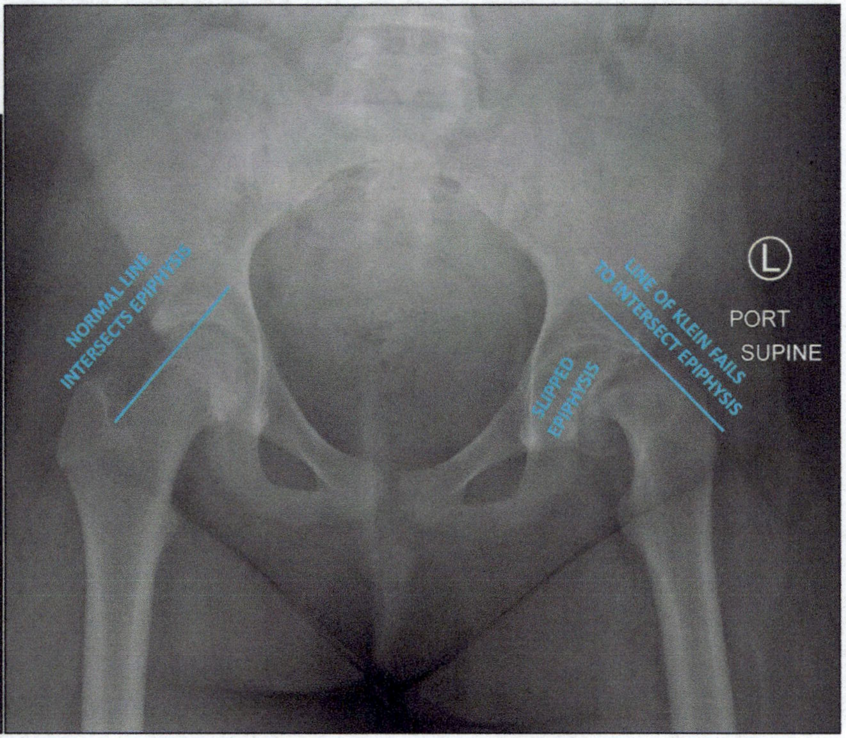

PEDIATRICS

LEGG-CALVE-PERTHES

IMAGING:

Osteonecrosis / collapse of the femoral epiphysis
Look for asymmetry if on radiograph

USMLE POINTS:

Age: 5 – 7 years old
Idiopathic → **Disruption of bone formation or blood supply to the femoral head**
Insidious onset of hip pain that may result in limping
More common in males (4:1 ratio)
Idiopathic avascular necrosis of femoral head
Normal ESR / CRP
Gait disturbances → Trendelenburg sign (weakness in the hip abductor muscles)

MODALITIES:

XR → MRI WO

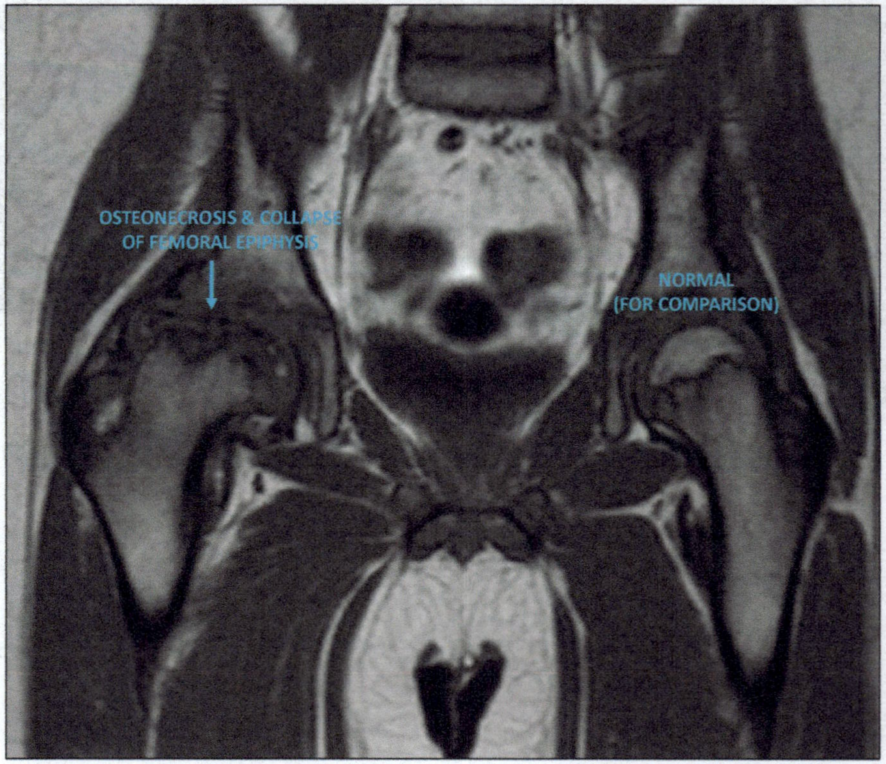

PEDIATRICS

DIAPHRAGMATIC HERNIA

IMAGING: **Multiple bubbly lucencies within the thorax**

USMLE POINTS:
Pulmonary hypoplasia is cause of morbidity / mortality
Left posterolateral side
Bowel sounds in thorax
Infants: Congenital defect of pleuroperitoneal membrane results in left-sided herniation (diaphragm develops 4-12 weeks of gestation)
Adults: Traumatic (diaphragmatic rupture)

MODALITIES: XR → CT

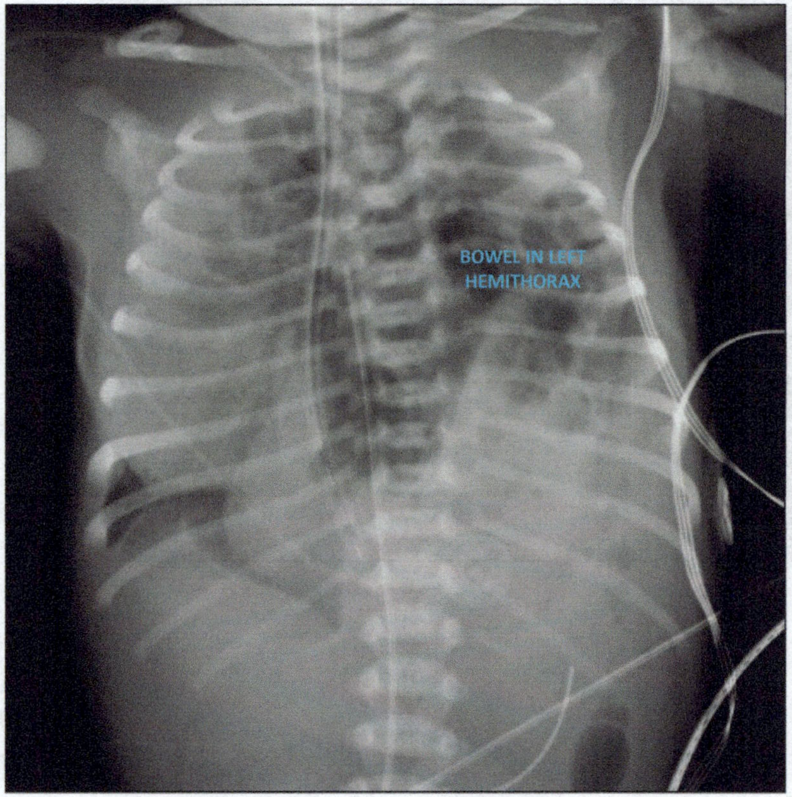

PEDIATRICS

CROUP

IMAGING: **Steeple Sign:** AP radiographs of the neck → **Uniform narrowing of the subglottic airway**
Lateral radiograph of the neck → Narrowing of the subglottic region

USMLE POINTS: Acute laryngotracheobronchitis
Children < 6 years old
Parainfluenza virus
"Seal-like" barking cough and inspiratory stridor
Treatment: Supportive care
Single dose steroids
Nebulized epinephrin

MODALITIES: XR → CT W

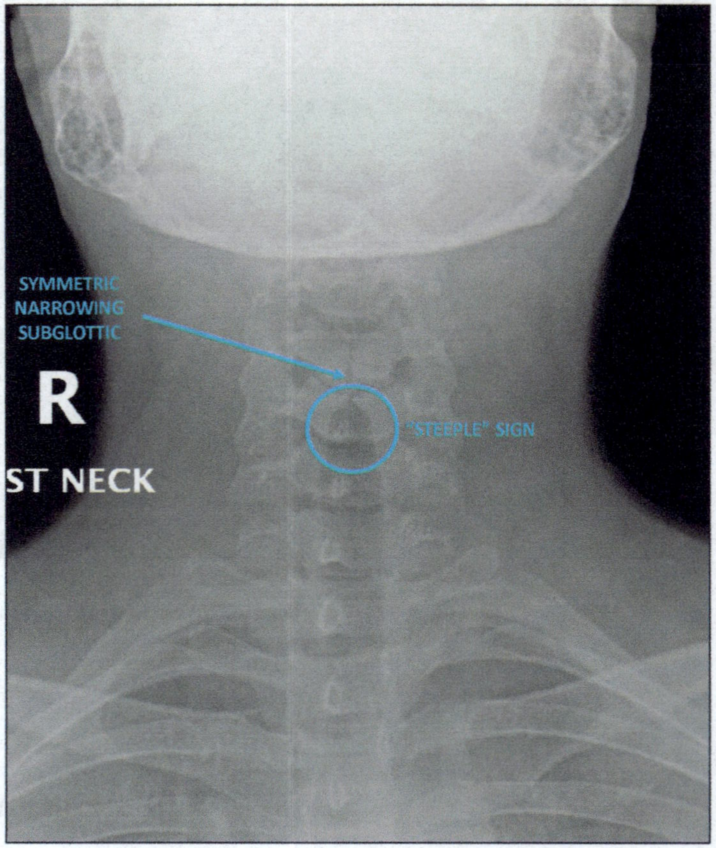

EPIGLOTTITIS

IMAGING: **Thumbprint Sign: Lateral radiographs of the neck → Thickening of the epiglottis and aryepiglottic folds**

USMLE POINTS: **Haemophilus influenzae type b**
Commonly affects young children

Appear very ill → **"Tripod stance": sit and lean forward to improve airway diameter**

Presentation: **Acute onset fever, drooling, sore throat, respiratory distress (severe)**

Risk factors: **Lack of immunization**
Immunodeficiency

MODALITIES: XR → CT W

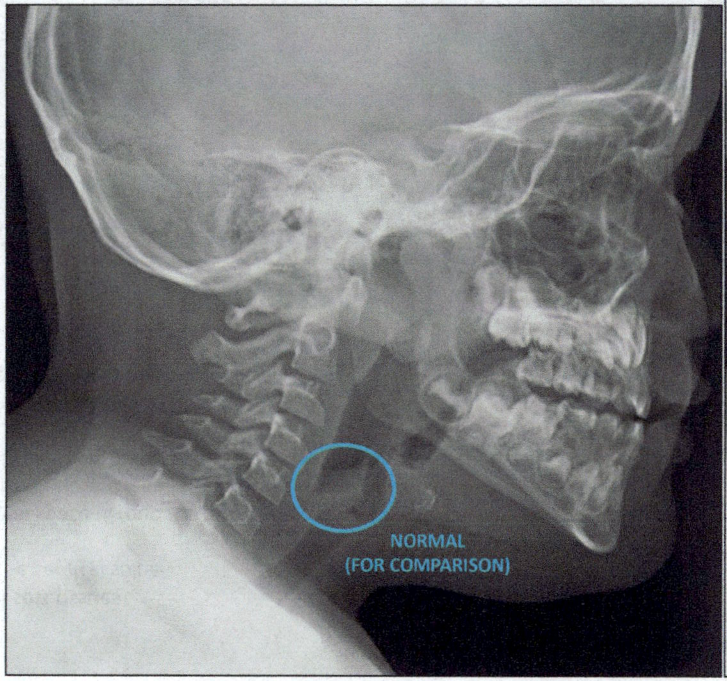

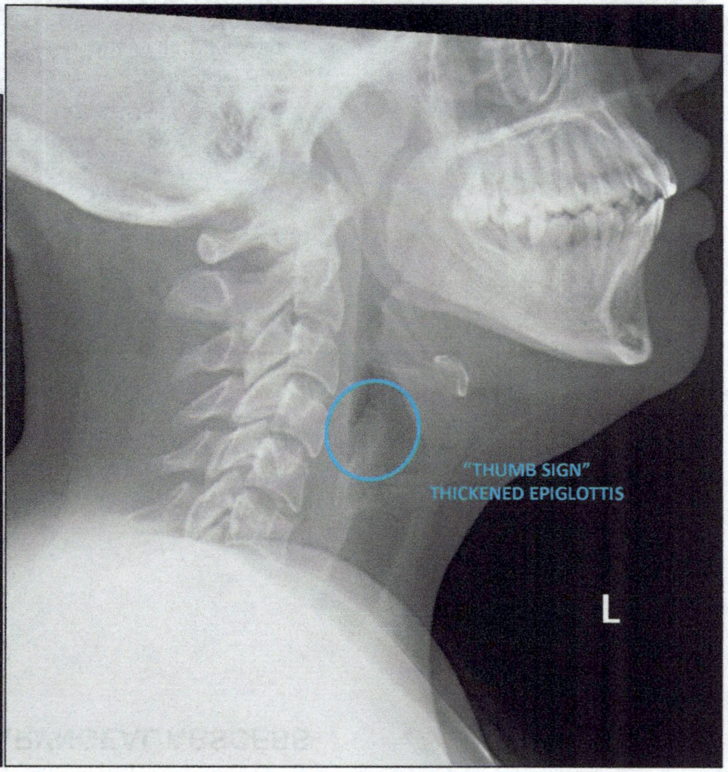

RETROPHARYNGEAL ABSCESS

IMAGING: **Widening of the prevertebral soft tissues**
Trachea should be overlying the cervical spine

USMLE POINTS: Infection of the retropharyngeal space (Group A strep, S. aureus, and Bacteroides)
Appear very ill → "Tripod stance": sit and lean forward to improve airway diameter
Infection → superior mediastinum and cause acute necrotizing mediastinitis
Children < 5 years old
Triad: Stiff neck + Fever + Odynophagia
May require surgical draining (airway compromise)

MODALITIES: XR → CT W

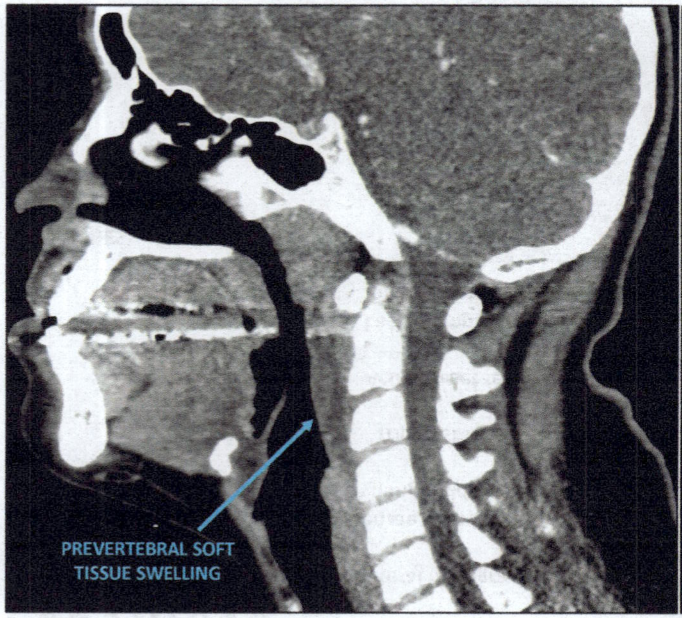

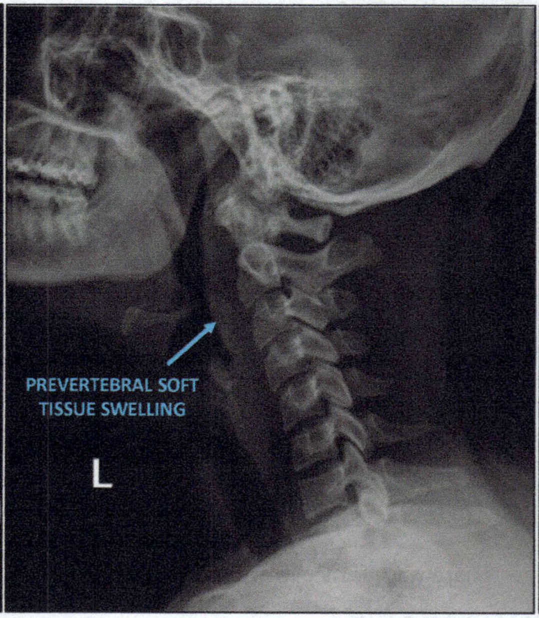

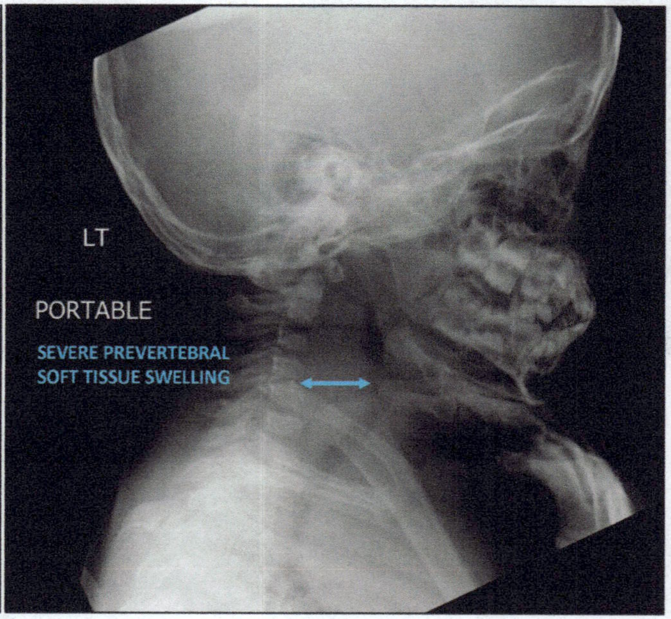

PEDIATRICS

DUODENAL ATRESIA

IMAGING: **Double-bubble (dilated stomach and proximal duodenum)**

USMLE POINTS:
Failure of duodenum to recanalize
Bilious vomiting and abdominal distension within first days of life
Down syndrome

Differential for "double-bubble"
- Duodenal atresia
- Duodenal web
- Annular pancreas
- Malrotation / Midgut volvulus
- Ladd's bands

MODALITIES: XR → FLX

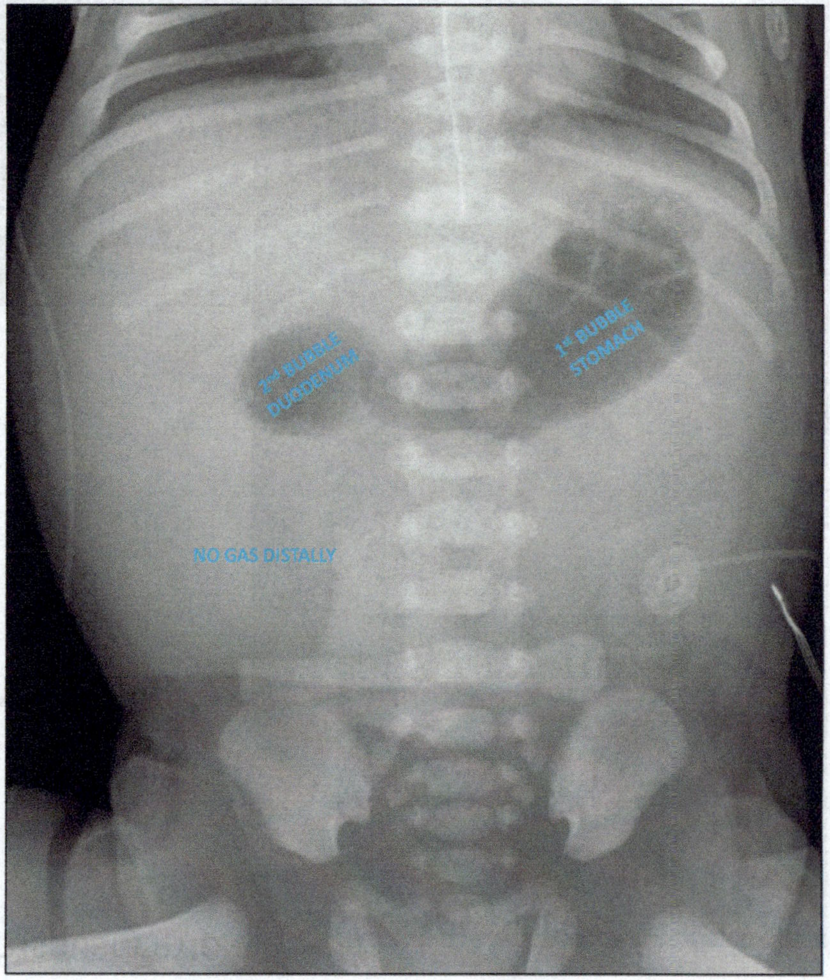

PEDIATRICS

INTUSSUSCEPTION

IMAGING:

XR: **Elongated soft tissue mass → Bowel obstruction**

US: **Target-Sign: concentric alternating echogenic and hypoechoic bands**

CT: **Bowel-within-bowel configuration**

Layers of the bowel are duplicated forming concentric rings

USMLE POINTS:

Age: **6 months to 2 years**

Telescoping of proximal bowel segment into distal segment (ileocecal junction)

Compromised blood supply → periodic, severe abdominal pain **with "currant jelly" dark red stools**

Usually idiopathic, but may result from lead point

In children: **Meckel diverticulum, viral illness/IgA vasculitis (adenopathy)**

In adults: Intraluminal mass/tumor

Physical exam shows sausage-shaped mass in right abdomen

Treatment: Emergent **air enema** (contraindicated if free air)

MODALITIES: XR / US

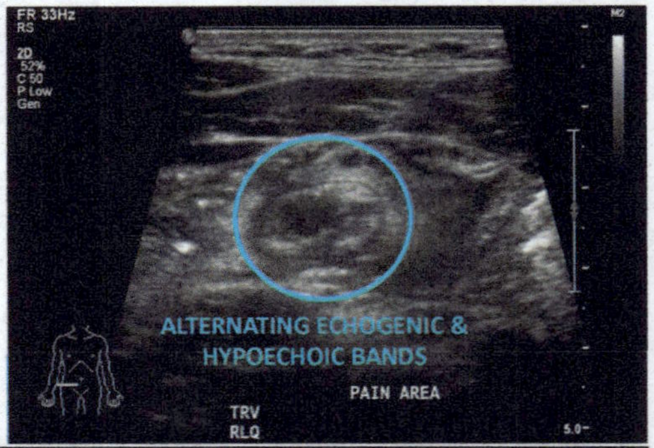

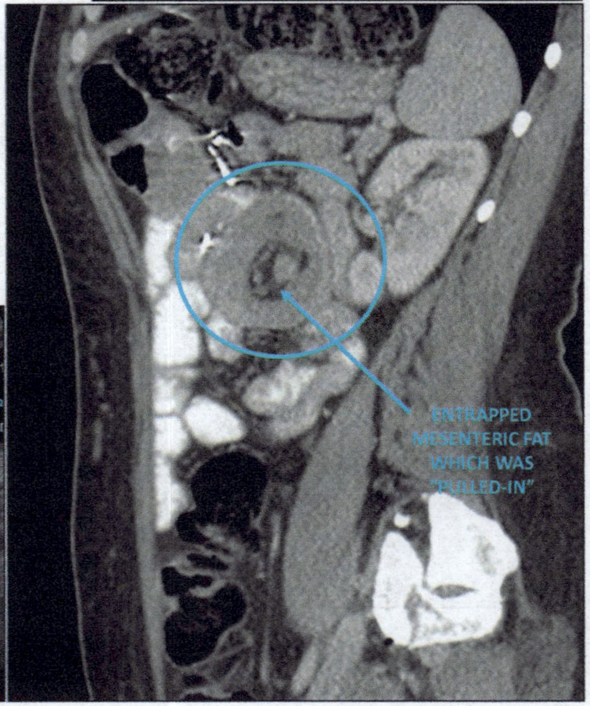

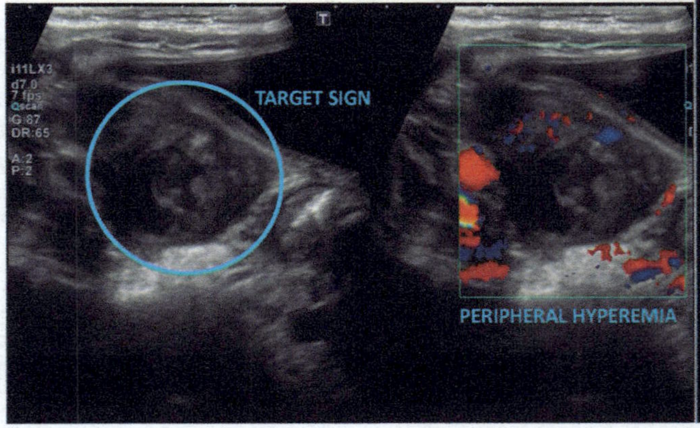

PEDIATRICS

RICKETS

IMAGING:

Metaphyseal Fraying:	**Indistinct margins of the metaphysis**
Metaphyseal Splaying:	**Widening of metaphyseal ends**
"Rachitic rosary":	Expansion of the anterior rib costochondral junctions

USMLE POINTS:

Vitamin D deficiency in children
Genu varum (bowlegs)
Risk Factors:
- Malabsorption
- Decreased sun exposure
- Chronic kidney disease (CKD)

MODALITIES: XR

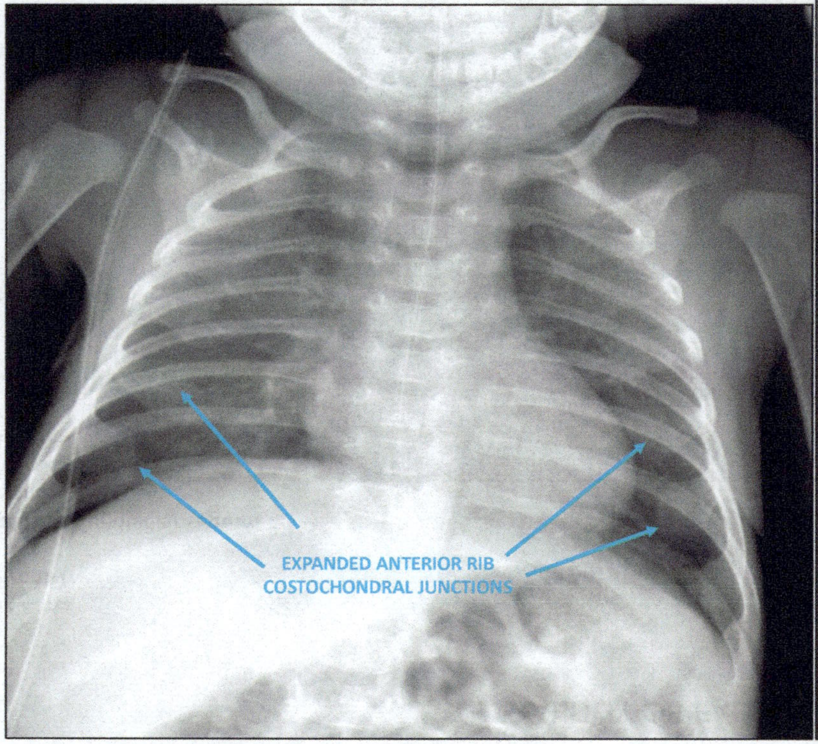

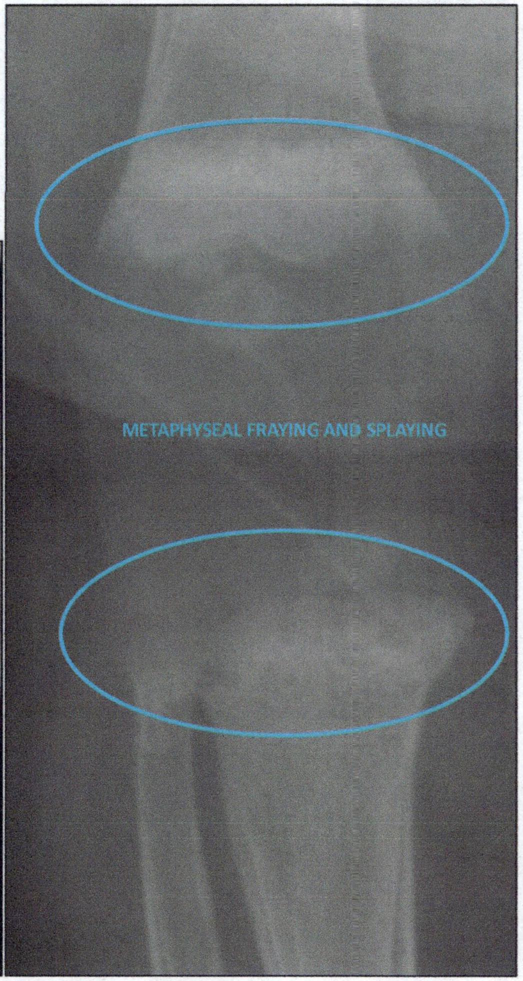

PEDIATRICS

TETRALOGY OF FALLOT

IMAGING: "Boot-Shaped" Heart:
VSD
RVOTO
Overriding Aorta
RV Hypertrophy

USMLE POINTS: Caused by **anterosuperior displacement of the infundibular septum**
Most common cause of early childhood **cyanosis**
Pulmonary stenosis forces right-to-left flow across VSD
Neonates rely on a patent ductus arteriosus for survival (prostaglandins)

Associations: **DiGeorge Syndrome**
Trisomy 21

Auscultation: Loud & harsh systolic ejection murmur

MODALITIES: XR / ECHO

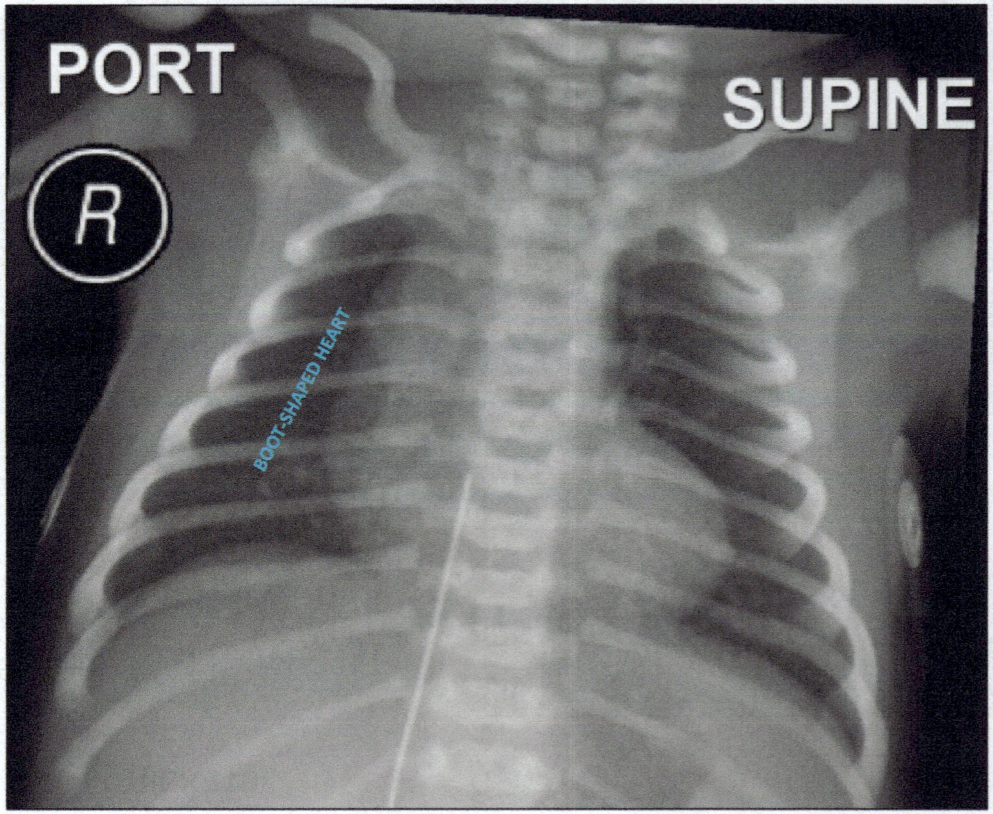

PEDIATRICS

HIRSCHSPRUNG DISEASE

IMAGING: Involved segment is of small caliber with proximal dilatation

Normally:	Rectum larger than sigmoid	→	Rectum : Sigmoid > 1
Hirschsprung:	**Rectum smaller than sigmoid**	→	Rectum : Sigmoid < 1

USMLE POINTS: Lack of ganglion cells/enteric nervous plexuses in distal colon
Failure of neural crest cell migration
Gold standard for diagnosis: Rectal suction biopsy

Presentation: **Bilious emesis**
Abdominal distension
Failure to pass meconium within the first 48 hours

Treatment: **Resection**

MODALITIES: FLX

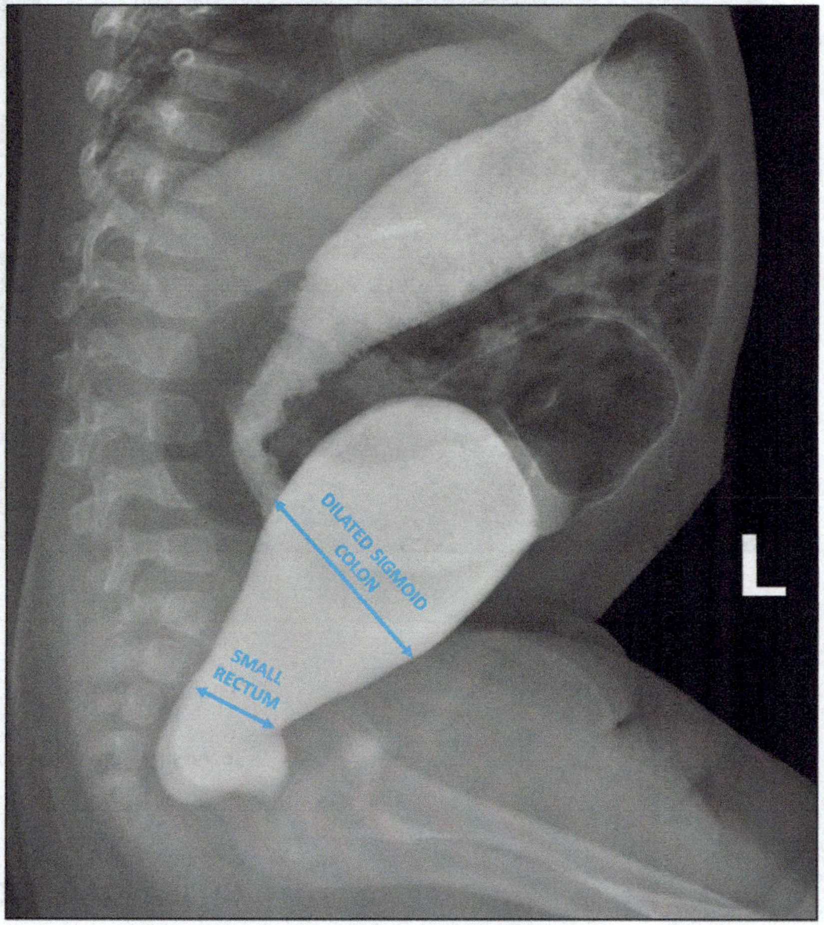

PEDIATRICS

MIDGUT VOLVULUS

IMAGING: **Malrotation: Duodenal sweep fails to cross the midline to the left of the left-sided vertebral body pedicle**

USMLE POINTS: **One third of children with malrotation → volvulus**
Anomaly of midgut rotation during fetal development → Improper positioning of bowel and formation of fibrous bands
Can lead to volvulus and duodenal obstruction

Treatment: **Malrotation without volvulus → Ladd procedure**
Malrotation with volvulus → Emergent surgical decompression

MODALITIES: FLX

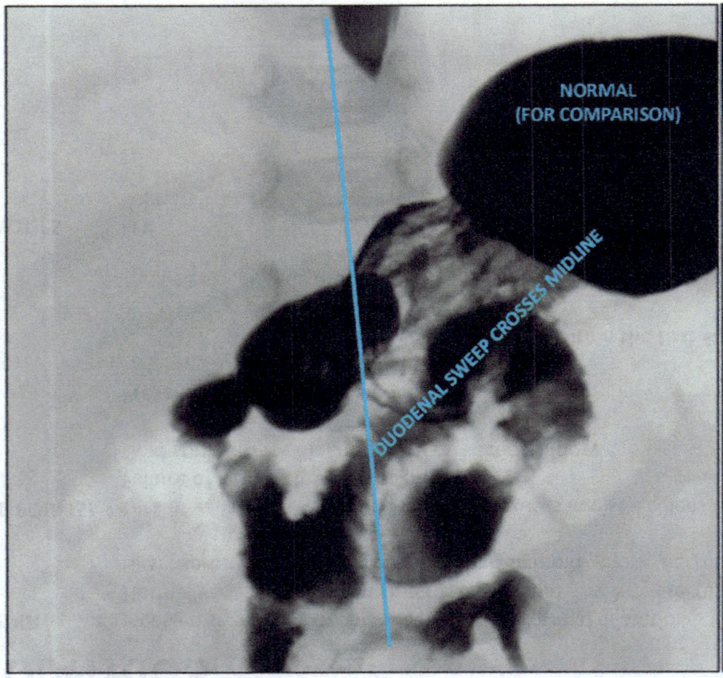

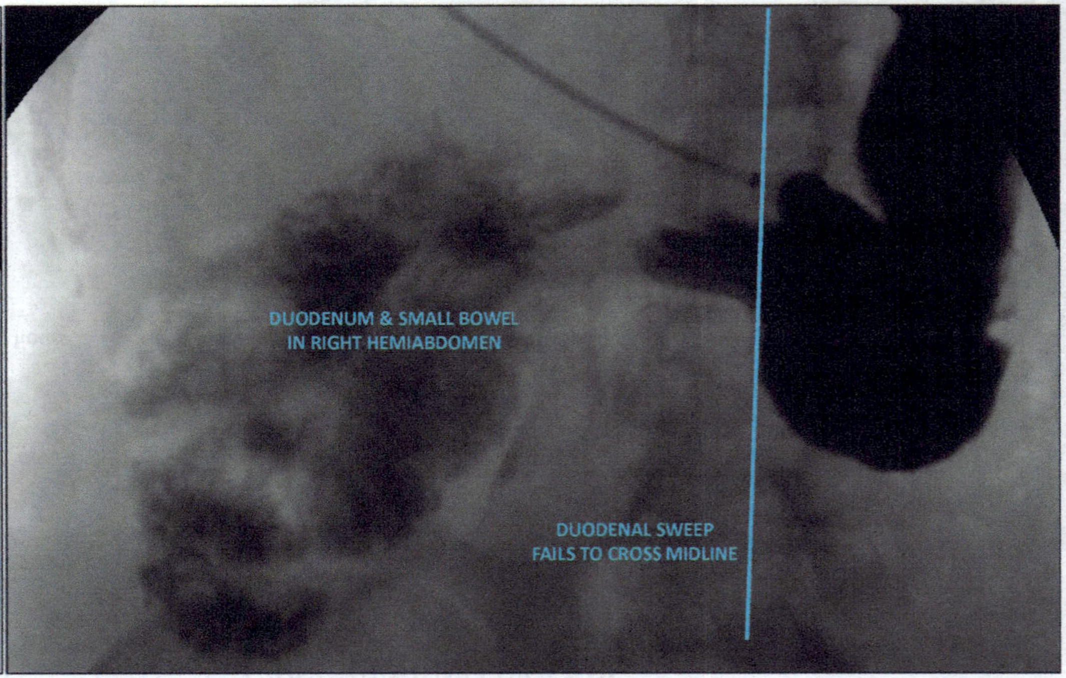

PEDIATRICS

TRACHEOESOPHAGEAL FISTULA

IMAGING: **NG tube which won't pass the proximal esophagus → usually sufficient for diagnosis**

USMLE POINTS: **VACTERL**
Incorrect division of tracheoesophageal septum

Most common:
Blind-ending upper esophagus
Lower esophagus connected to trachea

Presentation:
Food can pass into lungs and cause cyanosis
Choking and vomiting food causes pneumonitis
Air passes into stomach
Nasogastric tubes cannot be used

MODALITIES: XR / FLX

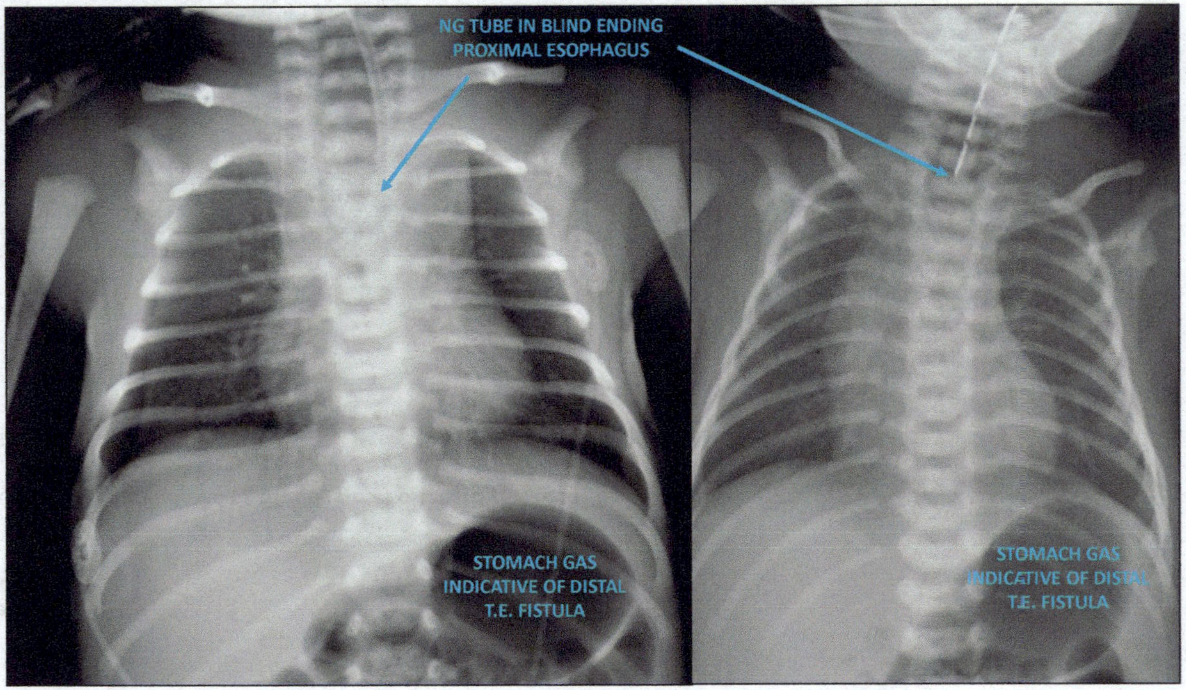

PEDIATRICS

HIP DYSPLASIA

IMAGING: **Upper femoral epiphysis should be in the inferior-medial quadrant**
Acetabular angle, alpha angle, etc... beyond scope of USMLE

USMLE POINTS: **Ortolani / Barlow**
Gradual misalignment or dislocation of the hip, wearing down cartilage and leading to **early-onset osteoarthritis of** the hip

Presentation: Pain in groin and/or side or back of hip joint

Treatment: **Bracing if treated early**
Periacetabular osteotomy in mature teenager or young adult in serious cases

MODALITIES: XR / US

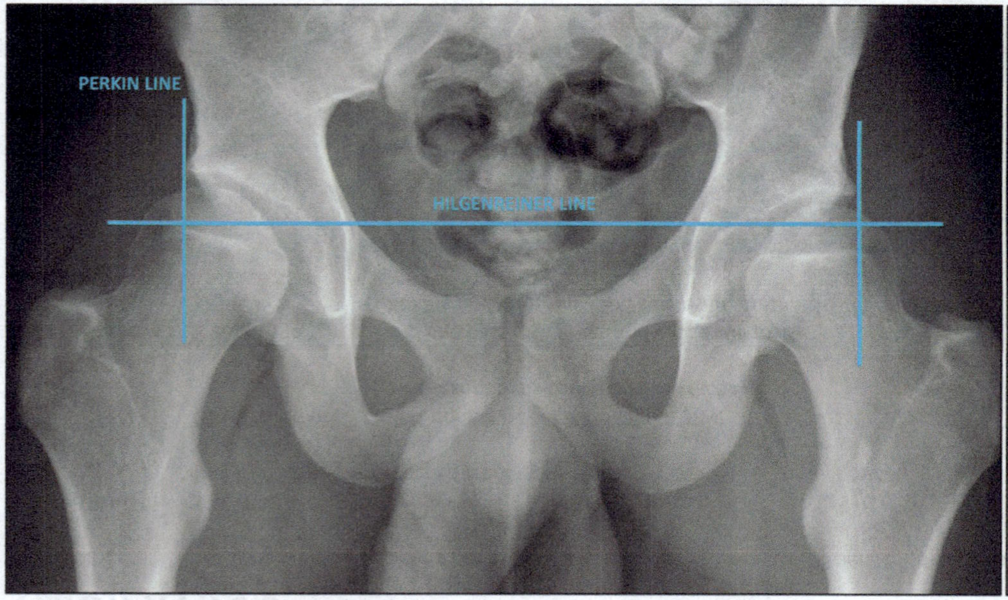

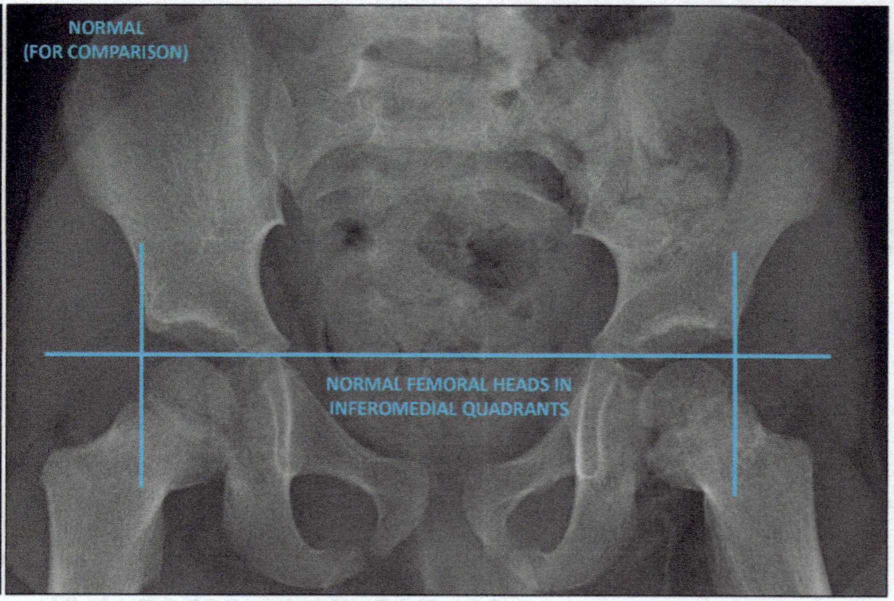

PEDIATRICS

SALTER I

IMAGING: **Fracture plane passes through growth plate without osseous fracture**

USMLE POINTS: Longitudinal force applied to the physis
Can only occur in unfused growth plate

Salter 1	**Slipped**
Salter 2	Above
Salter 3	Lower
Salter 4	Through
Salter 5	Ruined/rammed

MODALITIES: XR → CT

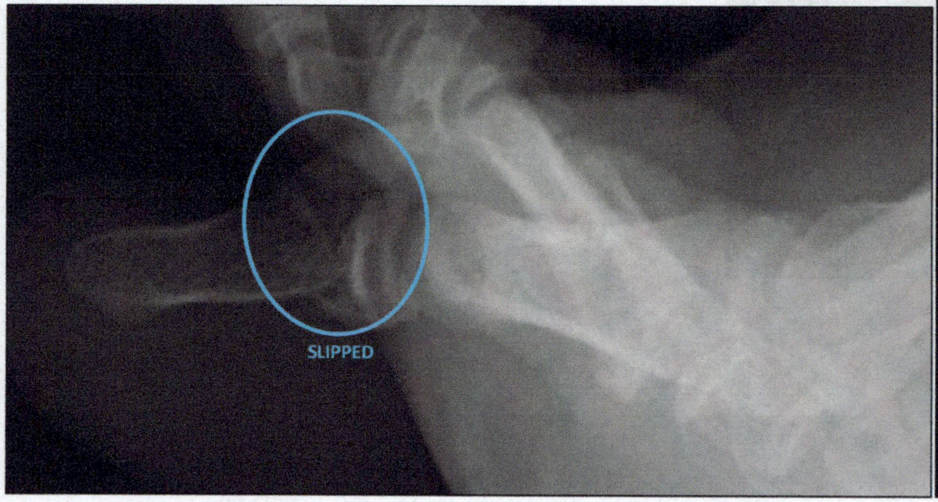

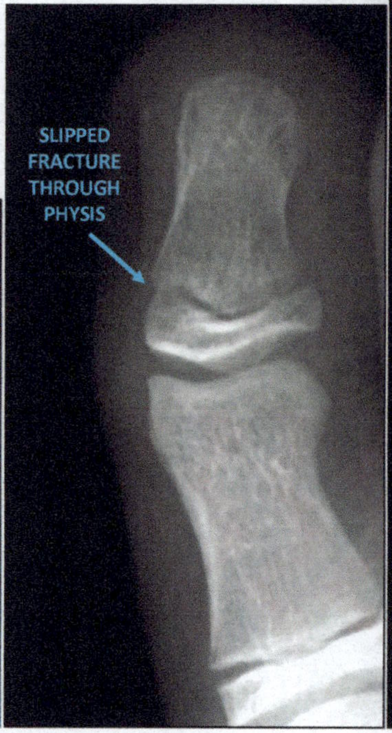

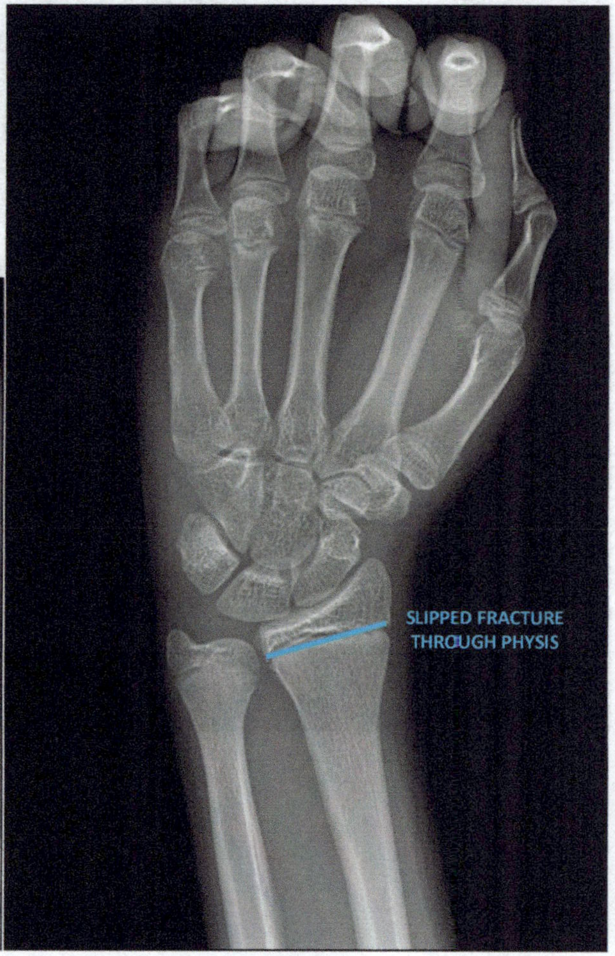

PEDIATRICS

SALTER II

IMAGING: Metaphysis → Physis

USMLE POINTS: Most common Salter fracture

Salter 1	Slipped
Salter 2	**Above**
Salter 3	Lower
Salter 4	Through
Salter 5	Ruined/rammed

MODALITIES: XR → CT

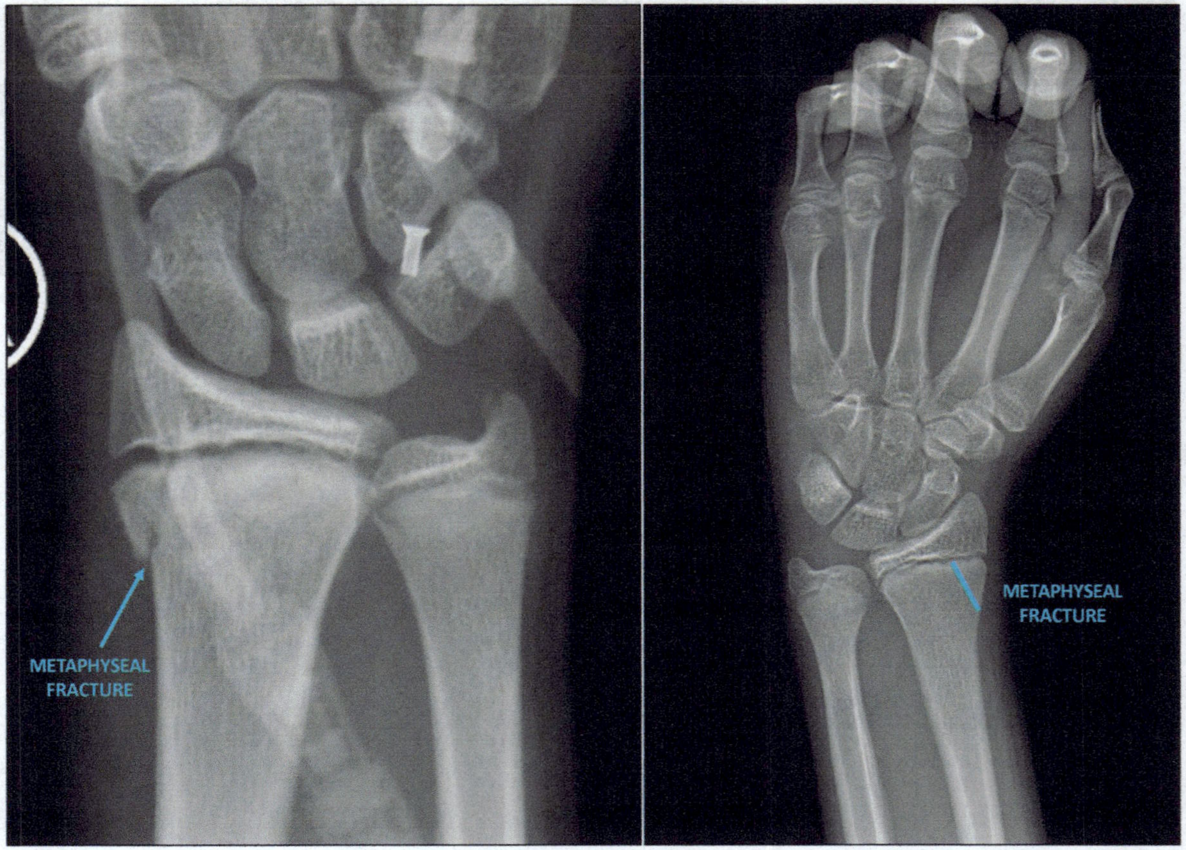

PEDIATRICS

SALTER III

IMAGING: **Epiphysis → physis**

USMLE POINTS: Fracture extends from physis into the epiphysis, thus **separating it from the metaphysis**
Usually seen in **older children with** partially-closed growth plate

Salter 1	Slipped
Salter 2	Above
Salter 3	**Lower**
Salter 4	Through
Salter 5	Ruined/rammed

MODALITIES: XR → CT

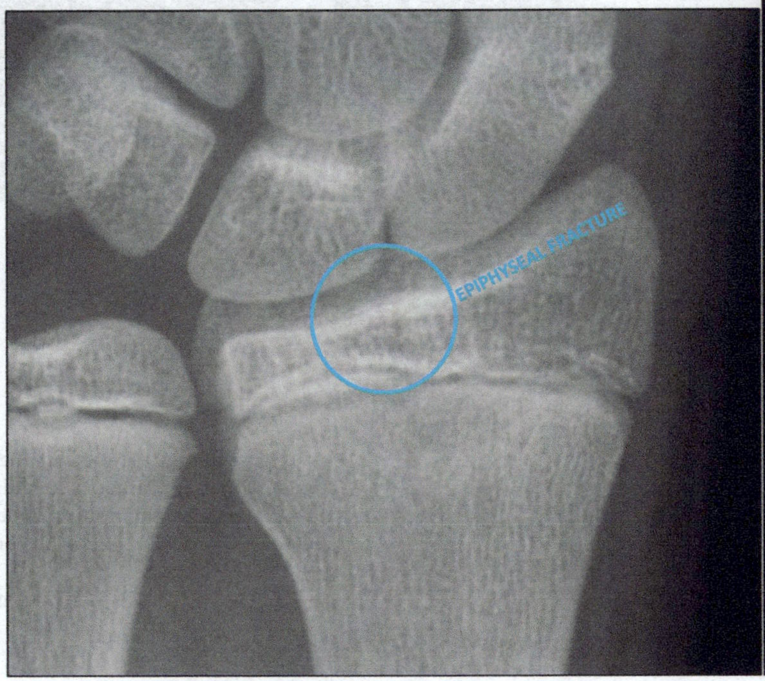

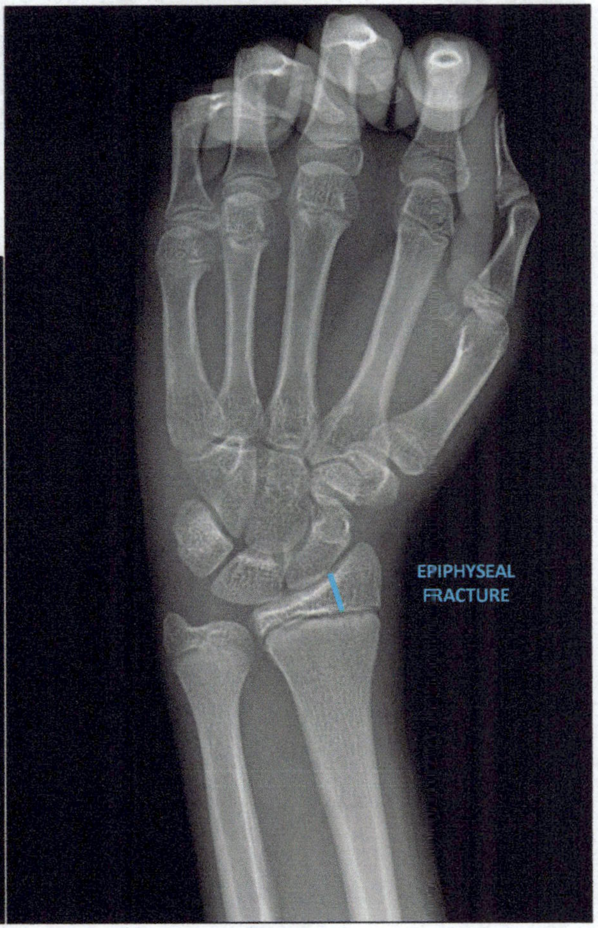

PEDIATRICS

SALTER IV

IMAGING: **Metaphysis → Epiphysis (Crosses the physis)**

USMLE POINTS: Intra-articular fracture that passes through epiphysis, physis, and metaphysis

"Triplane" fracture
- **Vertical component through epiphysis**
- **Horizontal component through the growth plate**
- **Oblique component through metaphysis**

Salter 1	**S**lipped
Salter 2	**A**bove
Salter 3	**L**ower
Salter 4	**Through**
Salter 5	**R**uined/rammed

MODALITIES: XR → CT

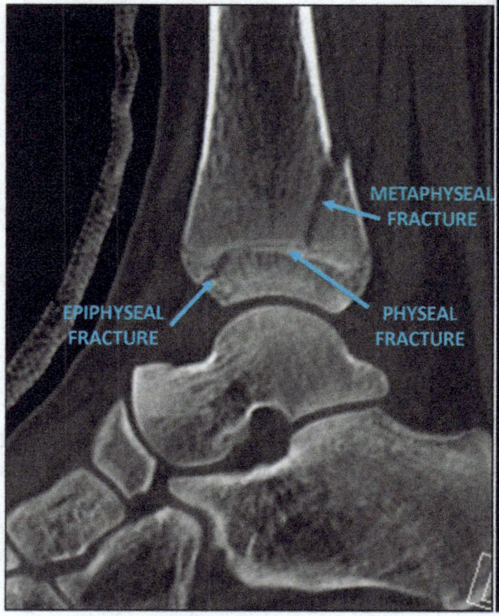

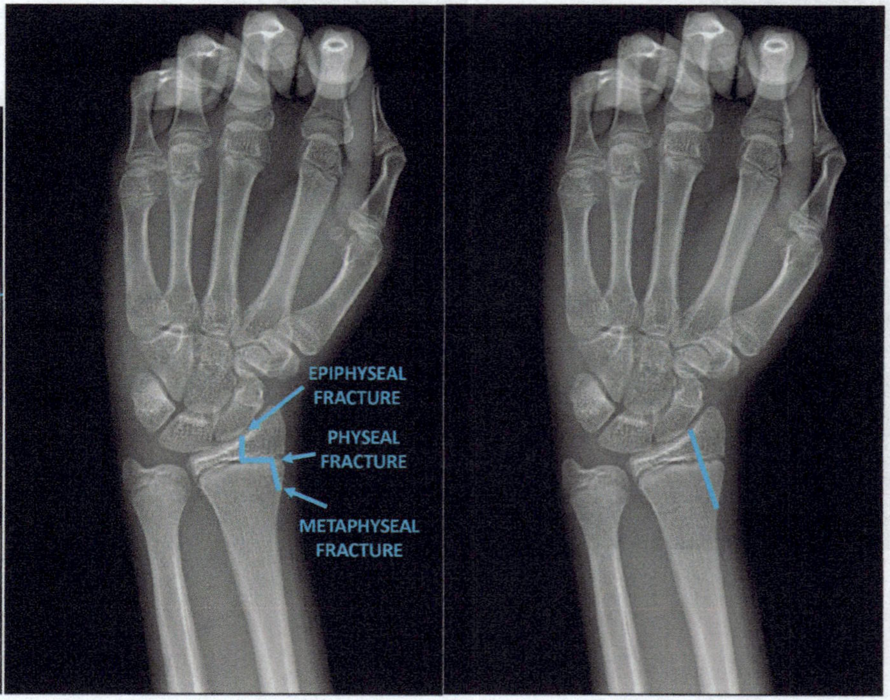

PEDIATRICS

SALTER V

IMAGING:
Crush injury
May not displace the growth plate

USMLE POINTS:
Type of physeal (growth plate) fracture (rare)
Fracture due to **compression of growth plate → can** disrupt germinal matrix and vascular supply
May require surgical resection of bone bridges and later treatment to restore alignment

Salter 1	**S**lipped
Salter 2	**A**bove
Salter 3	**L**ower
Salter 4	**T**hrough
Salter 5	**Ruined/rammed**

MODALITIES: XR → CT

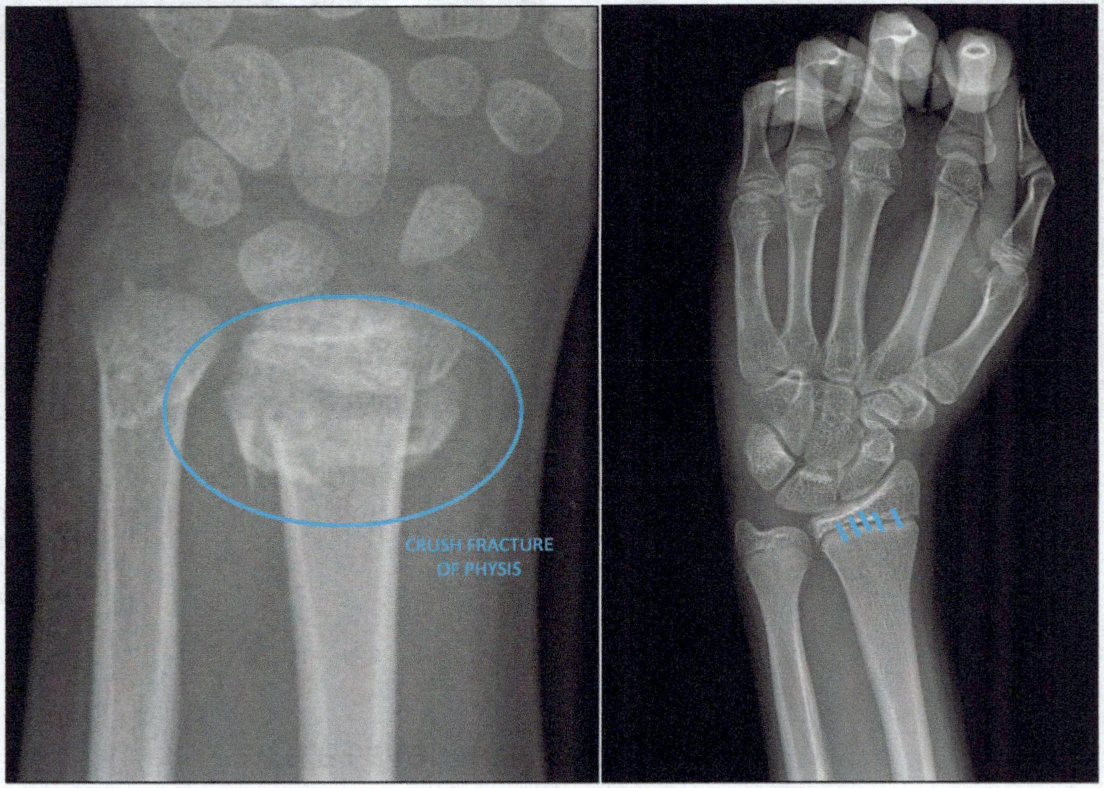

PEDIATRICS

LITTLE LEAGUER'S ELBOW

IMAGING: Medial epicondyle avulsion
XR: **Widening of the physis + adjacent sclerosis**
MRI: Increased fluid signal and widening of the physis

USMLE POINTS: Damage to **growth plate** that results from **repetitive throwing motions**
May result in ligaments and tendons tearing
Pain on **inner side of elbow when throwing a ball (pain with valgus stress)**
For the ortho gunners: Can use a palmaris longus autograft for UCL reconstruction

MODALITIES: XR → MRI WO

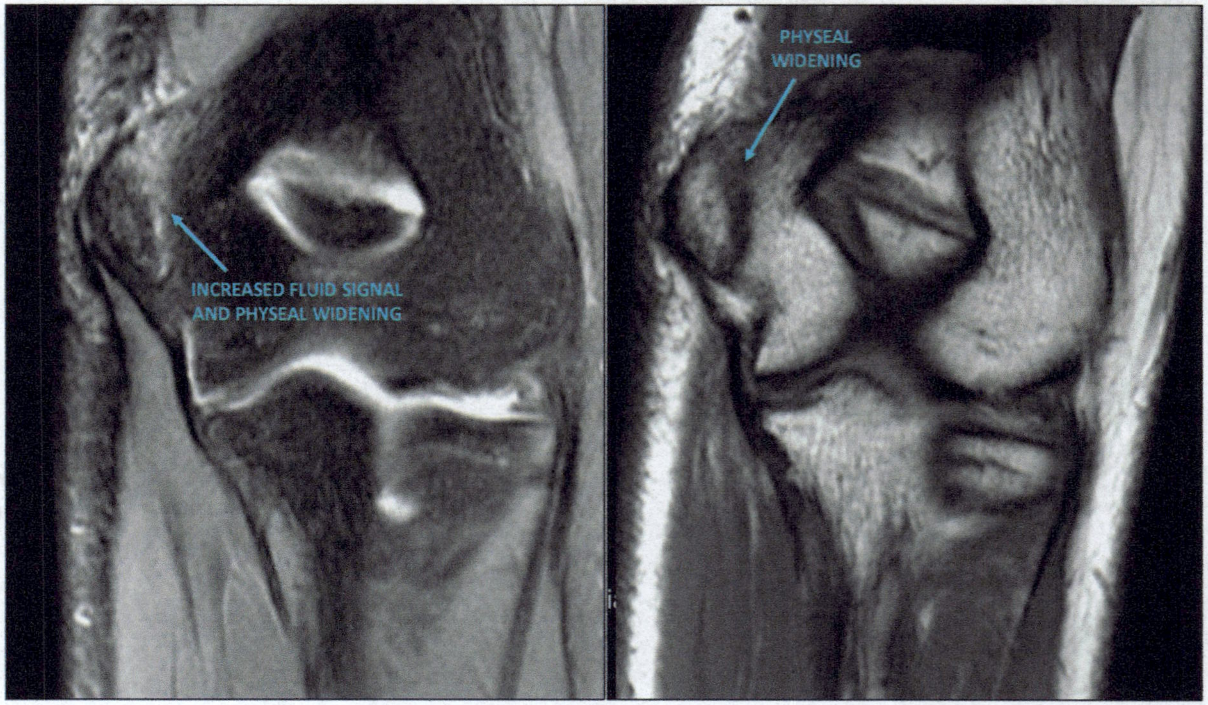

PEDIATRICS

ACUTE OSTEOMYELITIS

IMAGING:

XRAY:
- **Regional osteopenia from focal osteolysis**
- **Periosteal reaction**
- May occur at the physis

MRI:
- **Marrow edema** → High T2 signal intensity
- **Marrow infiltration** → Low T1 signal intensity

USMLE POINTS: **Hematogenous in children**

Sexually active:	**Neisseria gonorrhea (rare)**
Sickle cell disease:	**Salmonella and Staph aureus**
Prosthetic joint replacement:	**Staph aureus and S epidermidis**
Vertebral involvement:	**Staph aureas, Tuberculosis (Pott disease)**
Cat and dog bites:	**Pasteurella multocida**
IV drug use:	**Staph aureus, Pseudonomas, Candida**

Elevated ESR / CRP

Biopsy/Aspiration may be required

Treatment: IV antibiotics

MODALITIES: XR → MRI WO

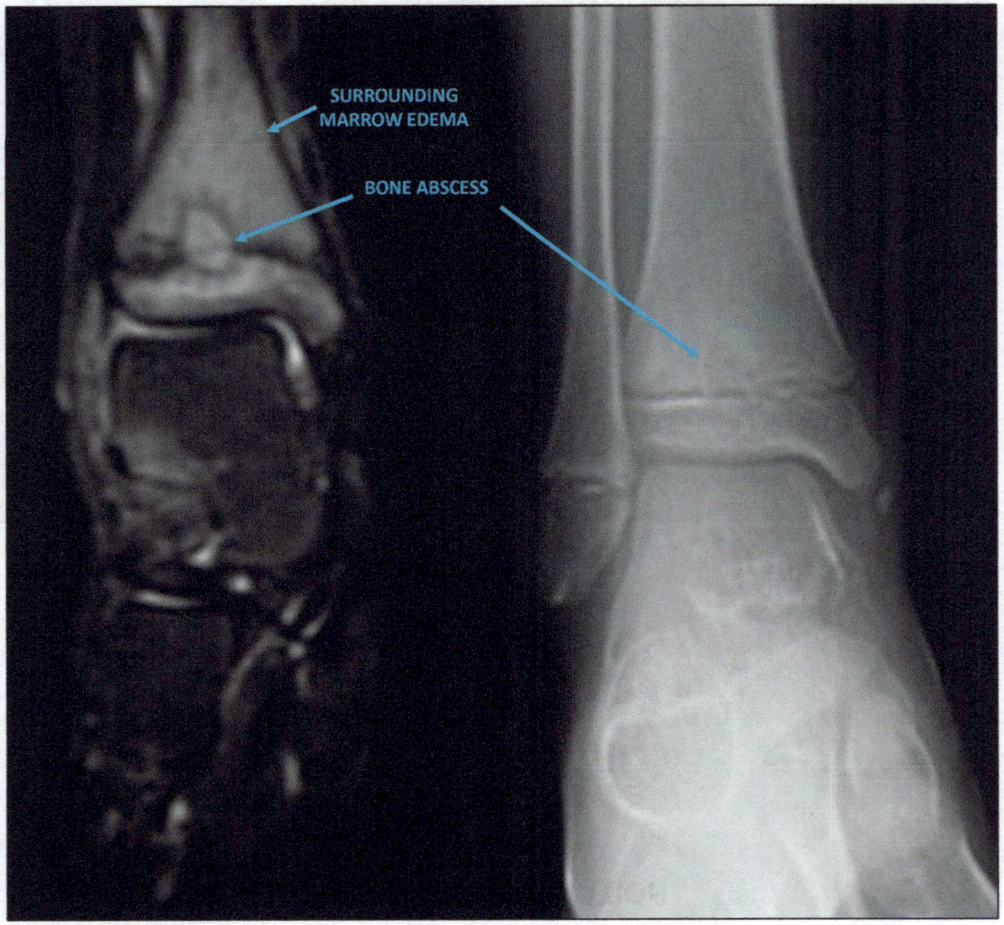

TRANSIENT PATELLAR DISLOCATION

IMAGING: Contusion pattern within the **medial patella and anterolateral aspect of the lateral femoral condyle**
Tearing of the medial retinaculum and MPFL

USMLE POINTS:

Associations:
- **Patella alta**
- **Shallow trochlear groove**
- Abnormal TT-TG distance

Presentation:
- Knee instability and anterior knee pain
- May be acute, chronic, or habitual

MODALITIES: MRI WO

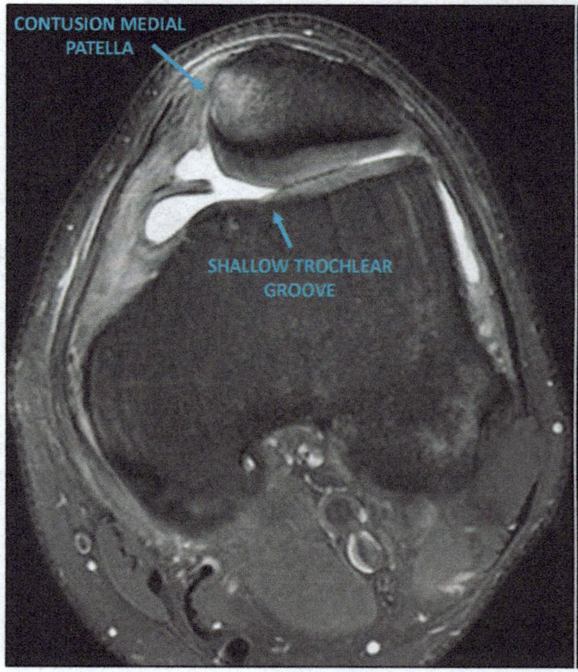

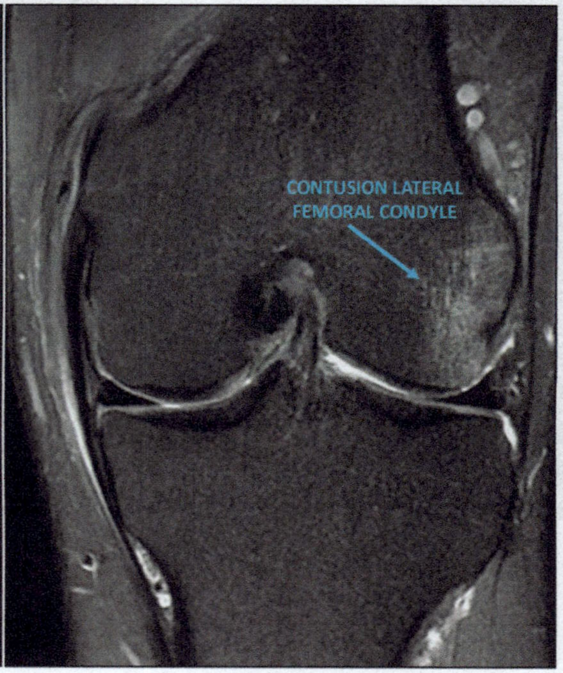

PEDIATRICS

IN-UTERO ZIKA / TORCH

IMAGING:
Periventricular calcifications (CMV) germinal matrix and periventricular regions
Ventriculomegaly / Cerebral atrophy / **Microcepahly**
Migrational abnormalities: Lissencephaly, pachygyria, cortical dysplasia, polymicrogyria

USMLE POINTS: **TORCH syndrome:**
Toxoplasmosis
Other agents
Rubella
Cytomegalovirus
Herpes simplex

CMV:
Biopsy reveals cells with intranuclear (owl eye) inclusion bodies
Linear ulcers on endoscopy
Cotton-wool spots on fundoscopy
Periventricular calcifications

Zika virus: **Most recent member of TORCH infections → Mosquito bites in topical and subtropical zones**
Mild fever, Rash, Joint pain (hands/feet), Conjunctivitis

MODALITIES: US IN UTERO / CT / MRI WO

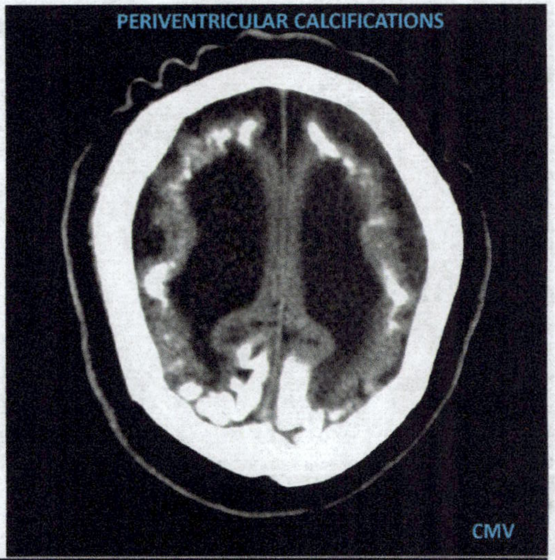

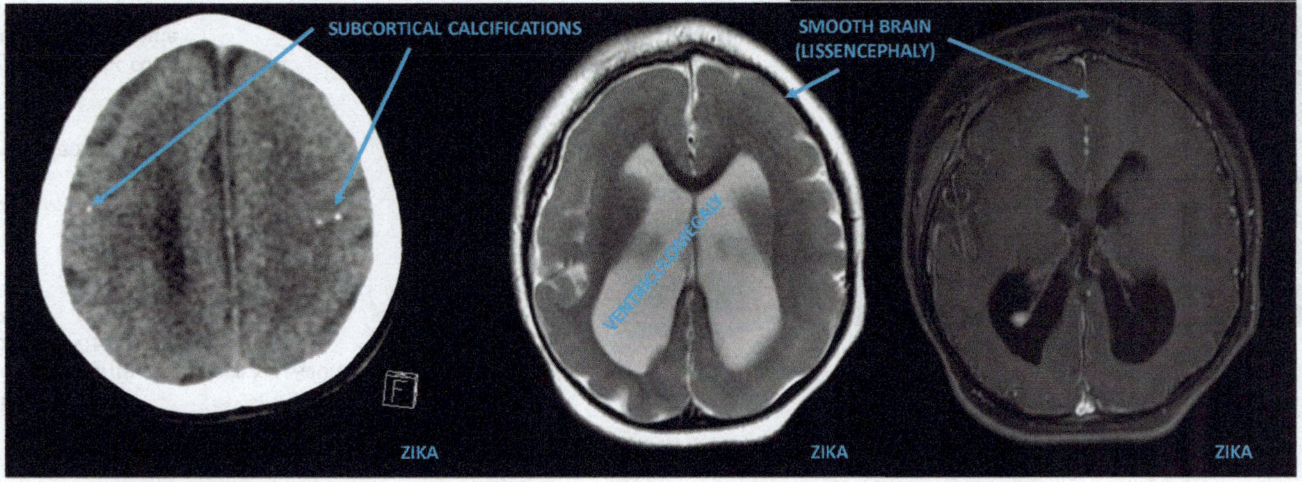

PEDIATRICS

PEDIATRIC BRAIN TUMORS

IMAGING:

Glioma (pontine)	→	Within the **brain stem**
Astrocytoma	→	Posterior fossa (**Cyst with a nodule** in kid. Adult = Hemangioblastoma)
Medulloblastoma	→	**Posterior fossa** (DWI+)
Ependymoma	→	**Posterior fossa**

USMLE POINTS: Childhood tumors are often infratentorial

Glioma
- H3-K27M-mutation
- Low grade
- Ataxia, CN palsy, hydrocephalus

Pilocytic Astrocytoma
- **GFAP+**
- Rosenthal fibers / eosinophilic corkscrew fibers
- **Cystic with enhancing mural nodule**

Medulloblastoma
- **Most common malignant intracranial tumor of childhood**
- Highly malignant / **PNET**
- Cerebellum → compress 4th ventricle → **hydrocephalus**
- Rosettes with small blue cells

Ependymoma
- Poor prognosis
- **Cerebellum** → compress 4th ventricle → **hydrocephalus**
- Perivascular pseudorosettes

MODALITIES: MRI WWO

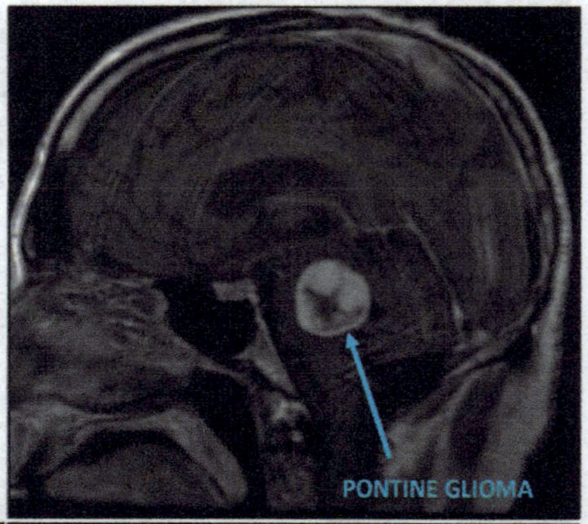

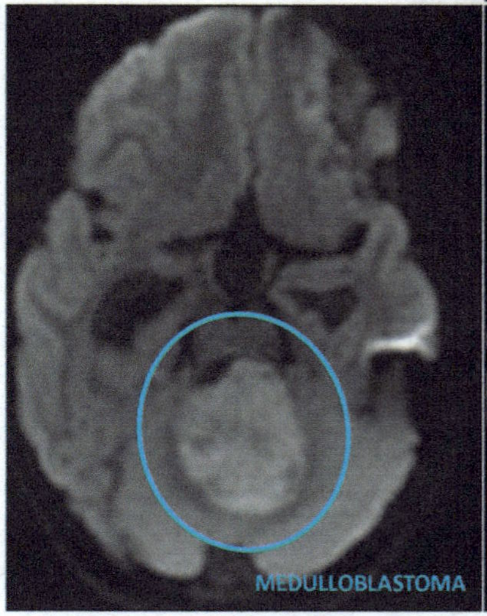

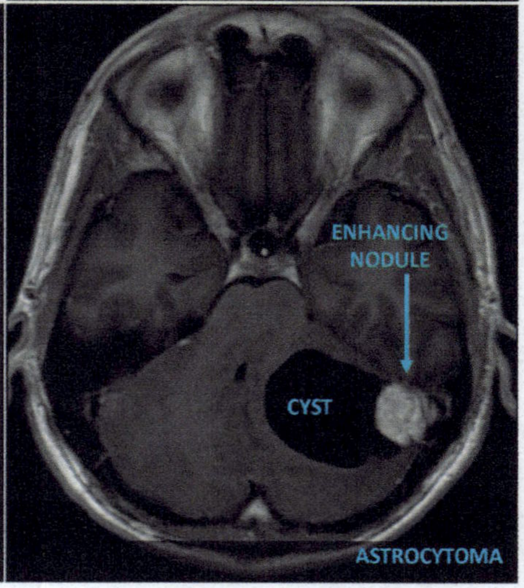

PEDIATRICS

NECROTIZING ENTEROCOLITIS

IMAGING:

Rounded cystic "bubbly" collections
Pneumatosis intestinalis
Portal venous gas (always look over liver on every pediatric abdominal x-ray)

USMLE POINTS: Inflammation, ischemia, and permeability of the neonatal bowel wall to bacteria

Risk Factors: **Formula-fed** with immature immune system
Premature → **≤ 35 weeks gestation**
Birth weight < 1000g

MODALITIES: XR → CT W

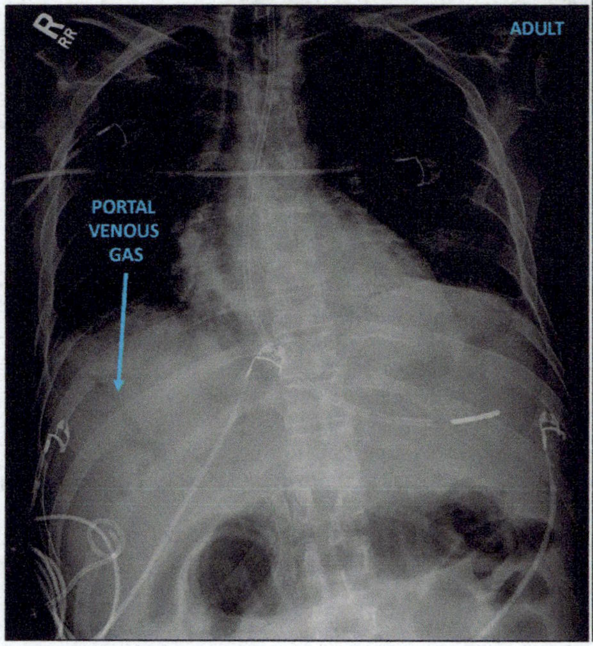

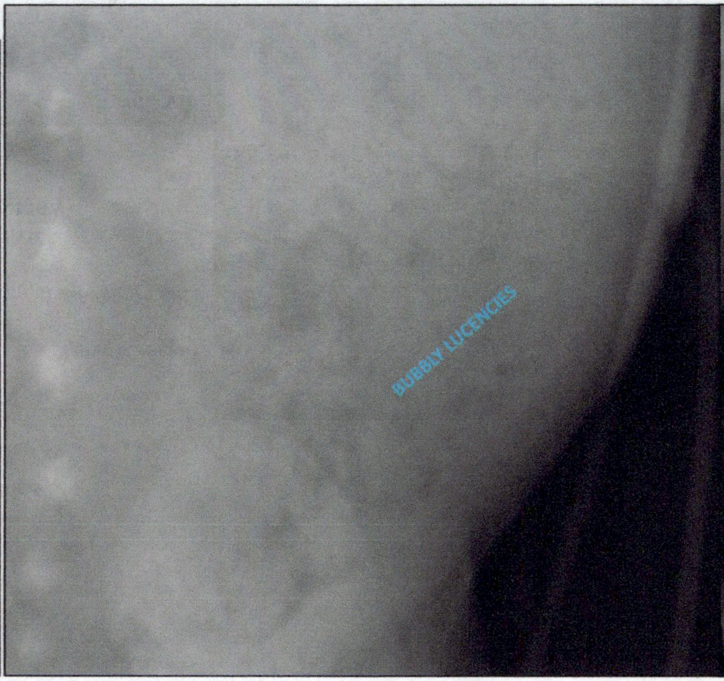

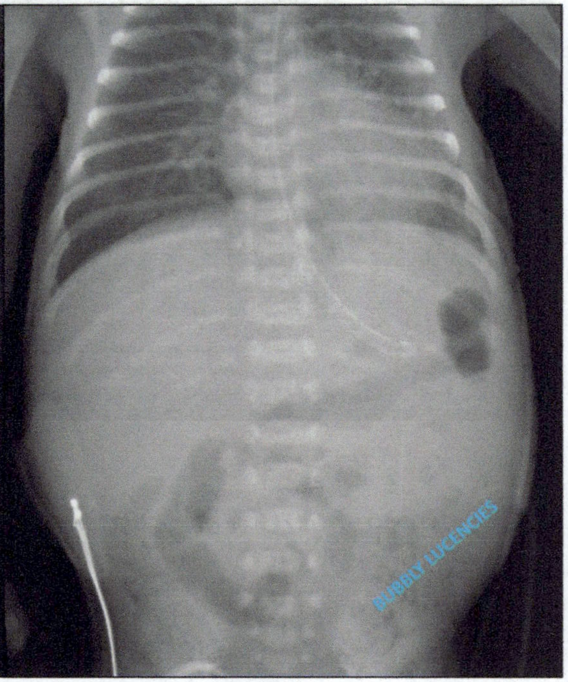

PEDIATRICS

HYPERTROPHIC PYLORIC STENOSIS

IMAGING: **Single muscular wall > 3 mm**
Length > 15-17 mm

USMLE POINTS: **Most common cause of gastric outlet in infants**
Hypokalemic, Hyperchloremic metabolic alkalosis

Risk factors: **First born male**
Macrolide exposure (erythromycin)

Presentation: **Palpable olive-shaped mass in epigastric region**
Visible peristaltic waves
Nonbilious projectile vomiting at 2-6 weeks old

Treatment: **IV fluids and correct electrolytes**
Surgical incision (pyloromyotomy)

MODALITIES: US

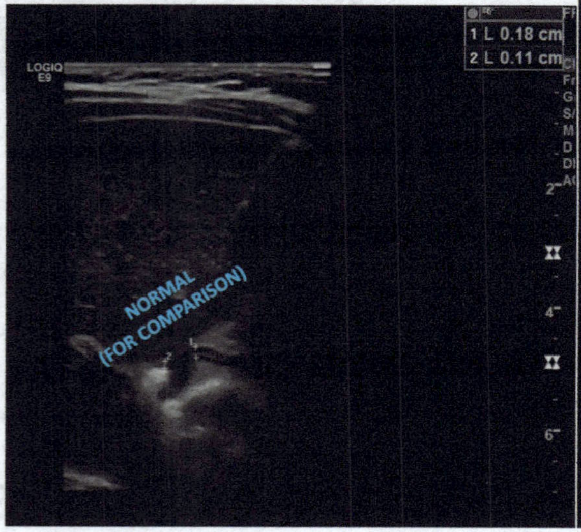

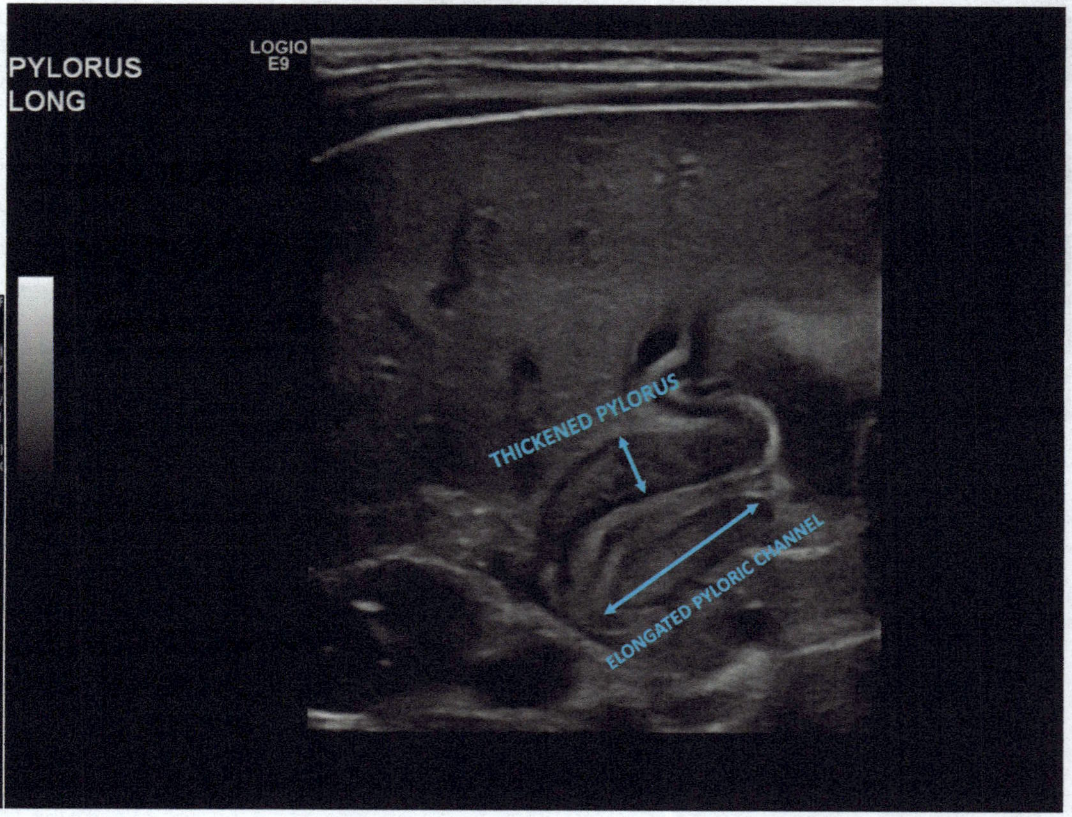

PEDIATRICS

VESICOURETERAL REFLUX

IMAGING: **Reflux of contrast from the urinary bladder → Ureters**

USMLE POINTS:
Abnormal or insufficient insertion of ureter within vesicular wall
Normal pinch-cock action of the vesicoureteral junction when bladder pressure increases is impaired
Abnormally high bladder pressure resulting in retrograde flow
Increases risk for UTI / Pyelonephritis
Common cause of UTI in children under 6 years old

Treatment:
Low-grade reflux → Prophylactic antibiotic
Higher-grade reflux → Surgical reimplantation

MODALITIES: FLX RETROGRADE CYSTOGRAM

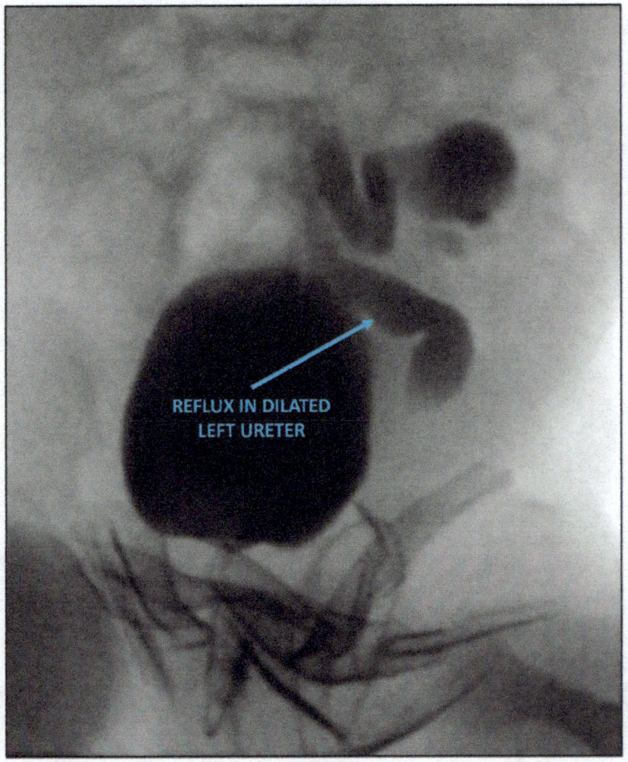

REPRODUCTIVE

REPRODUCTIVE

ECTOPIC PREGNANCY

IMAGING: **No IUP**
Any adnexal mass in pregnant women + Free fluid in the pelvis

USMLE POINTS: Implantation of fertilized ovum in a site other than the uterus (most often in fallopian tube)
Second leading cause of maternal mortality
β-hCG quantification: **≥ 1500 mIU/mL or failure to double after 48 hours**

Locations: **Fallopian tubes (96%), ampulla (75%), isthmus (12%)**
Risk factors: **Tubal pathologies, Previous ectopic, IUD, IVF, PID, TOA**
Presentation: **First trimester bleeding, hypotension/shock if ruptured**
Treatment: **MTX, Surgery**

MODALITIES: US / MRI

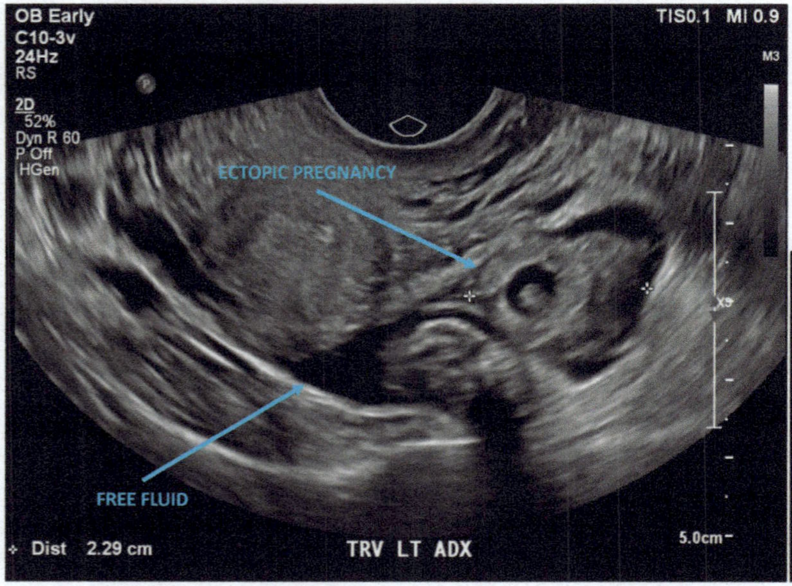

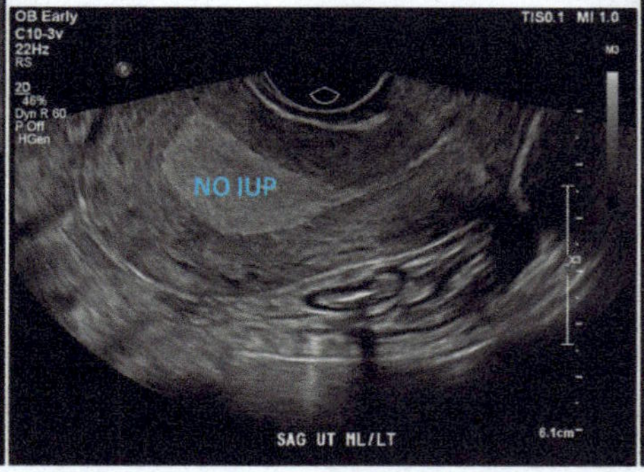

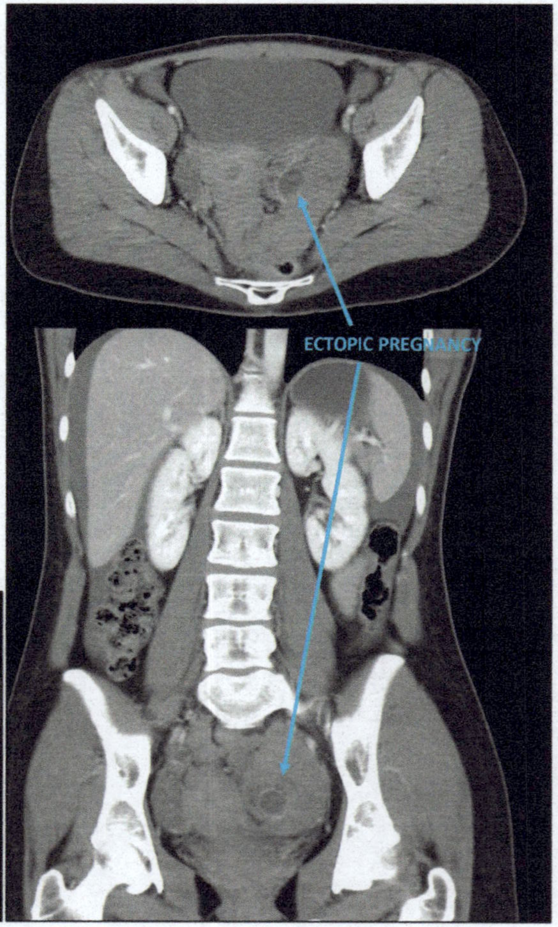

ECTOPIC PREGNANCY

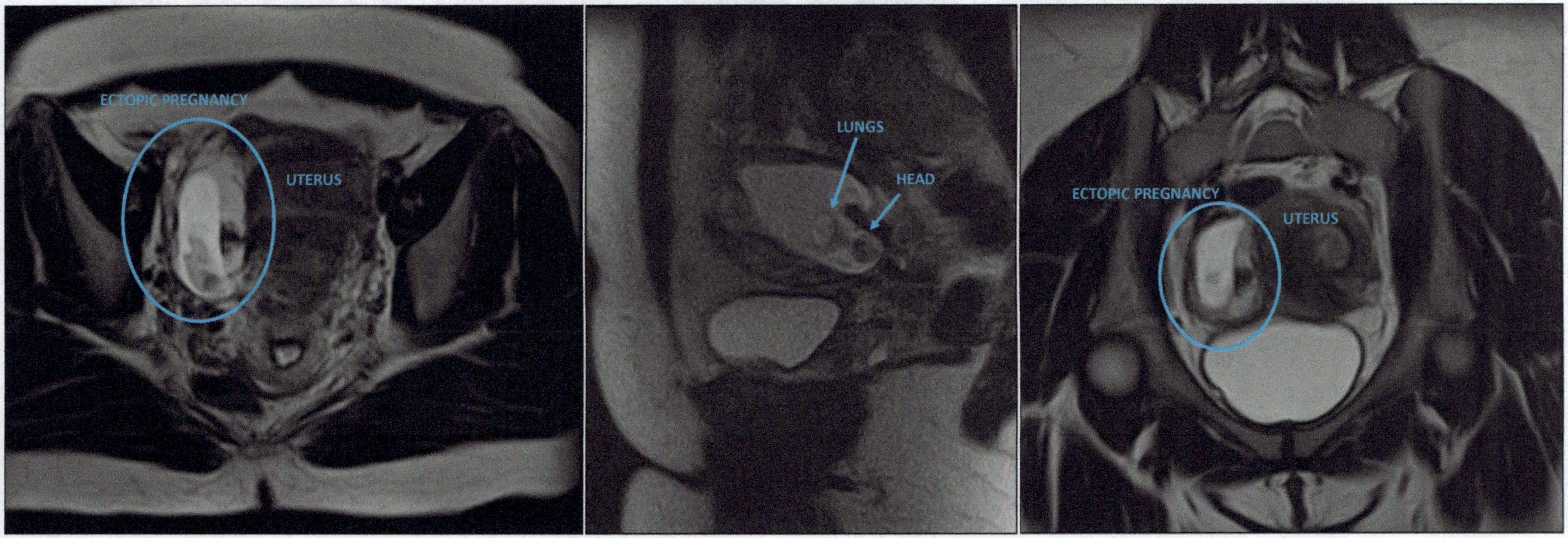

REPRODUCTIVE

MOLAR PREGNANCY

IMAGING: **"Snow-storm" appearance: multiple cystic structures**
Bilateral theca-lutein cysts from increased b-HCG

USMLE POINTS: Complete mole: **46,XX or 46,XY**
Empty egg fertilized by one or two sperm
All genetic material from father
DNA from mother is inactivated and father's is duplicated

Partial mole: **69,XXX, 69,XXY, or 69,XYY**
Mother's DNA remains, but father's is duplicated
Fetal parts

MODALITIES: US

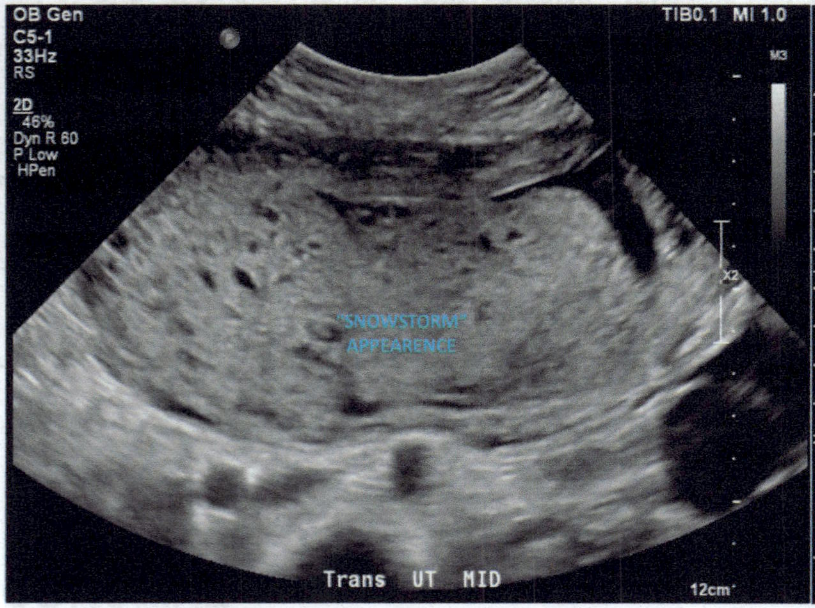

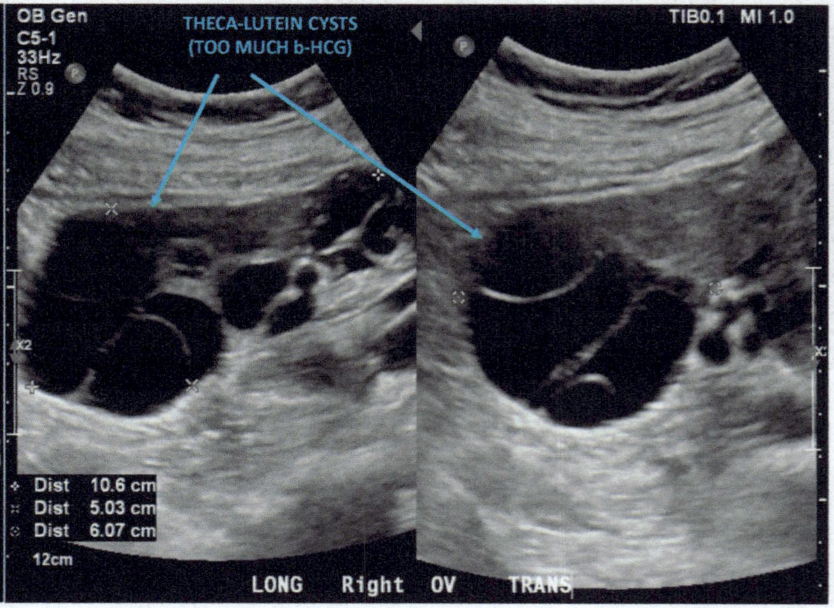

REPRODUCTIVE

OVARIAN TORSION

IMAGING:
- **Enlarged, edematous ovary**
- **Lack of spectral wave-form pattern**
- **Blood flow may be present → Intermittent torsion**

USMLE POINTS:
- **Sharp and usually unilateral lower abdominal pain**
- Risk factors: Ovarian cysts
  - Masses
  - Neoplasms

MODALITIES: US

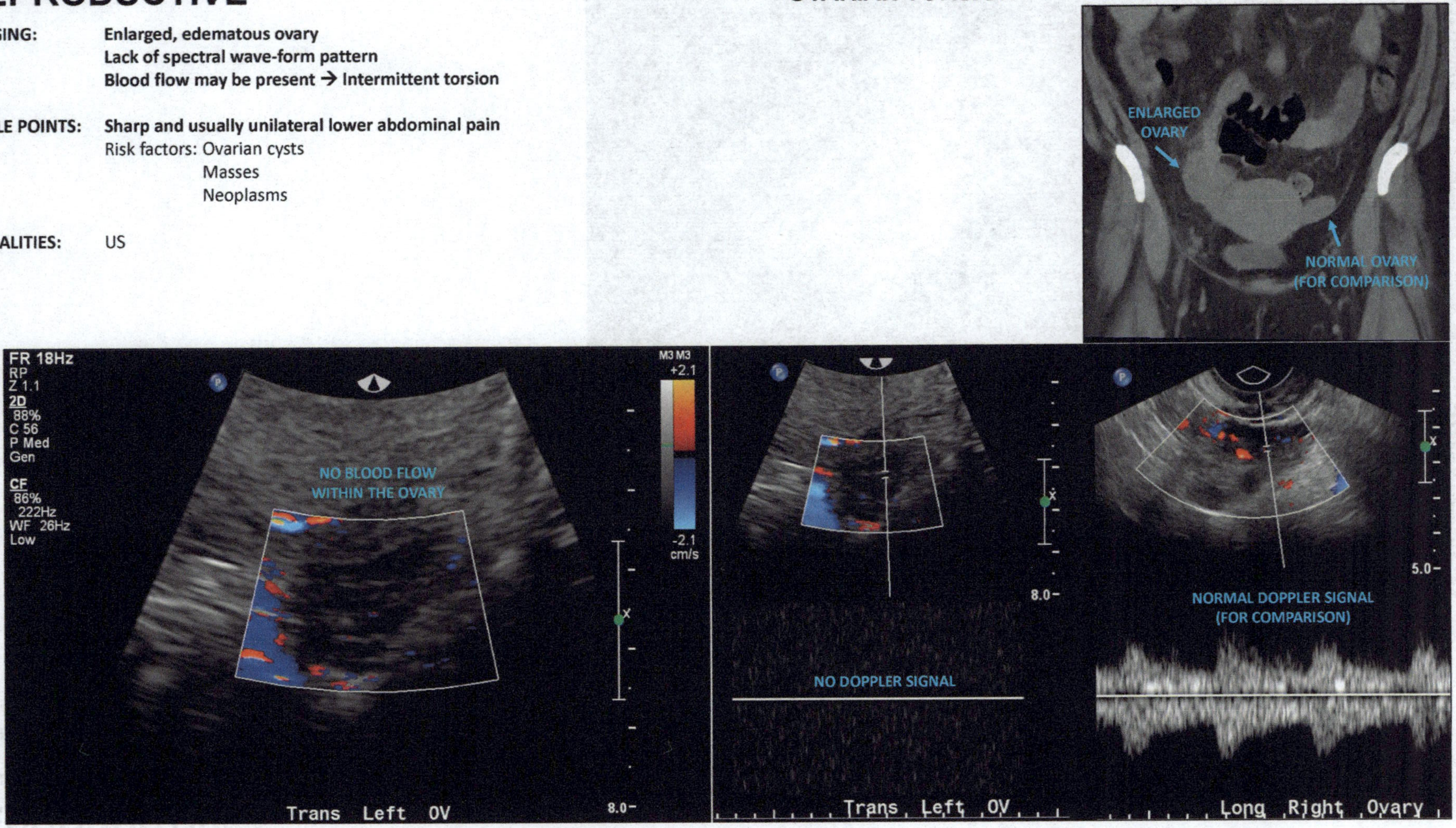

REPRODUCTIVE

PCOS

IMAGING: **Multiple peripheral follicles** (≥12 follicles) within the ovary

USMLE POINTS: **Hyperinsulinemia and/or insulin resistance**

Hypothalamic hormonal feedback → Increasing LH:FSH → Decreased rate of follicular maturation → Unruptured follicles and anovulation

Presentation:
- **Amenorrhea/oligomenorrhea**
- **Hirsutism**
- **Acne**
- **Decreased fertility**

Treatment:
- **Spironolactone**
- **Finasteride (hirsutism)**

MODALITIES: US

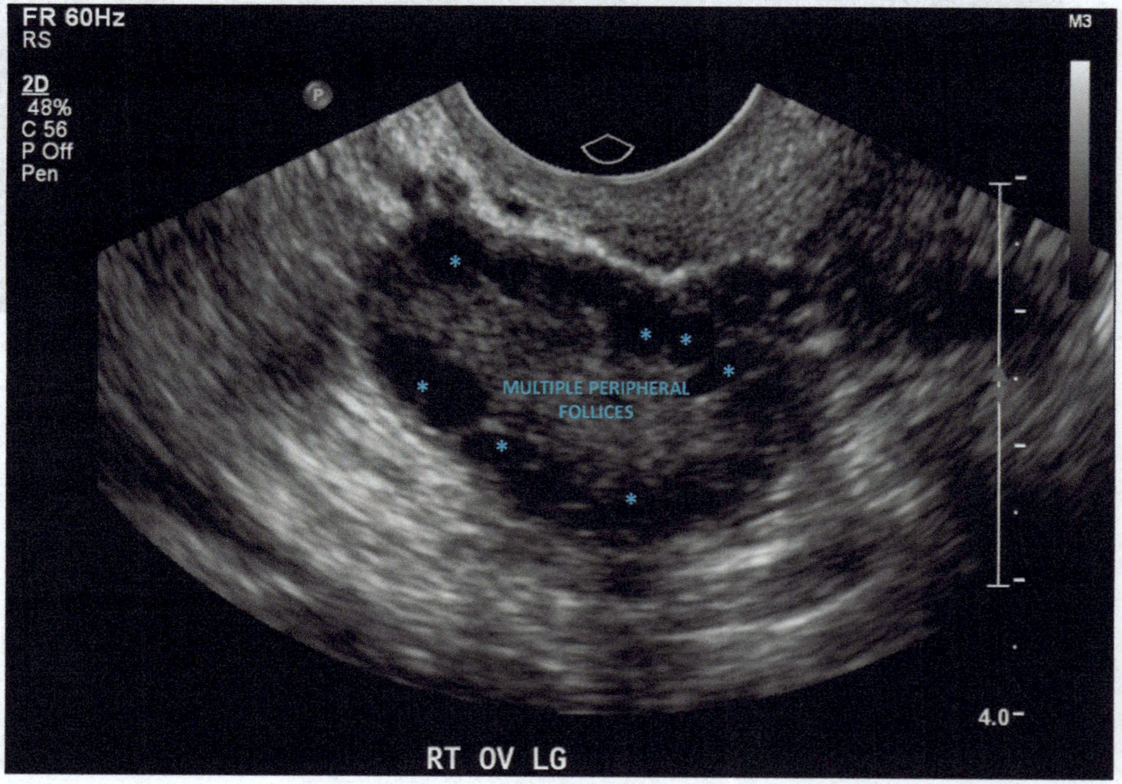

REPRODUCTIVE

HEMORRHAGIC OVARIAN CYST

IMAGING: **Ovarian cyst with "lace-like" internal echos**
May have adjacent free fluid indicating rupture
DDX: Endometrioma

USMLE POINTS: Hemorrhage into a corpus luteum or other functional cyst
Due to hormone response → corpus luteum has a vascularized, fragile granulosa layer
Presentation: **Sudden-onset pelvic pain**
Mittelschmerz → "middle-pain" AKA Ovulation pain

MODALITIES: US

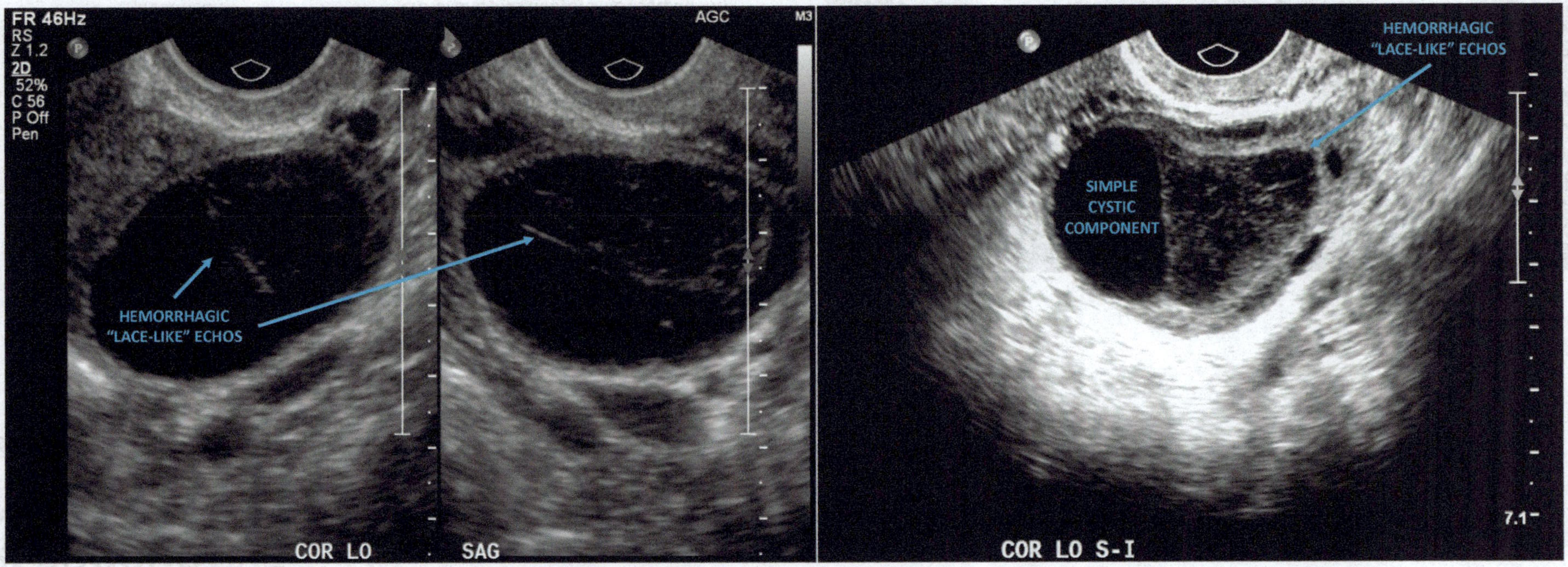

REPRODUCTIVE

TUBO-OVARIAN ABSCESS

IMAGING: **Multiloculated cystic collection** in the pelvis of a female
Thickened **fluid-filled tubes**

USMLE POINTS: **Due to pelvic inflammatory disease (PID)**
Sexually active women: 15-29 years old
Neisseria gonorrhoeae
Chlamydia trachomatis
10x higher risk for ectopic pregnancy

Fitz-Hugh-Curtis Syndrome: Infection of liver capsule + Peritoneal adhesions

Risk Factors:
Age < 25 years of age
High risk sexual behavior
Earlier age at first intercourse

Presentation:
Adnexal collection
Fever + Leukocytosis
Pelvic pain + Vaginal discharge
Septic shock
CMT → "Chandelier-sign"

Treatment: **Ceftriaxone plus doxycycline (outpatient)**

MODALITIES: US → CT W / MRI W

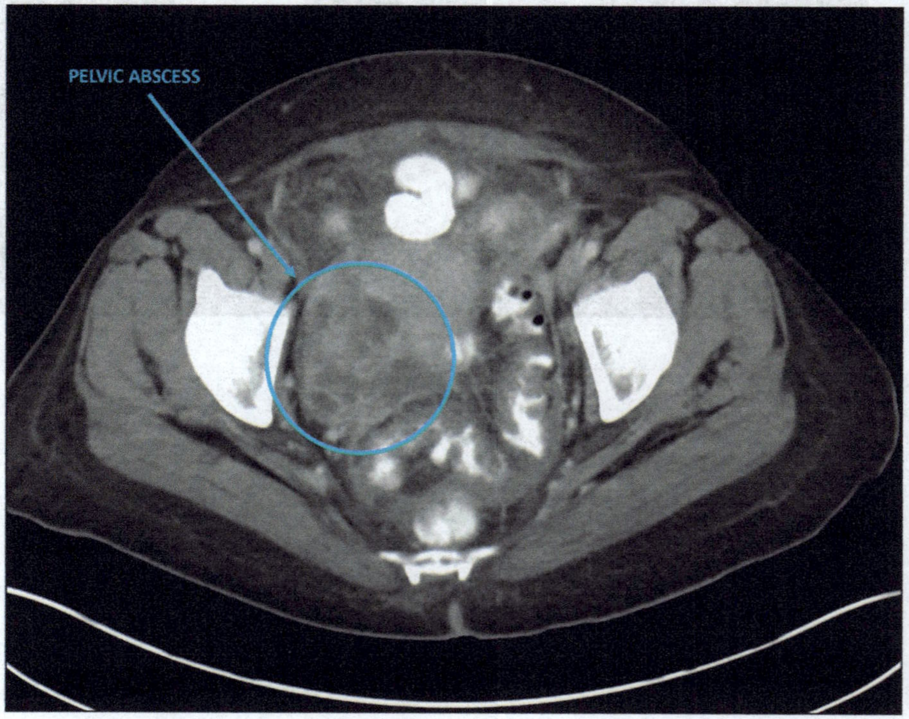

REPRODUCTIVE

PLACENTA PREVIA

IMAGING: Placental tissue extending **over or < 2 cm from the internal cervical os**

USMLE POINTS: Presentation: **Painless** bleeding (3rd trimester most common)
If persistent placenta previa → Cesarean delivery should be considered

Risk Factors:
- Multiparity
- **Prior C-section**
- Previous placenta previa

MODALITIES: US

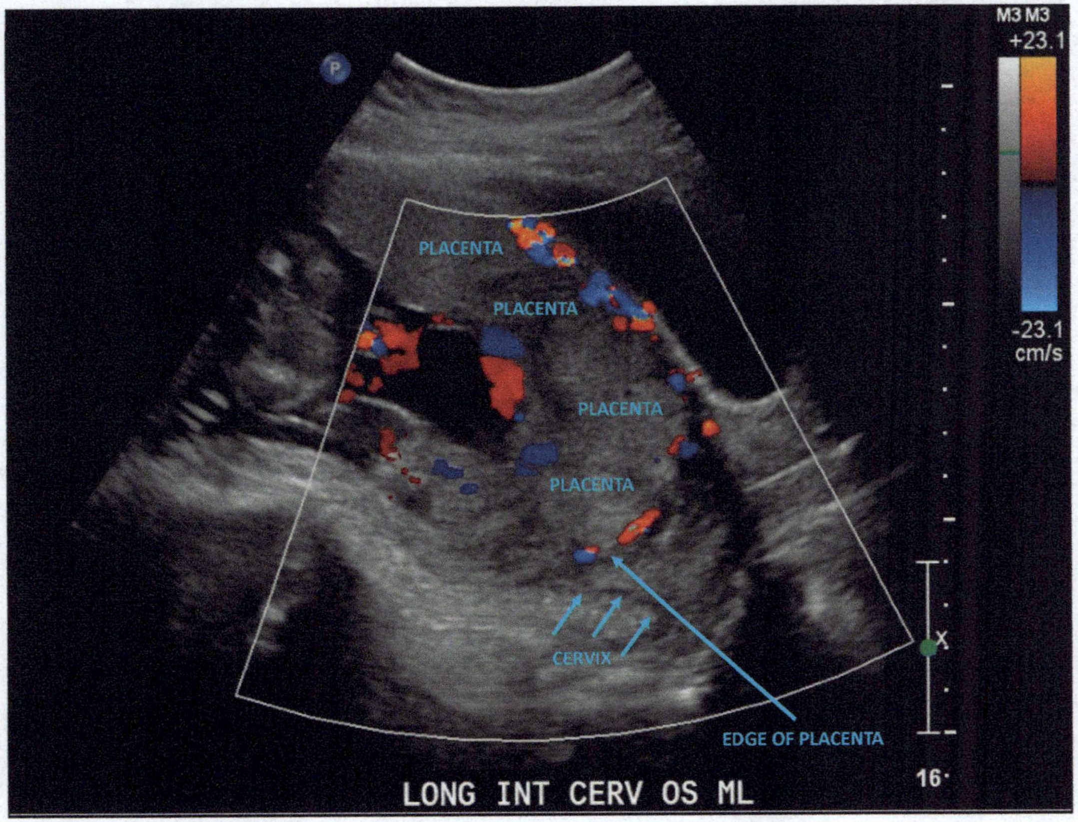

REPRODUCTIVE

IMAGING:

Retroplacental hematoma
Intraplacental anechoic areas
Separation and rounding of the placental edge
Rupture of maternal vessels in the decidua basalis

USMLE POINTS:

Placenta prematurely separates from uterine wall before delivery

Risk factors: Trauma, smoking, **hypertension, preeclampsia, cocaine**

Presentation:
- **Severe abdominal pain**
- **Abrupt, painful bleeding**
- **Pregnancies > 20 weeks of gestation**

Labs:
- Increased alpha fetoprotein
- Increased hCG
- Very low or very high levels of inhibin A
- Fibrinogen ≤ 200 mg/dL → Severe postpartum hemorrhage

MODALITIES: US

PLACENTAL ABRUPTION

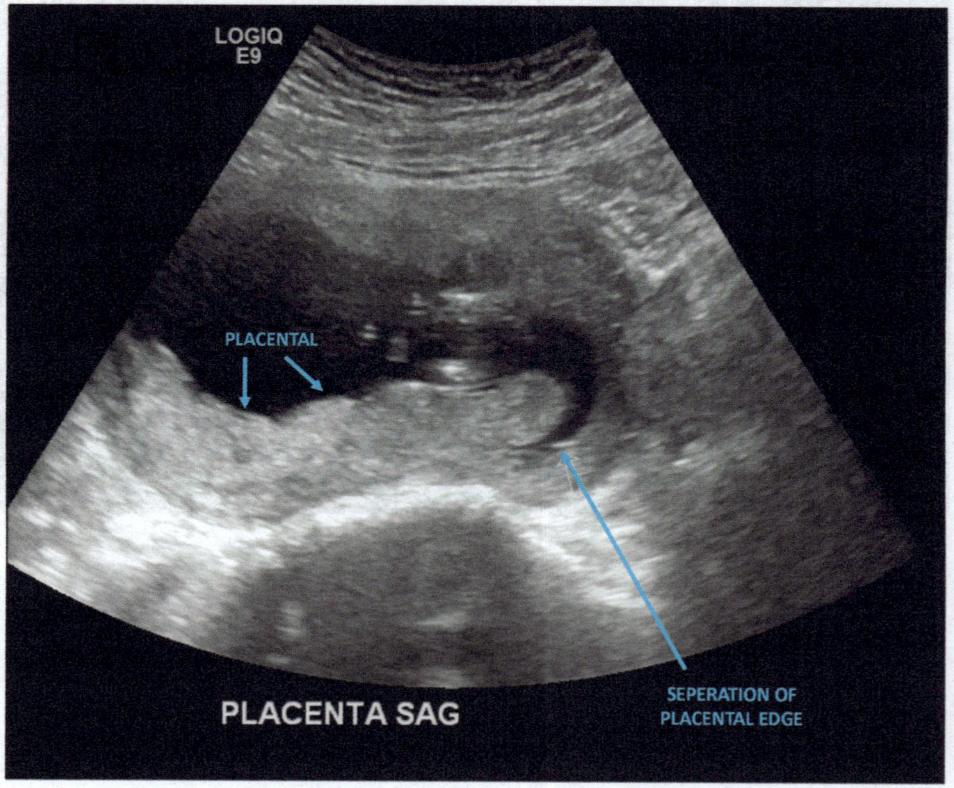

REPRODUCTIVE

FIBROIDS

IMAGING:
CT: **Uterine mass** may calcify – Often multiple
US: **Uterine mass** may be submucosal, intramural, subserosal

USMLE POINTS: Originate from **uterine smooth muscle** (excessive production of extracellular matrix)

Major risk factors: Increase in exposure to higher levels of endogenous **estrogen**
African Americans (5x more common)

Submucosal classification: Grow beneath the endometrium
Intermenstrual bleeding and menorrhagia (Tx: OCP)

Subserosal classification: Compression of bladder, rectum, or ureter

Presentation: **Abnormal menstruation, DUB, Enlarged uterus, Infertility**

MODALITIES: US / MRI WWO

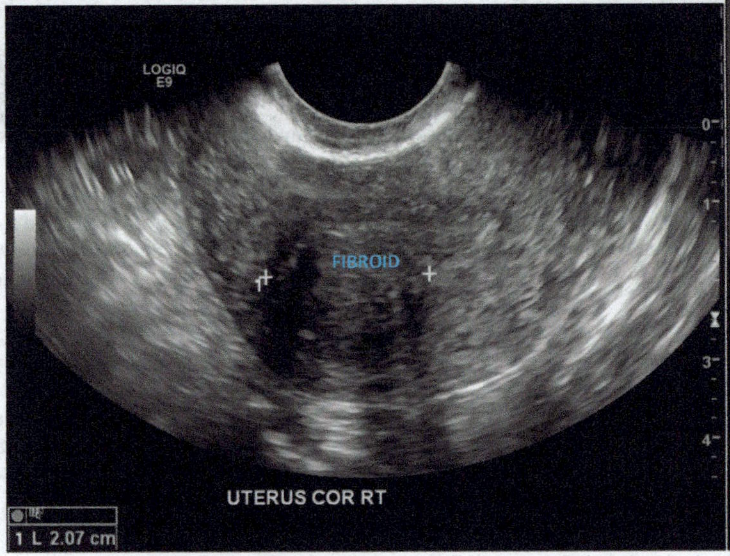

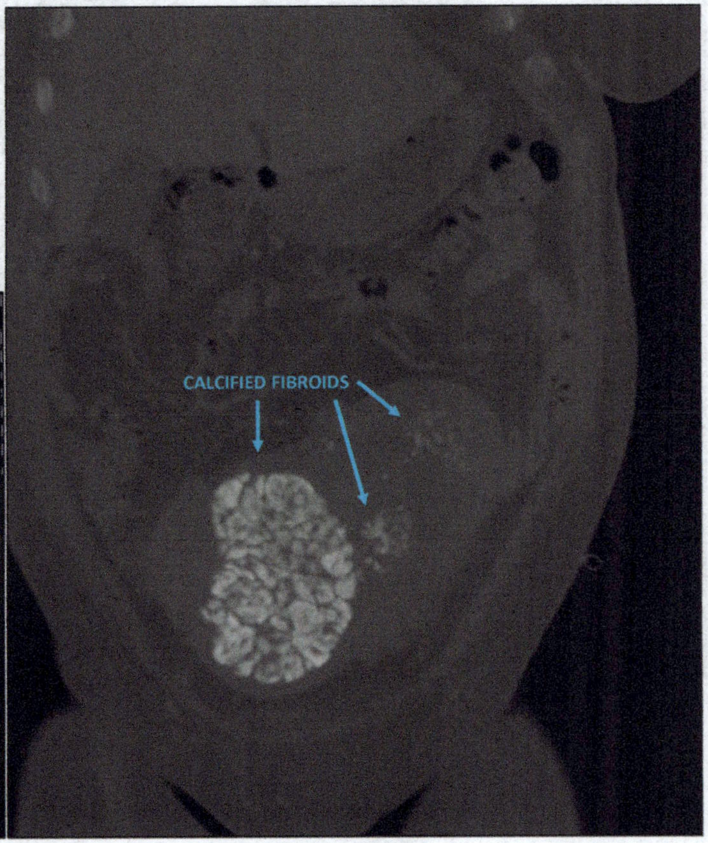

REPRODUCTIVE

OVARIAN HYPERSTIMULATION SYNDROME

IMAGING:

Multiple cysts of varying sizes (classic spoke-wheel appearance)
Ovaries may be severe enlarged
Ascites and pleural +/- pericardial effusion (capillary leak)

USMLE POINTS:

Ovarian stimulation treatment (ovarian induction therapy) for IVF
May progress to intravascular volume depletion

Presentation:

Abdominal distension
Potentially life-threatening capillary leak → Fluid sequestration in a third space
Acute pelvic pain may result from stretching of the ovarian capsule

MODALITIES: US → CT W + PO

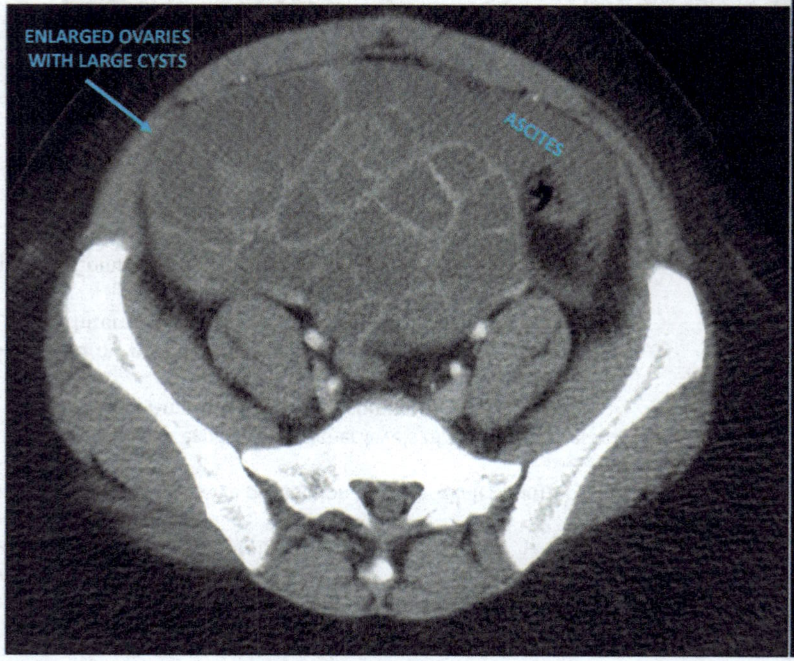

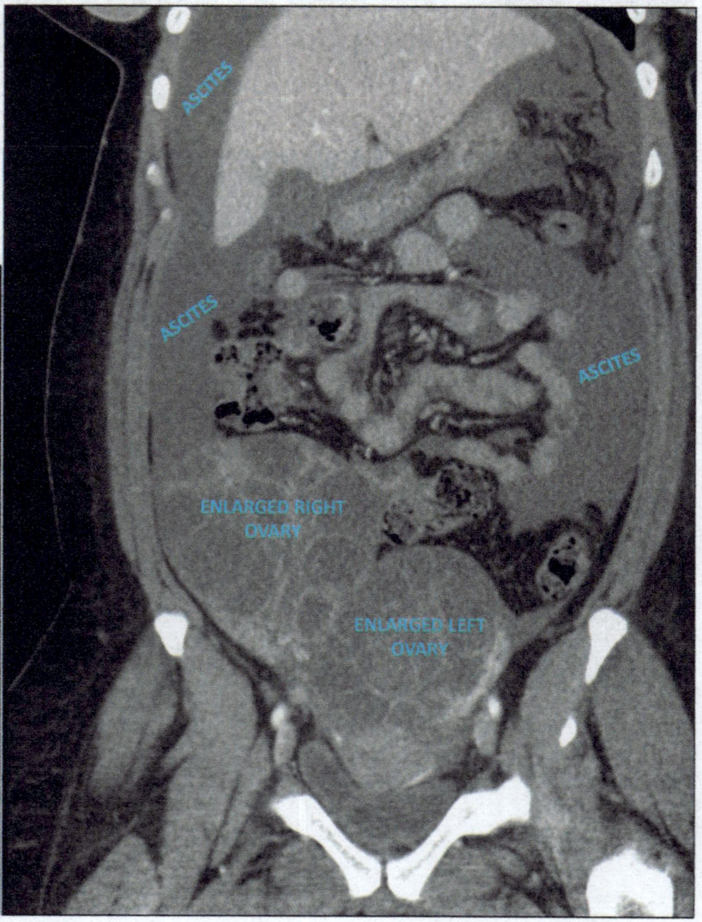

REPRODUCTIVE

PENILE FRACTURE

IMAGING: Tear in the **tunica albuginea of the corpus cavernosum**
Often accompanies adjacent hematoma
May be dorsal or ventral

USMLE POINTS: Due to sudden trauma
Requires surgery

MODALITIES: MRI WO

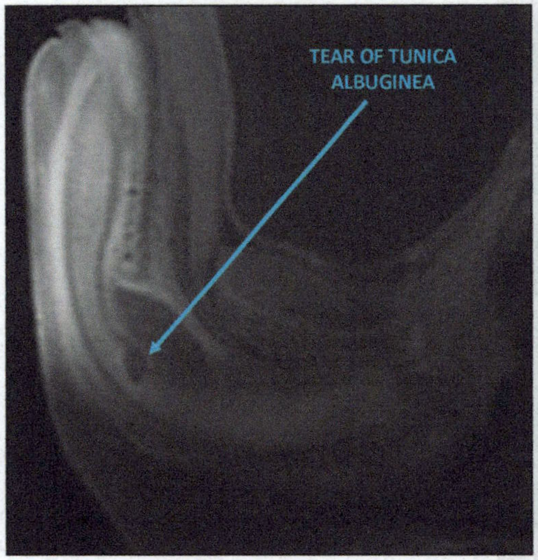

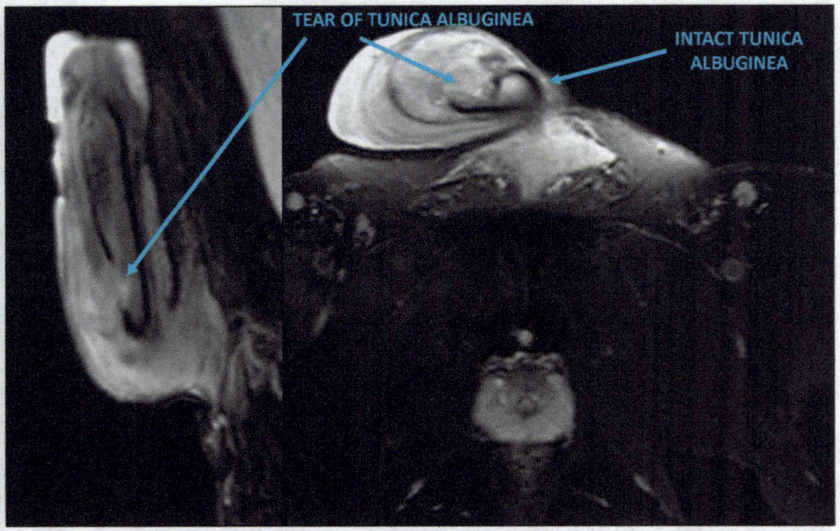

REPRODUCTIVE

ADENOMYOSIS

IMAGING: **Thickening of the junctional zone ≥12 mm**
Uniformly enlarged, globular uterus

USMLE POINTS: **Ectopic endometrial tissue in the myometrium (similar to endometriosis)**
Hyperplasia of basal layer of endometrium
Presentation: Dysmenorrhea, DUB
Treatment: GnRH agonists, Aromatase inhibitors Hysterectomy

MODALITIES: US / MRI WO

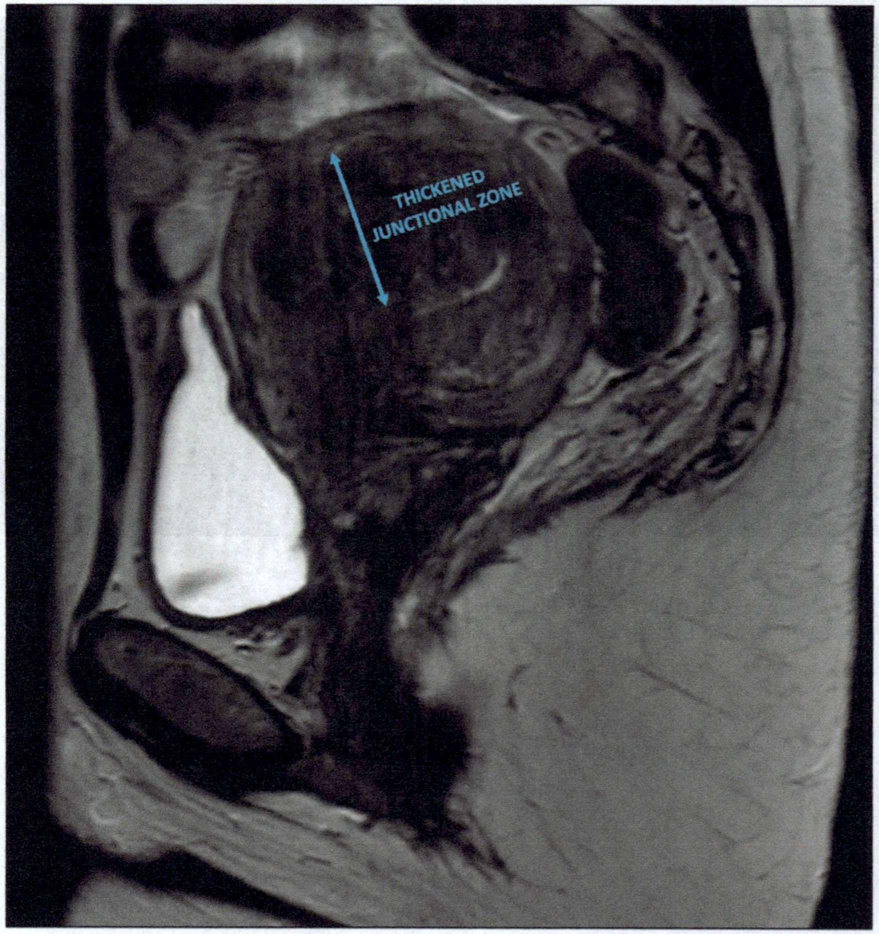

REPRODUCTIVE

ENDOMETRIOSIS

IMAGING: US: **Uniform low level internal echos** (endometrioma → "chocolate cyst")
MRI: T1: Increased SI
T2: "Shading" (hypointense)

USMLE POINTS: Endometrium-like glands/stroma outside endometrial cavity, most commonly in ovary, pelvis, peritoneum

Presentation: Cyclic pelvic pain, Bleeding, **Dyspareunia**, Infertility

Treatment: NSAIDS, OCP, Progestins, GnRH Agonists, Laparoscopic removal

MODALITIES: US / MRI WWO

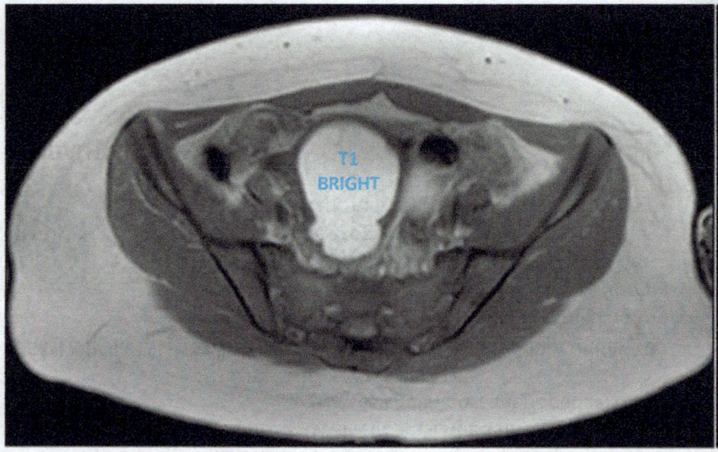

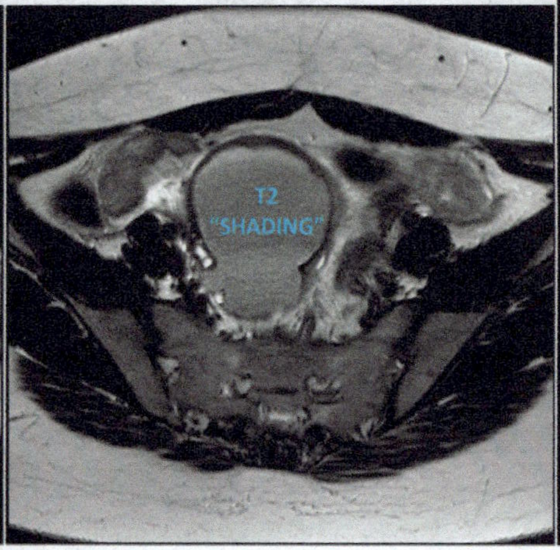

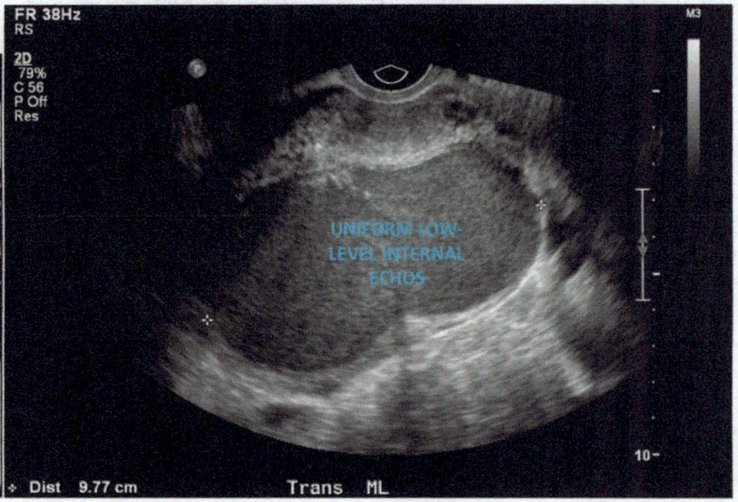

REPRODUCTIVE

FIBROADENOMA

IMAGING:

US: **Well-circumscribed**
Uniform hypoechogenicity

Mammo: Well-circumscribed discrete oval mass hypo- or isodense
May calcify in post-menopausal period

USMLE POINTS:

Most common breast tumor in women under 30
Presentation: Small, firm, mobile, & non-tender breast lump
Excess proliferation of connective tissue → Composed of fibrous tissue and glands
Does not change with menstrual cycle
Responds to estrogen
Intact basement membrane on histology (benign)

MODALITIES: US / MAMMO

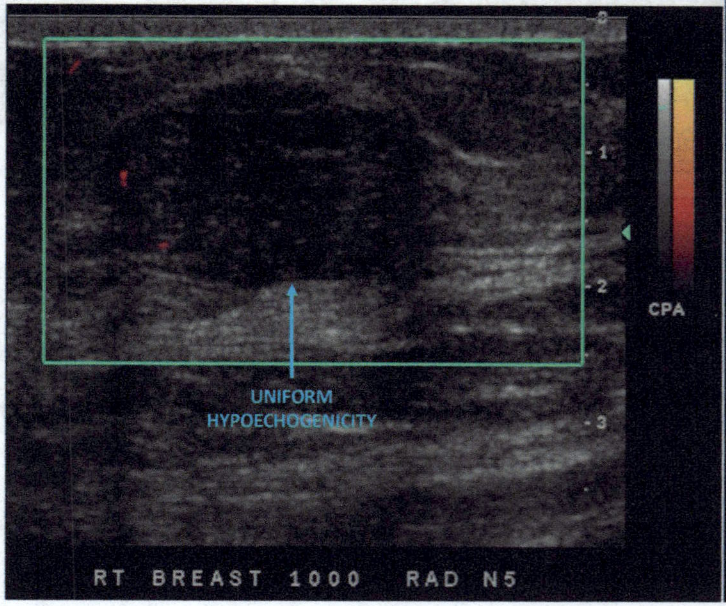

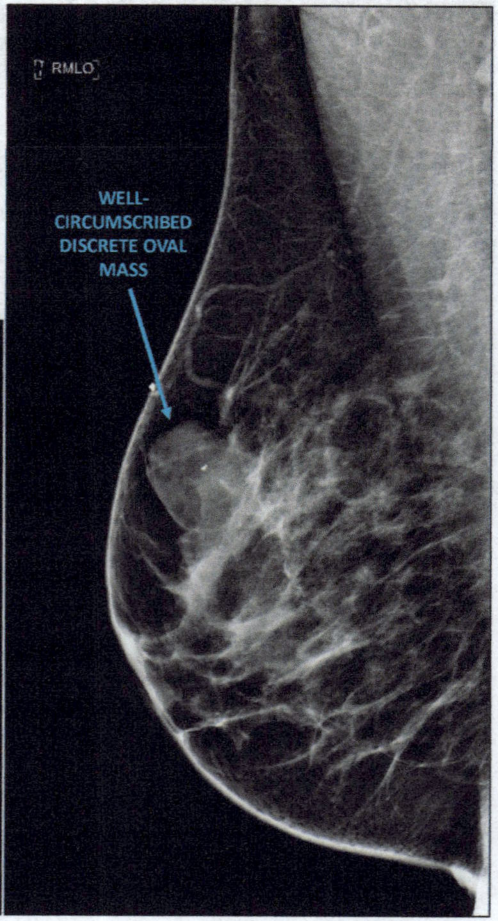

GENITOURINARY

GENITOURINARY

ADPKD

IMAGING: **Diffuse cystic changes** throughout the kidneys
Cysts may be hyperdense (blood) and/or calcify
Often has accompanying hepatic cysts

USMLE POINTS: Mutations in PKD1 or PKD2 → Most common inherited cause of kidney disease
Associated with **Berry (saccular) aneurysm**
Autosomal Dominant
Often results in ESRD

Presentation: Abdominal pain
Low back pain
Hematuria
UTI

Treatment: ACE-Inhibitors (treatment of hypertension)

MODALITIES: US / CT W

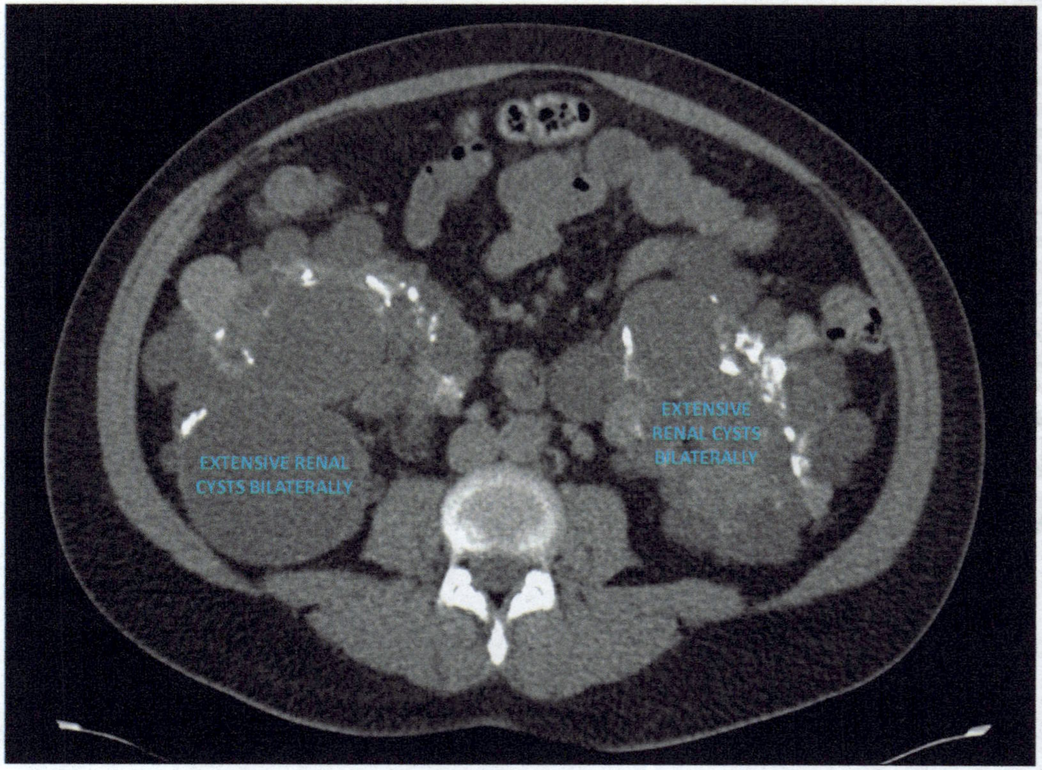

GENITOURINARY

HORSESHOE KIDNEY

IMAGING: **Fused kidney in the midline**

USMLE POINTS:
Inferior poles of both kidneys fuse abnormally
IMA prevents superior ascent of the horseshoe kidney
Kidneys can still function normally
Higher incidence in chromosomal aneuploidy

Associations:
- Hydronephrosis
- Nephrolithiasis
- Infection
- Renal cancer

MODALITIES: CT W

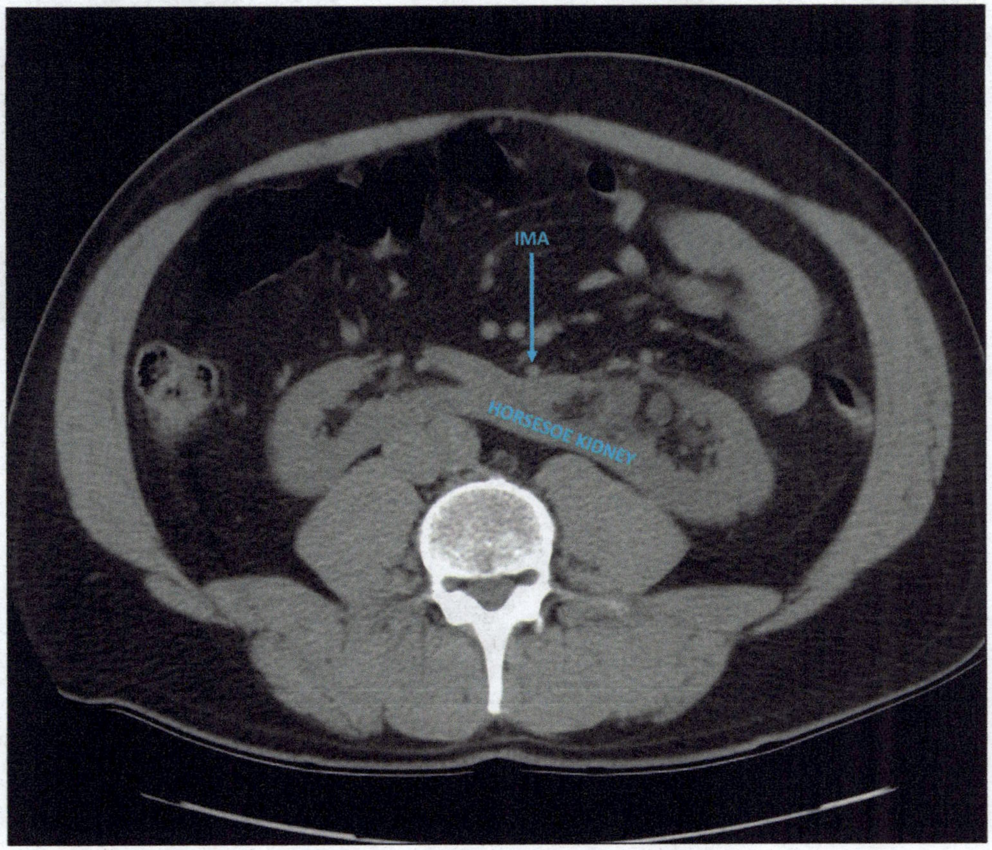

GENITOURINARY

RENAL CELL CARCINOMA

IMAGING: **Large, aggressive renal mass**
Assessment of the extent of local and regional involvement (IVC involvement)

USMLE POINTS: Originates from proximal convoluted tubule → invades renal vein → IVC
Metastasis are often lytic

Associations: **Von Hippel-Lindau**
Tuberous sclerosis

Presentation: Palpable mass, hematuria, flank pain, weight loss
Hypercalcemia, hypertension, erythrocytosis

Treatment: **Surgery** (resistant to chemo/radiation)

MODALITIES: CT W (CT UROGRAM) / MRI WWO

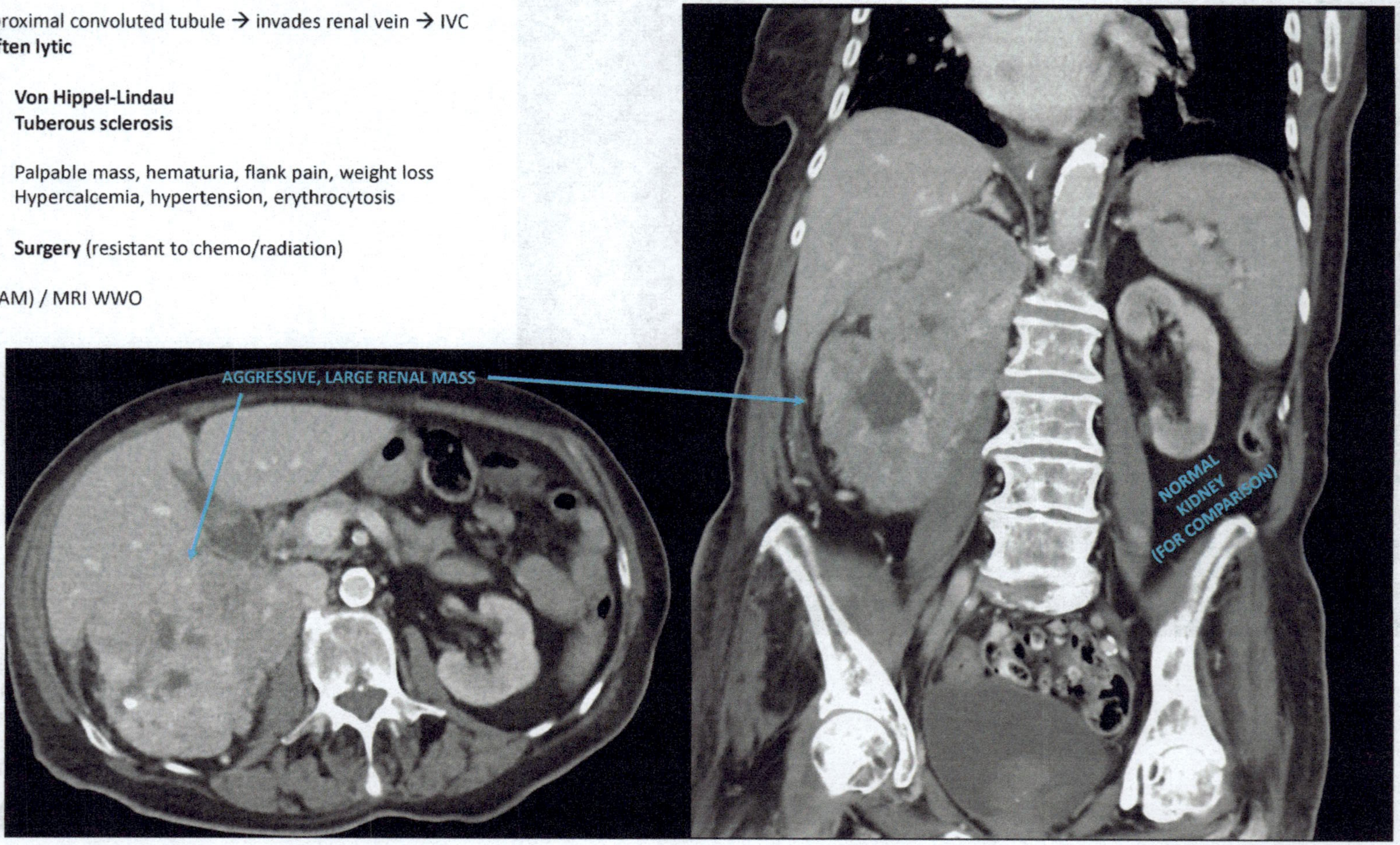

OBSTRUCTIVE UROPATHY

IMAGING: **Obstructing ureteral calculus**
Hydronephrosis, asymmetric enlargement, perinephric stranding/fluid

USMLE POINTS: Difficulty initiating urination
Acute urinary retention
Lower abdominal discomfort and distension

<u>Types of stones</u>

Calcium	Hypercalciuria / **Chron's**	Radiopaque	Envelope or dumbbell shaped	**HCTZ /** Low sodium diet
Cystine	Impaired cystine reabsorption	Radiopaque	Hexagonal	Dietary modification / Chelating agent
Struvite	**Urease-positive** organisms	Radiopaque	Coffin-lid	**Surgical removal**
Uric acid	Hyperuricemia (gout)	**Radiolucent**	Rhomboid	**Urine alkalinization / Allopurinol**

MODALITIES: CT **WO (MUST BE WITHOUT CONTRAST)**

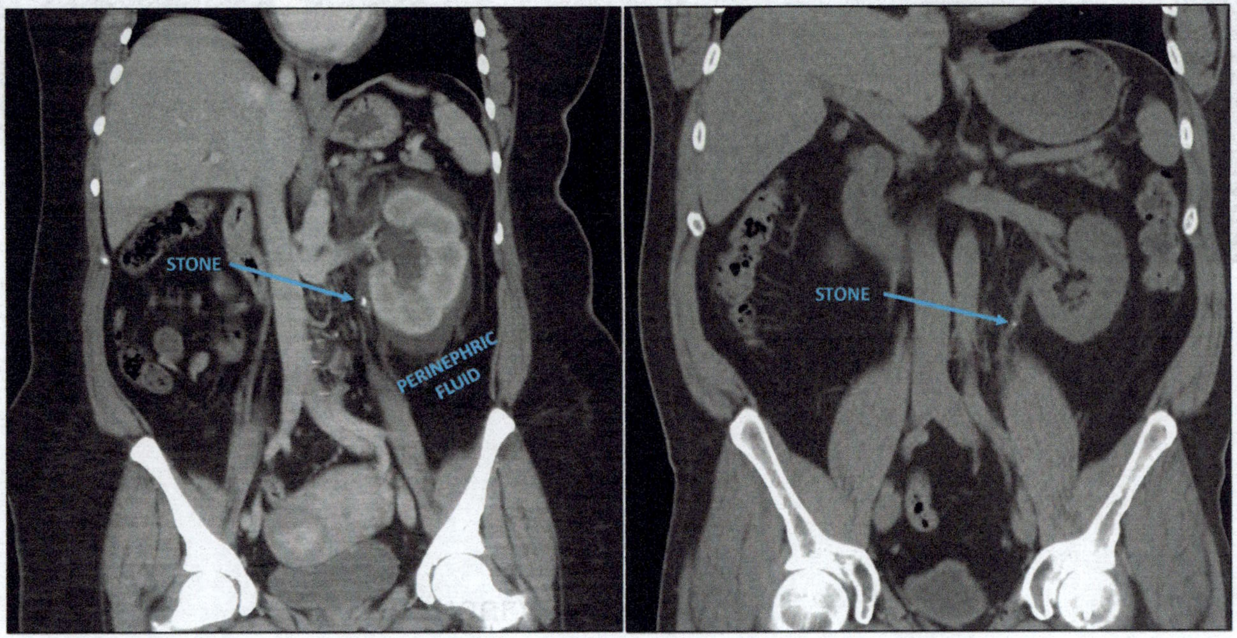

GENITOURINARY

TESTICULAR TORSION

IMAGING:
Avascular, heterogenous, enlarged testicle
Loss of low resistance spectral waveform
Flow may still be present in intermittent torsion

USMLE POINTS:
Males 12-18 years old
Bell-clapper deformity: Congenital horizontal positioning
Trauma or spontaneously
Absent cremasteric reflex

Treatment: Surgical correction: **6 hours**
Manual detorsion if surgical option unavailable

MODALITIES: US

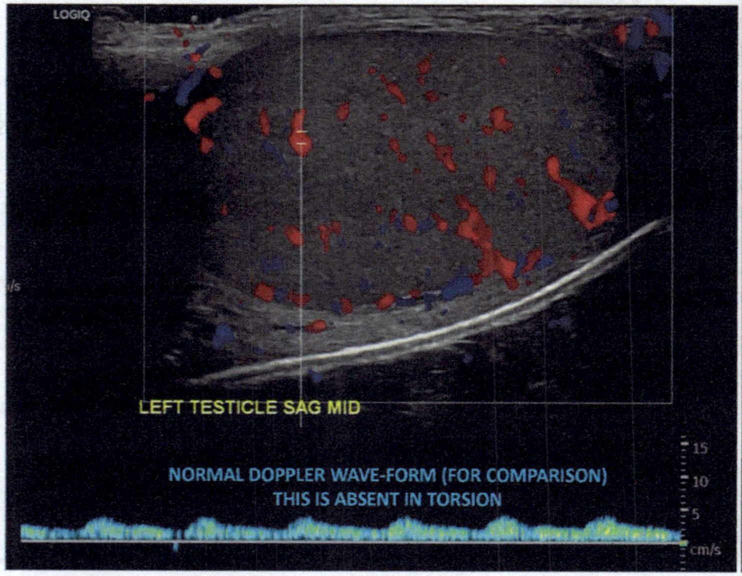

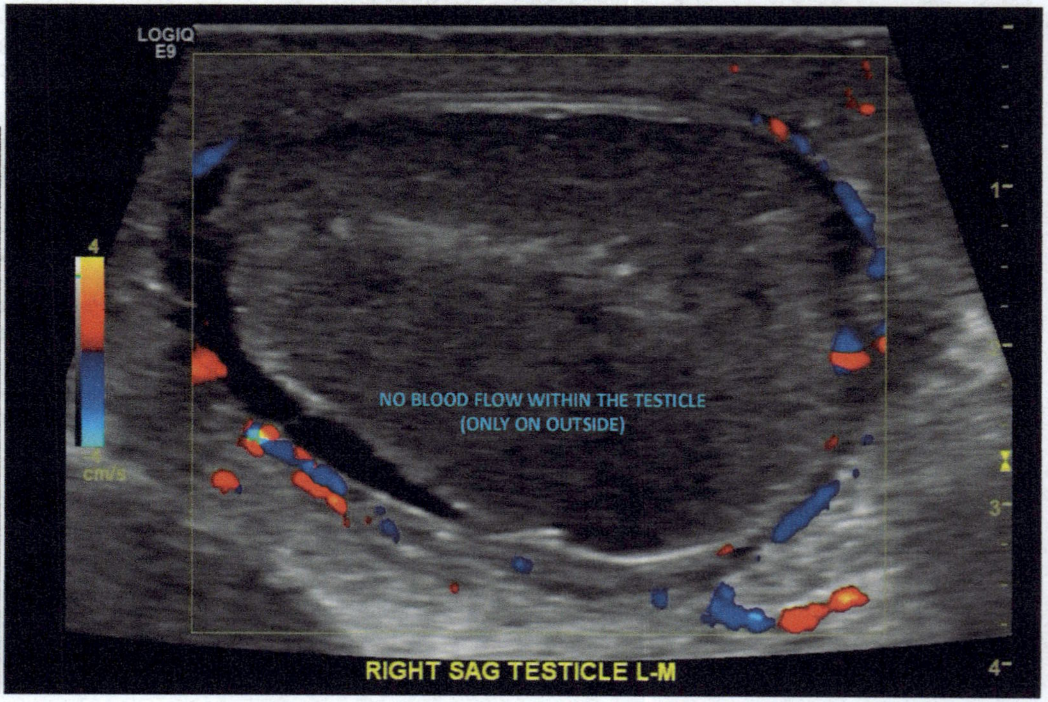

GENITOURINARY

IMAGING: **Air within the urinary bladder wall**
Bladder wall thickening + Induration surrounding the bladder

USMLE POINTS: Elderly **diabetic** and immunocompromised patients
Infection of the bladder wall by gas-forming bacteria: **E. coli**

MODALITIES: CT W

EMPHYSEMATOUS CYSTITIS

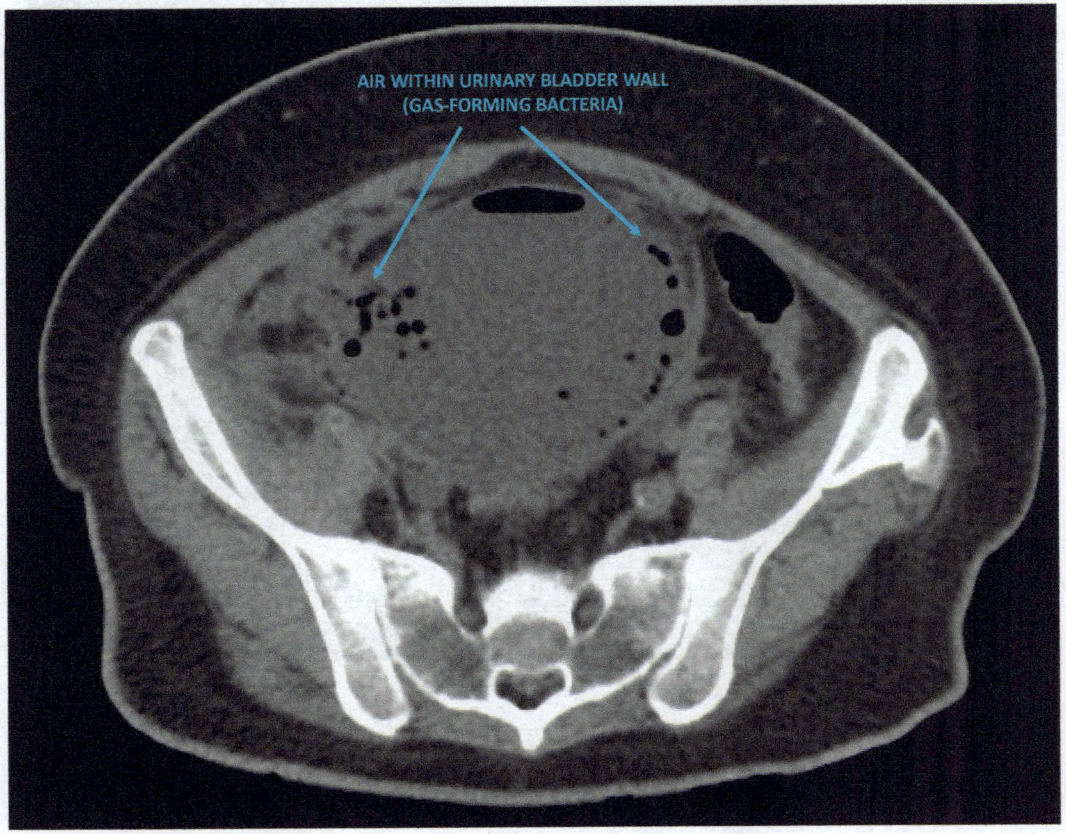

GENITOURINARY

IMAGING: Extraluminal **contrast into perivesical space**

USMLE POINTS: **Most common (80-90%)**
Result from **pelvic fractures**
Rupture is below peritoneal reflection and not on the dome
Treatment: **Foley catheter**

MODALITIES: CT **CYSTO**

BLADDER RUPTURE - EXTRAPERITONEAL

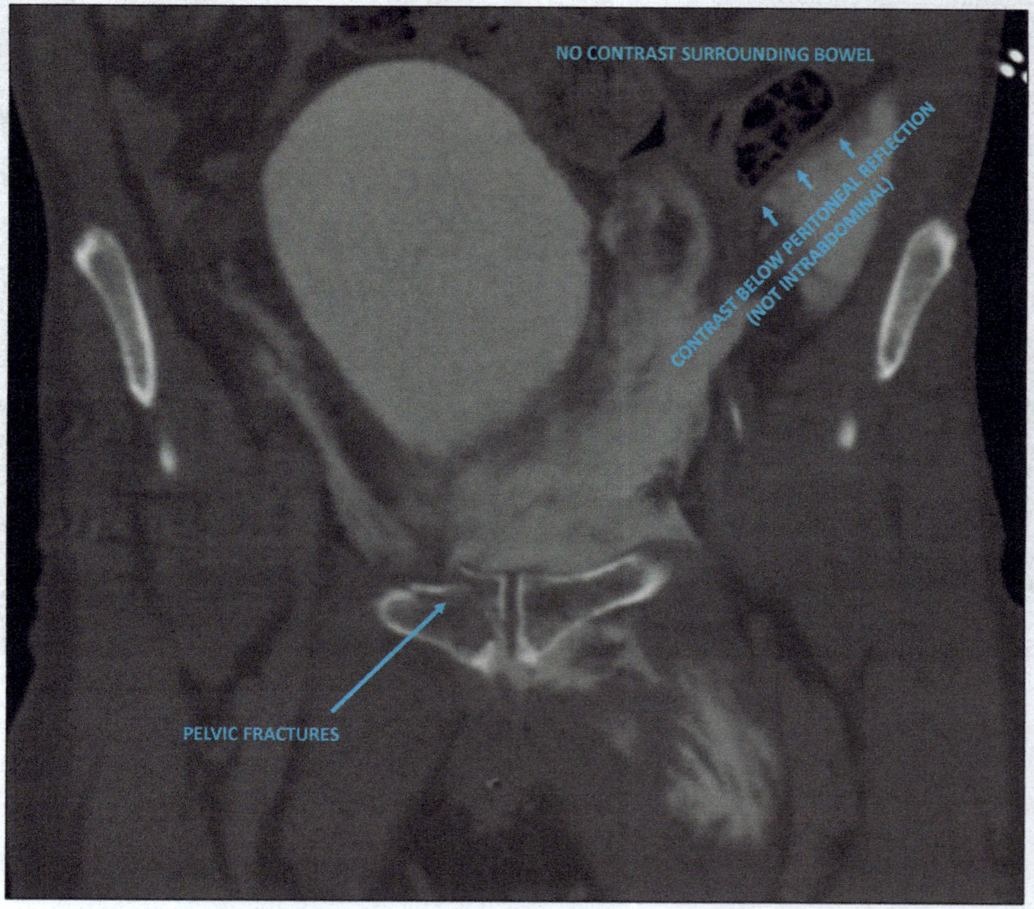

GENITOURINARY

BLADDER RUPTURE - INTRAPERITONEAL

IMAGING:
Bladder **dome** rupture
Urine within the **intraperitoneal space** → contrast in paracolic gutters and between loops of small bowel

USMLE POINTS:
MVA with full bladder (compressive forces)
Far less common than extraperitoneal (pelvic fractures)
More common in children
Treatment: **Requires surgical treatment**

MODALITIES:
CT CYSTO

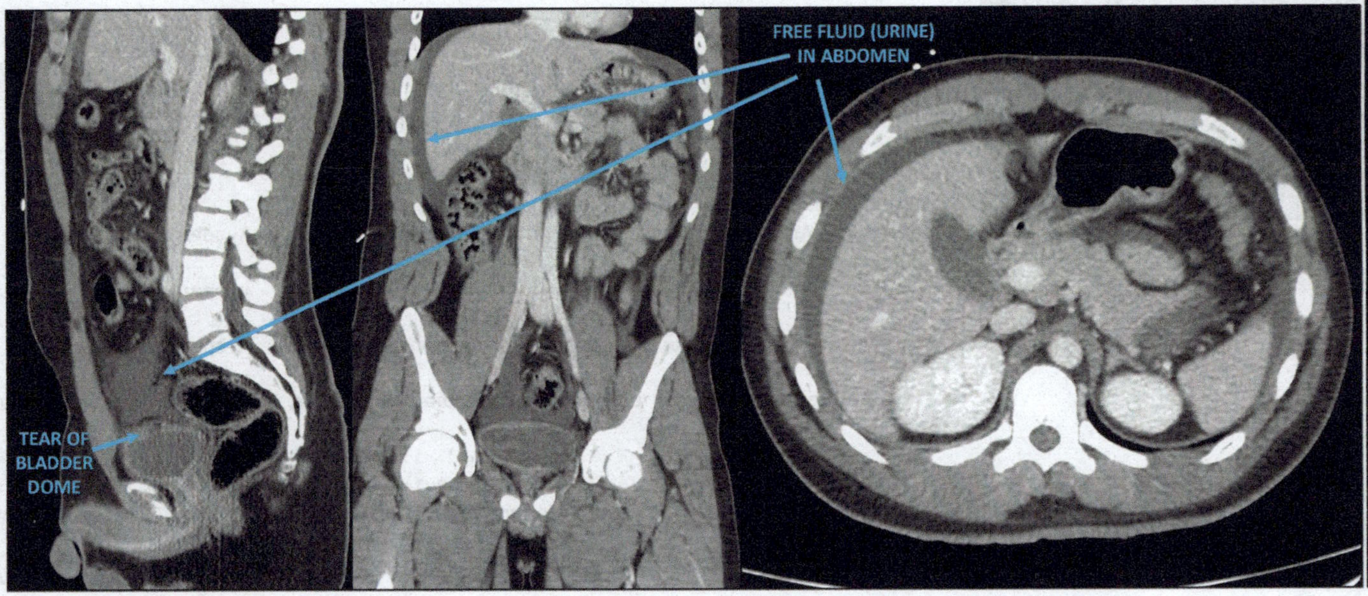

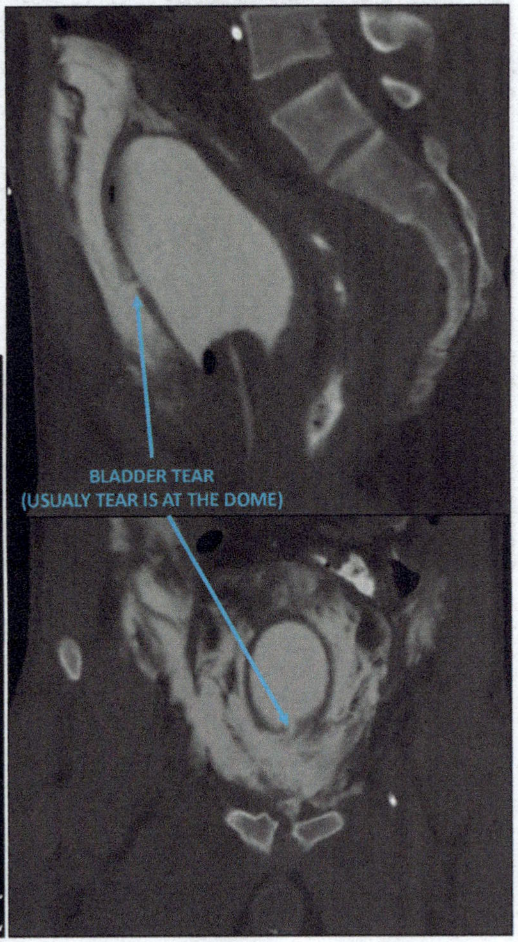

GENITOURINARY

RENAL LACERATION

IMAGING:

Renal laceration (linear hypoattenuation)
Devascularized portion of the kidney
Adjacent hemorrhage

USMLE POINTS:

Grade I	**Subcapsular hematoma or contusion, without laceration**
Grade II	Superficial **laceration ≤ 1 cm depth** not involving the collecting
Grade III	**Laceration > 1 cm** not involving the collecting system
Grade IV	Laceration **involving the collecting system with urinary extravasation** Laceration of the renal pelvis and/or complete ureteropelvic disruption Vascular injury to segmental renal artery or vein
Grade V	**Shattered kidney**

MODALITIES: CTA / CT W

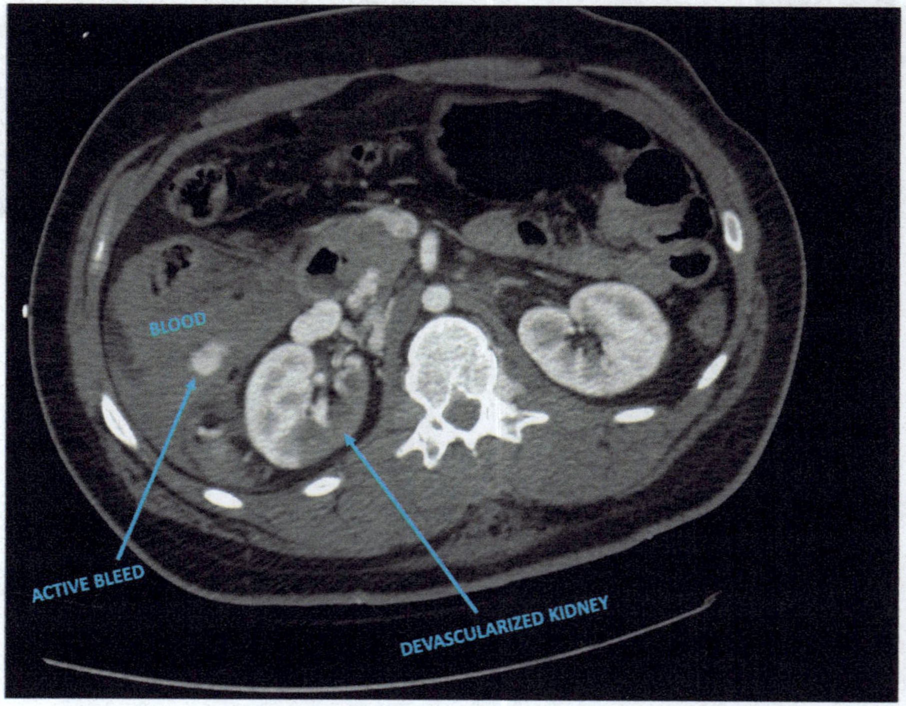

GENITOURINARY

PERSISTENT NEPHROGRAM

IMAGING: **Intravenous contrast is retained by both kidneys for** more than 3 minutes
Look for contrast in the kidneys on a noncontrast exam

USMLE POINTS: **Hypotension**
Bilateral intrarenal obstruction
Vascular causes
Bilateral obstructive uropathy

MODALITIES: Seen on CT WO

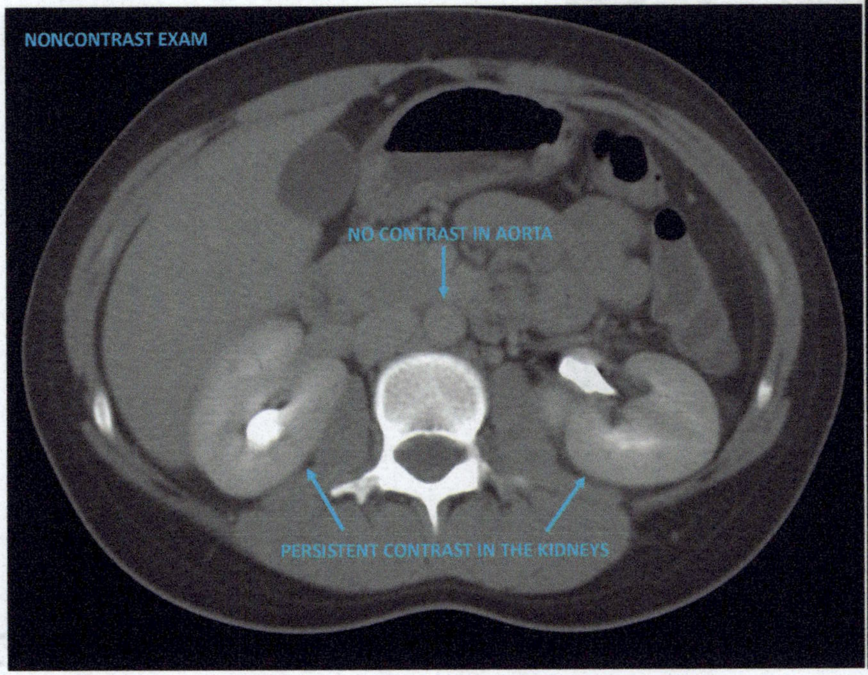

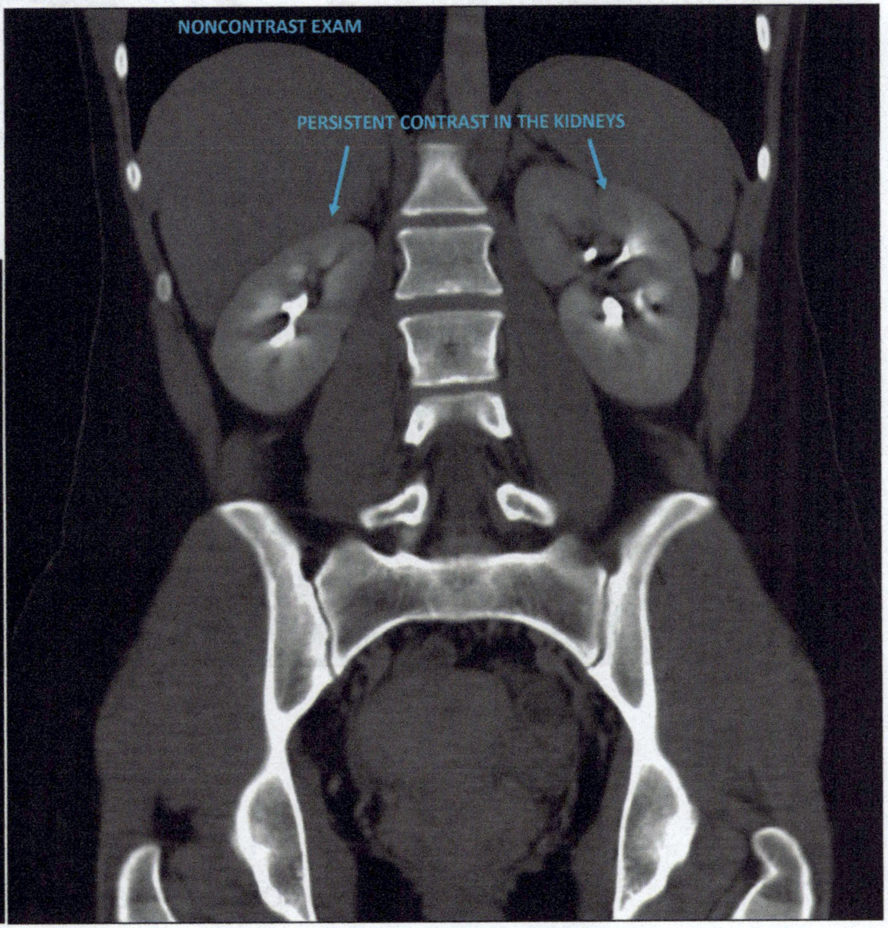

GENITOURINARY

DELAYED NEPHROGRAM

IMAGING: Absence or reduction of the normal renal parenchymal enhancement on nephrographic phase images.

USMLE POINTS: Etiologies:
Obstructive uropathy
Renal vein thrombosis
Renal artery stenosis
Extrinsic compression (Page kidney)

MODALITIES: Seen on CT WO

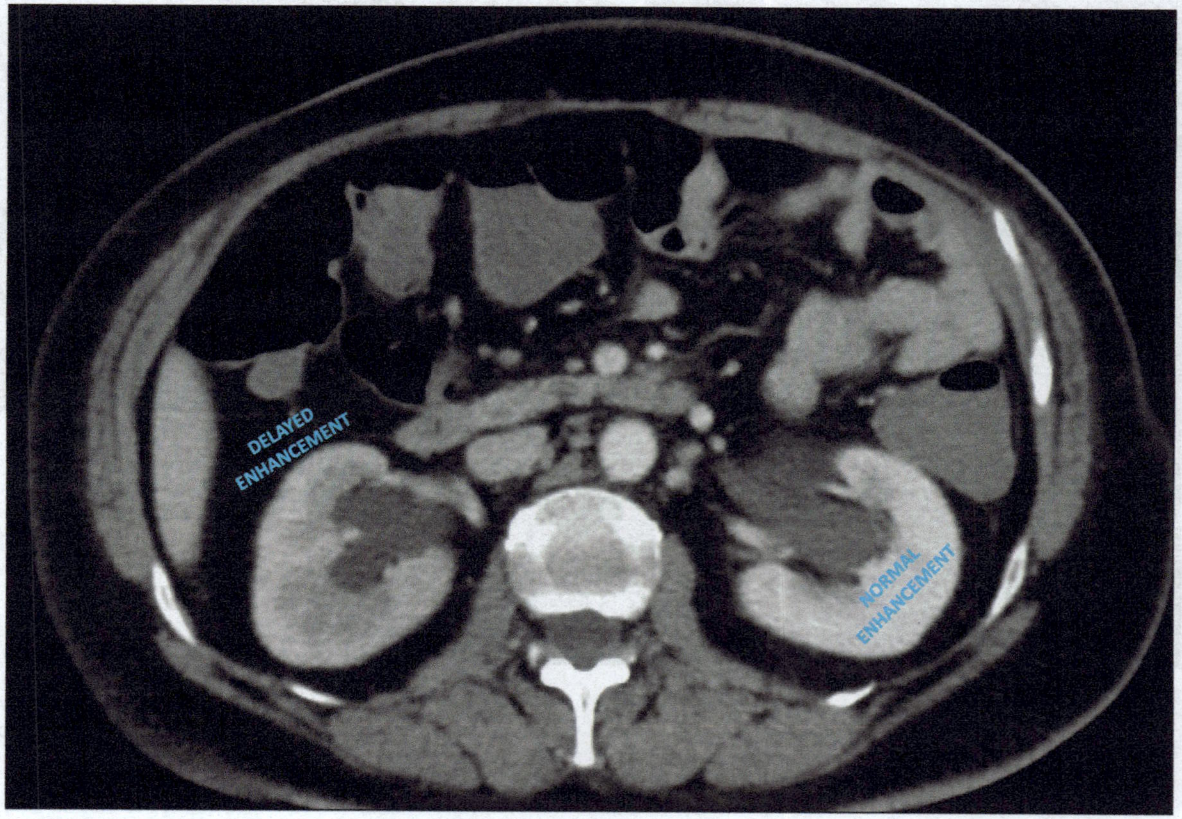

GENITOURINARY

PYELONEPHRITIS

IMAGING: **Striated or patchy nephrogram**
Asymmetric perinephric stranding

USMLE POINTS: **Fevers, flank pain (CVA tenderness), nausea/vomiting, chills**
Ascending UTI (most commonly E. coli)
Outpatient oral antibiotic therapy with a fluoroquinolone (uncomplicated)
Diabetics → Emphysematous pyelonephritis

MODALITIES: CT **W (MUST HAVE CONTRAST)**

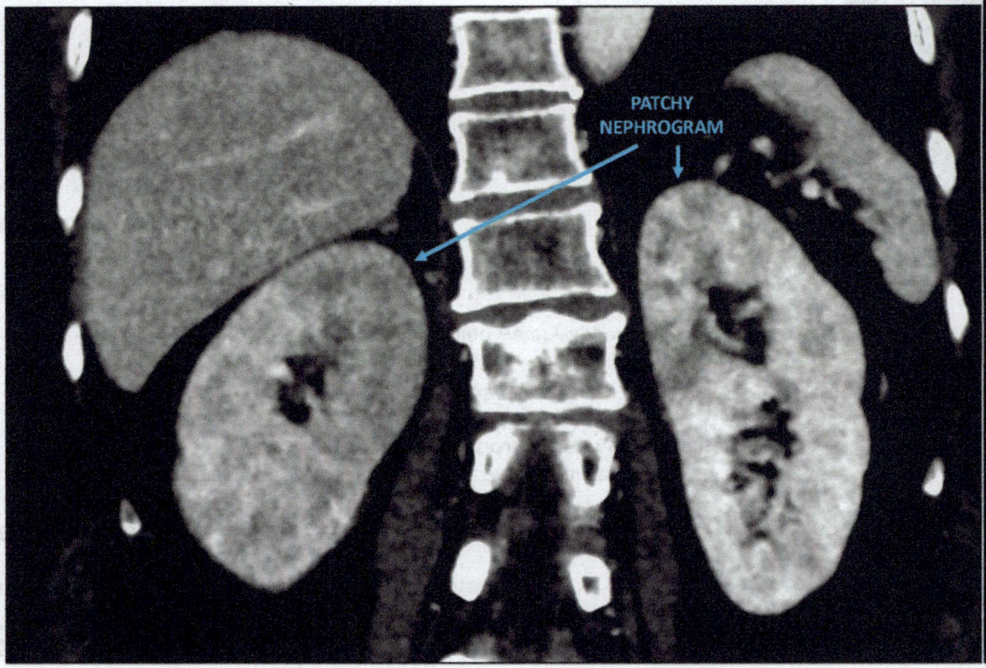

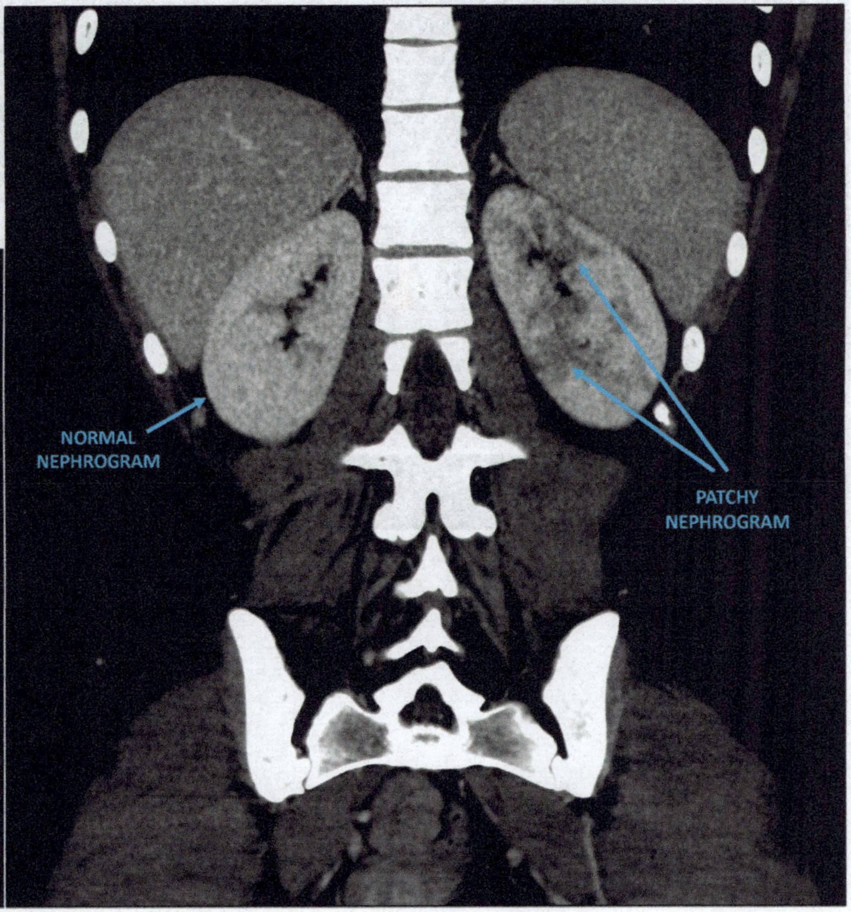

GENITOURINARY

TESTICULAR SEMINOMA

IMAGING: Homogenous **hypoechoic** mass in the testicle

USMLE POINTS: **Germ cell tumors (~95)**

Seminomas:
- Cells can resemble primordial germ cells
- **Most common testicular tumor (germ cell)**
- **Male 15 – 49 years old**
- **Increased placental ALP**
- **Painless**
- Histology: Clear and watery-appearing cytoplasm ("fried-egg")

Non-seminomas

MODALITIES: US

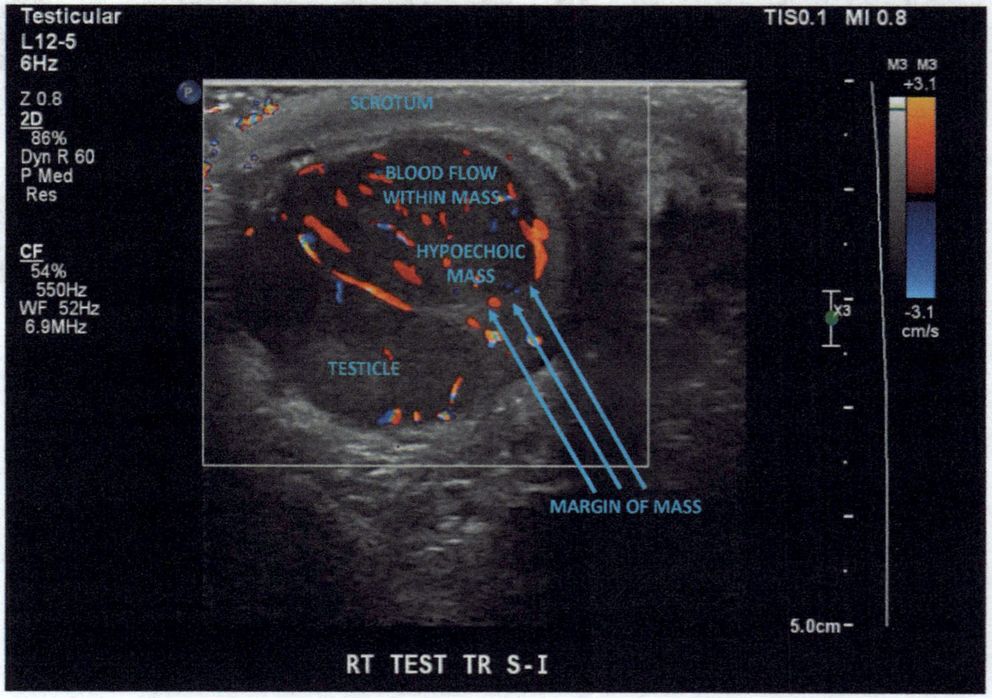

GENITOURINARY

VARICOCELE

IMAGING: **Dilatation of vessels of pampiniform plexus > 2 mm → "Bag-of-worms" appearance**
Augmentation to valsalva

USMLE POINTS: Dilated veins in pampiniform plexus due to increased venous pressure
Unilateral right-sided varicocele is worrisome → Requires evaluation of the retroperitoneum (exclude a mass)
Positive transillumination test

Associations:
- Pain
- **Infertility** (increased temperature impairs spermatogenesis)
- Nutcracker syndrome: Compression of Left renal vein between Aorta and SMA

Treatment:
- Surgical ligation
- Venous embolization

MODALITIES: US

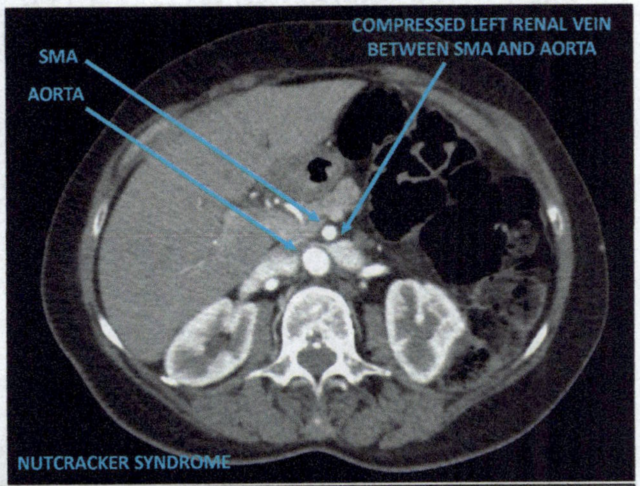

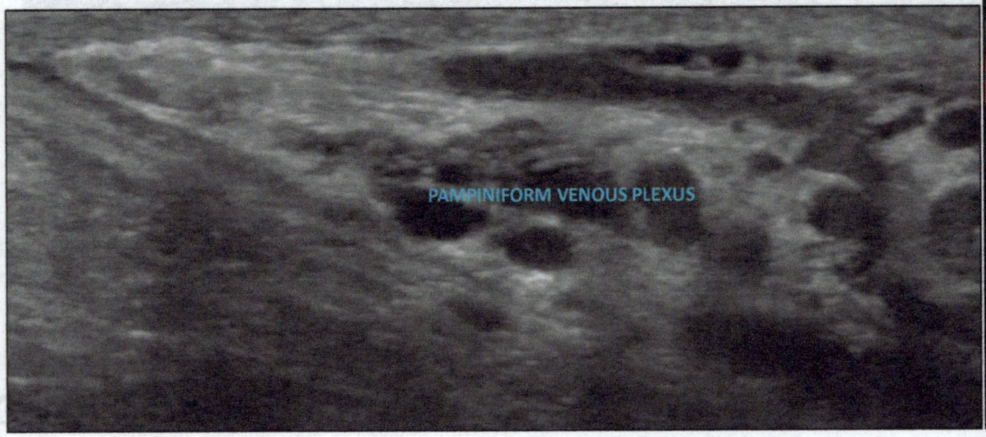

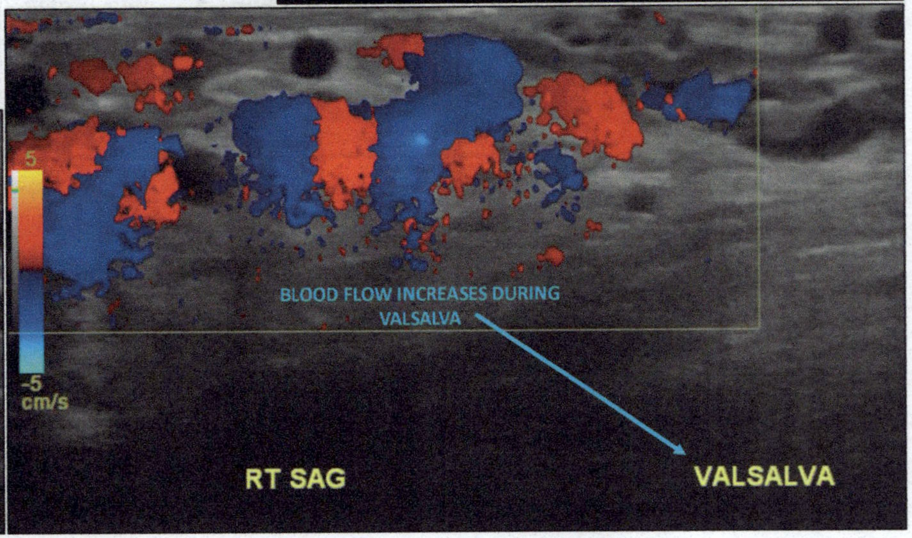

GENITOURINARY

HYDROCELE

IMAGING: **Congenital serous fluid collections**
Between the layers of the tunica vaginalis
Fluid collects in thin sheath surrounding testicle

USMLE POINTS: Congenital: Due to incomplete obliteration of **processes vaginalis**
Resolves within 1 year

Acquired: Infection, trauma, tumor

MODALITIES: US

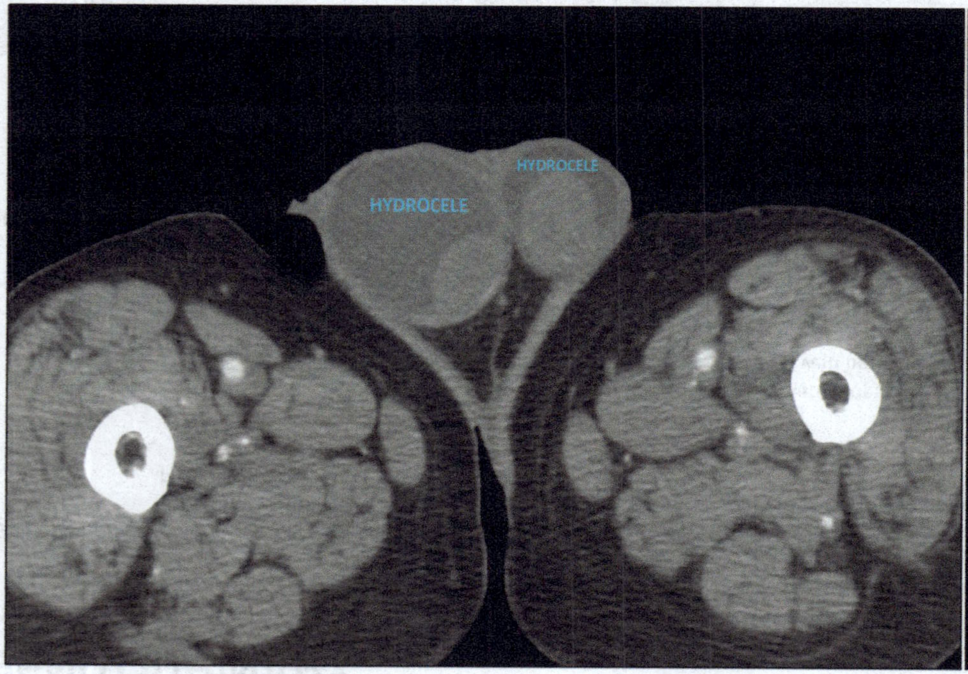

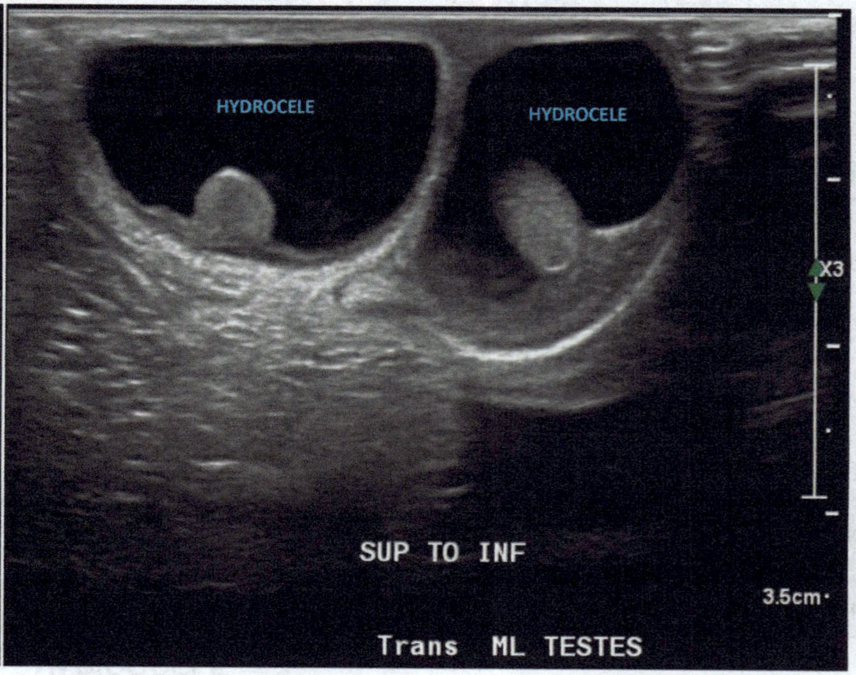

GENITOURINARY

IMAGING: Enlarged, nodular prostate gland
Narrowing of urethra → Bladder outlet obstruction / wall thickening

USMLE POINTS:

Risk factor: **Old age**

Urinary symptoms:
- Post-void dribbling
- Increased urgency and frequency
- Nocturia
- Weak urinary stream

Treatment:
- **Alpha blockers**
- **5-alpha reductase inhibitors**
- **Tadalafil**
- TURP

MODALITIES: US / MRI WWO

BENIGN PROSTATIC HYPERTROPHY

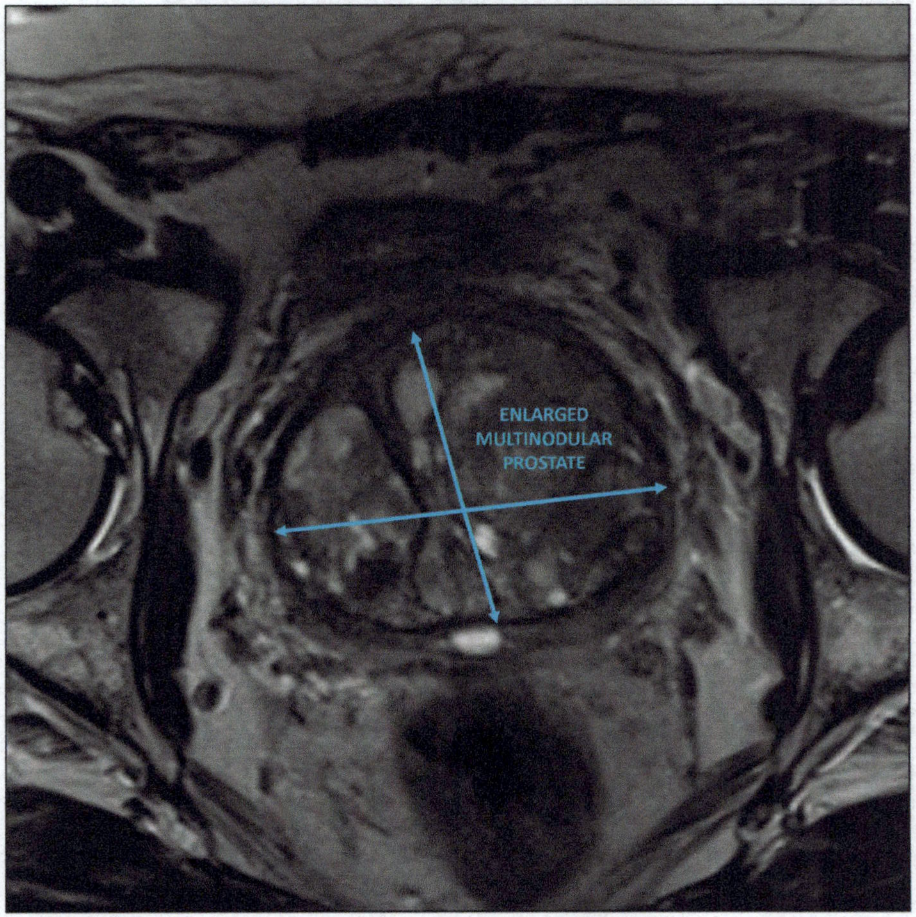

GENITOURINARY

IMAGING: Deposition of calcium salts in the medulla of the kidney

USMLE POINTS: Etiologies:
- **Hyperparathyroidism**
- Medullar sponge kidney
- RTA – Type 1
- Hypervitaminosis D

MODALITIES: US / CT WO

MEDULLARY NEPHROCALCINOSIS

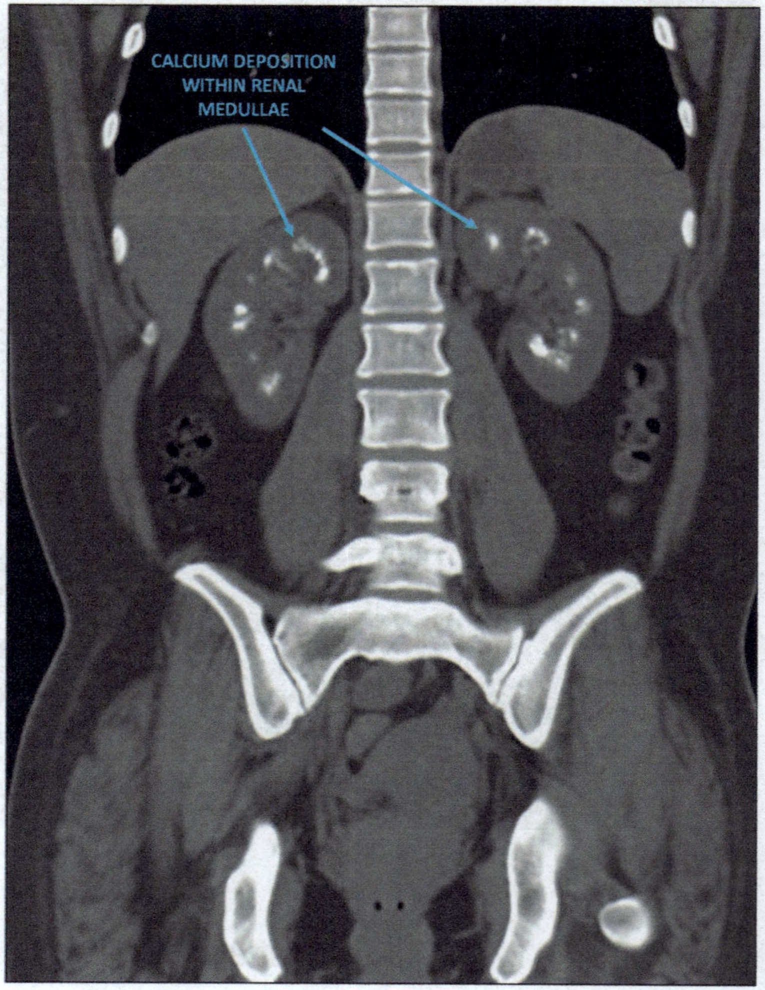

GENITOURINARY

PHEOCHROMOCYTOMA

IMAGING: Large, heterogeneous masses +/- areas of necrosis and cystic change
Know location of adrenal glands on CT

USMLE POINTS: **Rule of 10%**
- **10% familial**
- **10% malignant**
- **10% extra-adrenal**

Associations:
- **MEN 2A**
- **MEN 2B**
- **VHL**
- **NF1**
- **Sturge-Weber**
- **TS**

Increased catecholamines and metanephrines in urine and plasma

5 P's: Pressure (hypertension
- Pain (headache)
- Perspiration
- Palpitations
- Pallor

Treatment: **Irreversible alpha-antagonists → b-blockers prior to tumor resection**

MODALITIES: CT W / MRI WWO

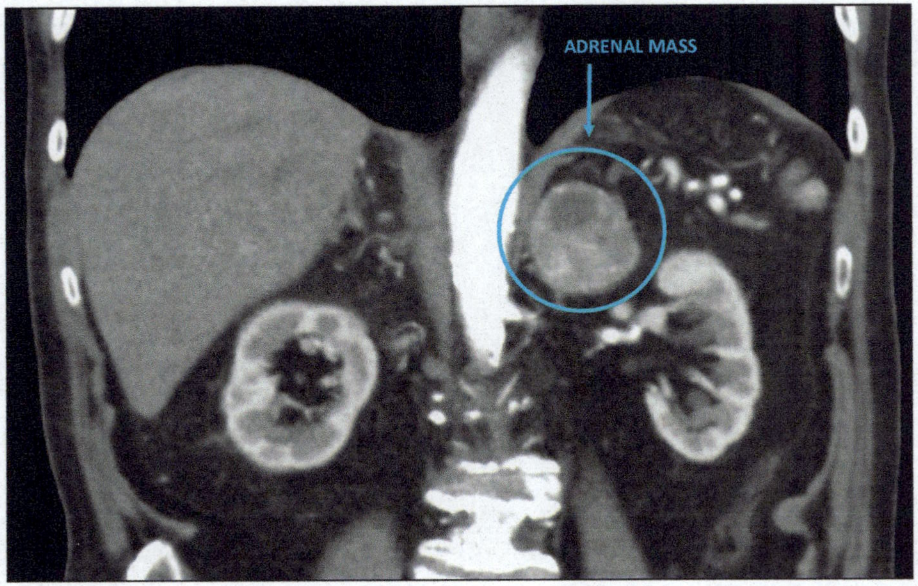

SECTION 2

CHAPTER 9: IMAGING MODALITIES

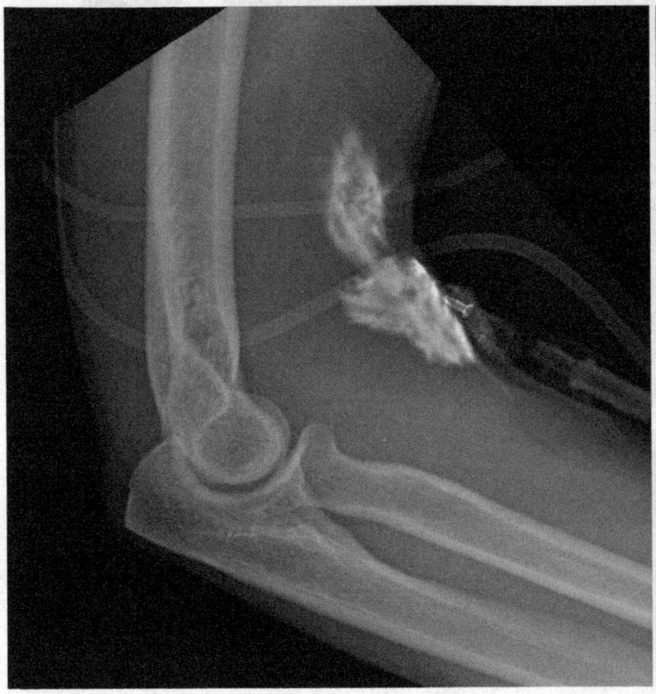
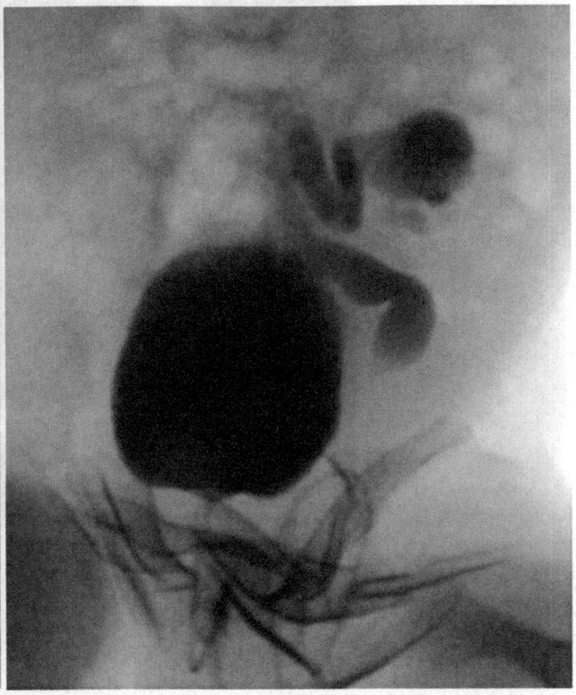

HEAD CT WITHOUT CONTRAST

Acute blood, skull fractures, loss of gray-white matter differentiation (stroke), or mass lesions which may explain clinical symptoms

COMMON INDICATIONS:

- **Stroke**
- **Acute Head trauma**
- Suspected acute **intracranial hemorrhage**
- **Acute Headache**
- Mental status change
- **Initial evaluation for acute neurologic deficits**
- Coma
- Immediate post-op eval following brain surgery
- Suspected shunt malfunction
- Suspected hydrocephalus
- Evaluating psychiatric disorders
- Suspected mass or tumor
- Brain herniation
- Skull lesions (MM)
- **Initial evaluation for seizures / syncope**
- Detection or evaluation of calcification (certain tumors)

NOT FOR:

- Infection
- Cancer

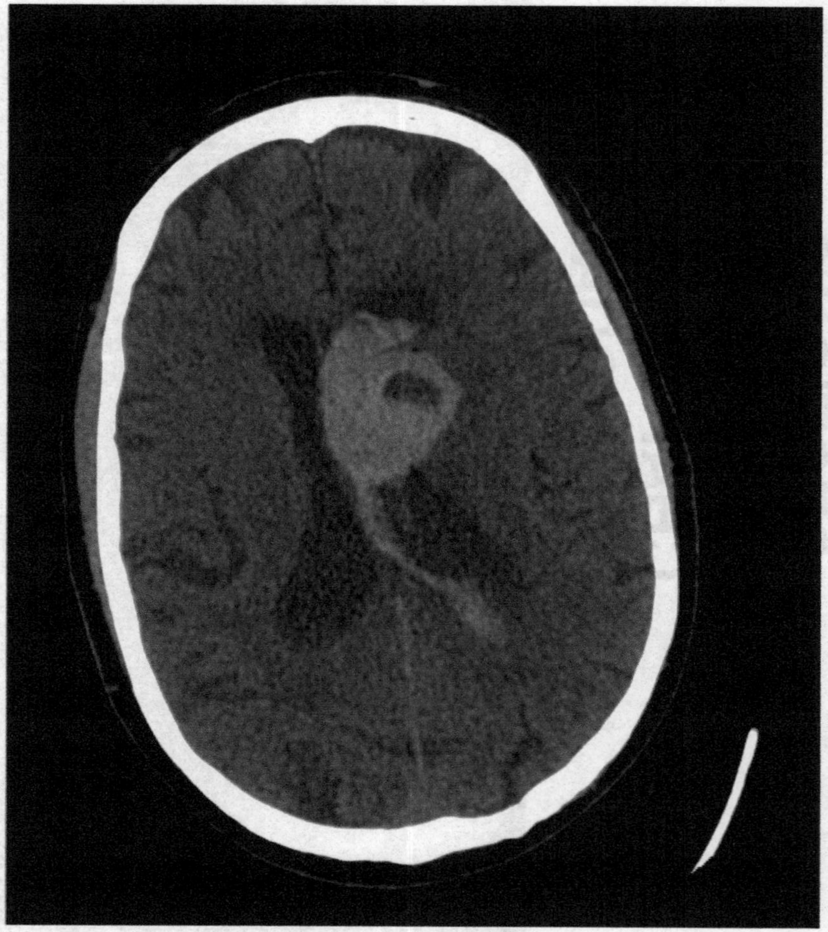

HEAD CT WITH AND WITHOUT VS. HEAD CTA

When MRI is contraindicated (NSF, metal, etc...)
Most indications are better evaluated on MRI
Almost never the answer!

COMMON INDICATIONS:	Suspected intracranial **infection**	(MRI better)
	Cancer	(MRI better)
	Seizures	(MRI better)
NOT FOR:	**Trauma**	
	Stroke	
	Acute or chronic headache	
	Dementia	
	Coma	
HEAD CTA:	Ordered with noncontrast Head CT to evaluation for arterial occlusion	

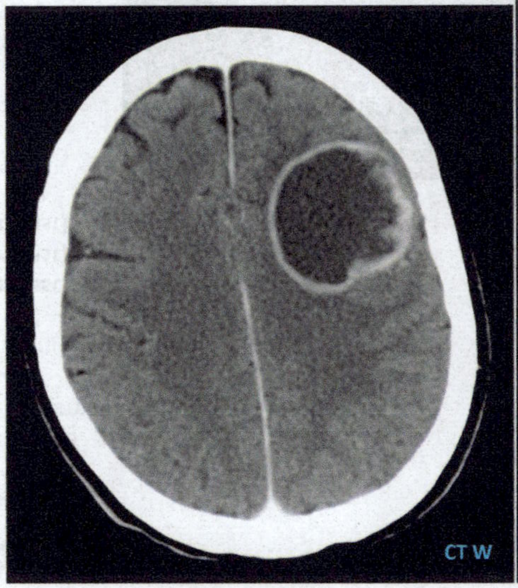

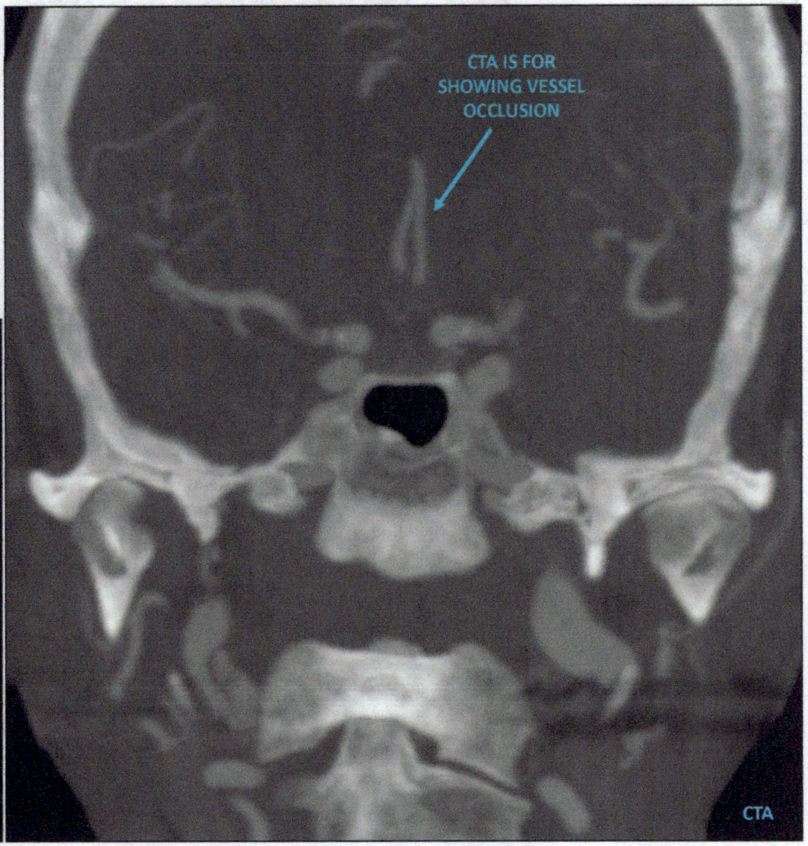

BRAIN MRI WITHOUT CONTRAST

COMMON INDICATIONS:

Acute ischemia and infarction (DWI)
Chronic headache
Neurodegenerative disorders / Dementia
Congenital disorders & anatomical abnormalities
Hemorrhage (GRE Sn = CT Sn)
MRI > CT: Detection of diffuse axonal injury, post-traumatic brain injury

Seizure	**(Better with contrast)**
Infection	**(Better with contrast)**
Cancer	**(Better with contrast)**

NOT FOR:

Trauma
Coma

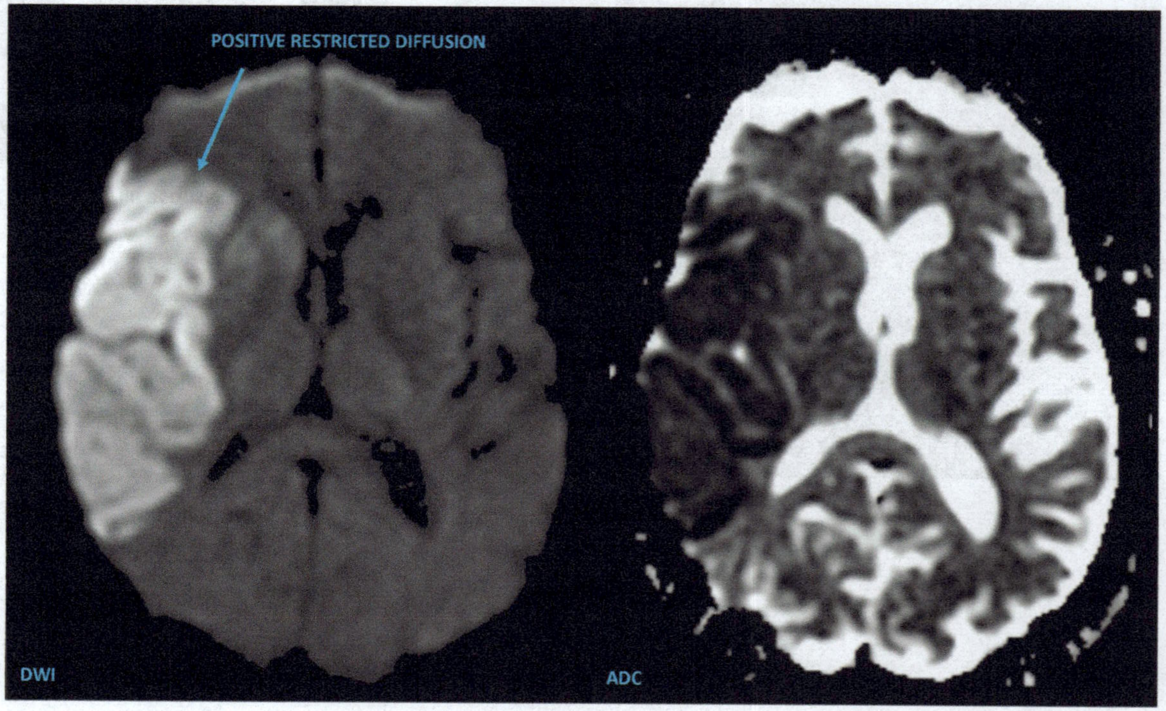

BRAIN MRI WITH AND WITHOUT CONTRAST

COMMON INDICATIONS:

Neoplastic conditions
Infectious disorders
Encephalitis
Meningitis
Abscess
Pituitary evaluation
Seizures
Inflammatory and autoimmune disorders including disorders of myelination (MS Protocol)

Vascular malformations: Developmental venous anomaly
Cavernous angioma
Arteriovenous malformation
Arteriovenous fistulas

Epilepsy and movement disorders
Follow-up of treatment/tumor resection

NOT FOR:

Trauma
Stroke
Acute headache
Chronic headache
Dementia

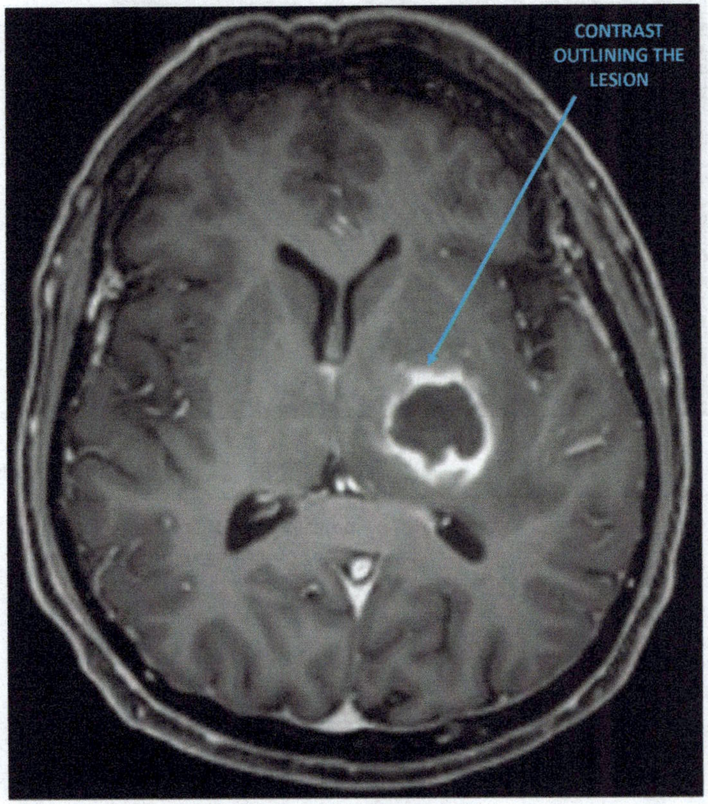

SPINE CT WITHOUT CONTRAST

COMMON INDICATIONS:

- Better for **fractures** than MRI (although MRI can show edema without obvious fracture)
- CT has largely been **replaced by MR for most screening examinations of the spine**
- **Traumatic** injuries (better for fractures than MRI)
- **Acute spine trauma in adults**
- Vertebral **compression/insufficiency fractures in both** acute and chronic clinical situations
- Degenerative conditions and osteoarthritis evaluation
- Lumbar stenosis or in evaluating **disc degeneration** and is the primary evaluation technique → **when MRI is contraindicated**
- Infectious processes of the spine and related paraspinal tissues/structures → **when MRI is contraindicated**
- Pre-surgical planning (complementary to MRI)
- Abnormalities related to alignment or orientation of the spine (scoliosis or spondylolysis +/- spondylolisthesis)
- Postoperative evaluations
- Marrow-replacing conditions such as multiple myeloma

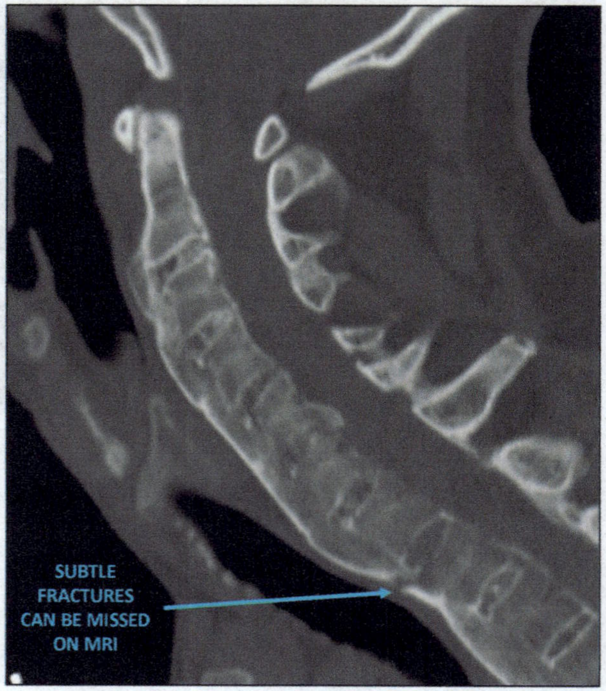

SPINE MRI

Better for water containing structures (ligamentous, spinal canal, disc, etc...)
Superior soft-tissue contrast (including the ability to evaluate the marrow compartment)
Lack of ionizing radiation

NONCONTRAST: Degenerative disk disease and its sequelae in the lumbar, thoracic, and cervical spine (Xray's first)
Disc herniations, nerve impingement

CONTRAST: Gadolinium is essential in the evaluation of **infection, inflammation, demyelination**

Neurodegenerative disorders: **Subacute** combined degeneration
Spinal muscular atrophy
ALS

Demyelinating disease: MS
ADEM
GBS
SLE

Infectious conditions: Spinal/disc infection
Vertebral osteomyelitis
Epidural abscess
Post-op infection

Neoplastic: Spinal cord tumors
Congenital spine and spinal cord malformations

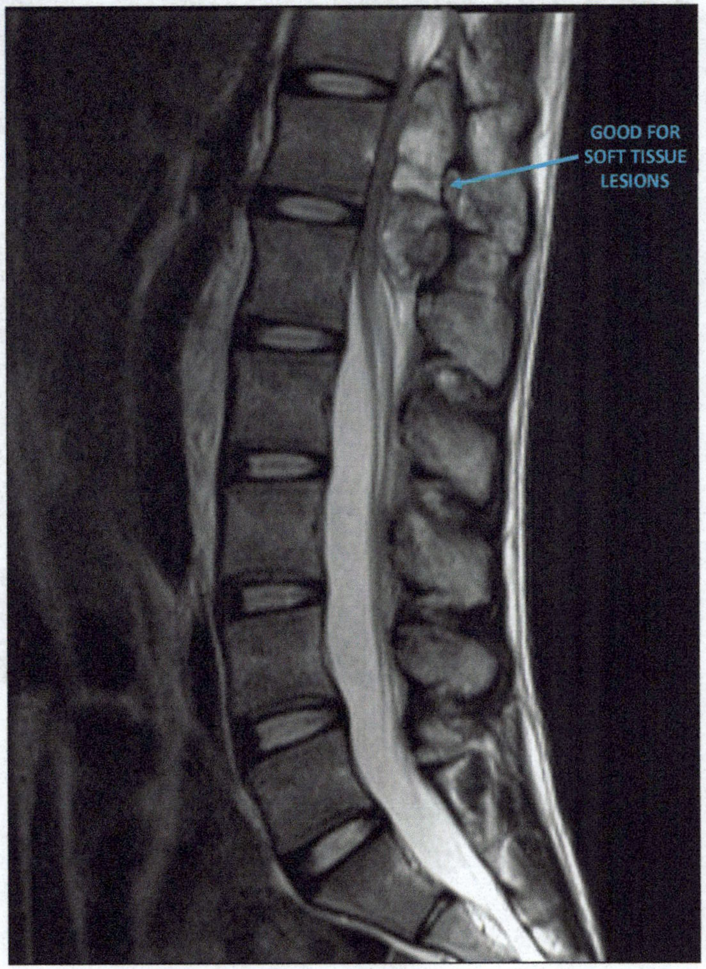

CT ABDOMEN & PELVIS WITHOUT CONTRAST

COMMON INDICATIONS: Evaluating for **urolithiasis** → Renal, ureteral and urinary bladder stones
Non-contrast exam can used to evaluate bowel **pathology if there is a contraindication to IV contrast**

NOT FOR:
Abdominal visceral trauma
Abdominal fluid collections/abscesses
Abdominal infections and inflammatory processes
Trauma patients (unless only osseous trauma)

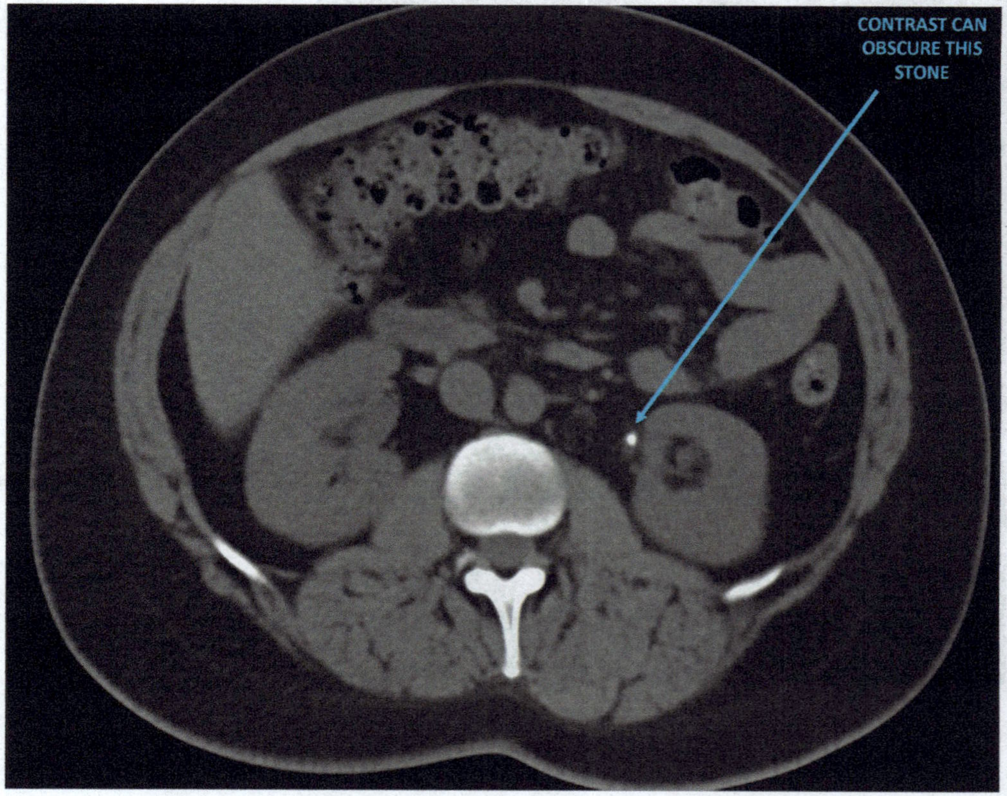

CT ABDOMEN & PELVIS WITH CONTRAST (PORTAL VENOUS PHASE)

COMMON INDICATIONS:

Abdominal or pelvic pain
Abdominal and pelvic trauma
Evaluation for **bowel obstruction**
Abdominal or pelvic **masses or fluid collections**
Evaluation of primary or metastatic malignancies

Post surgical complications:
- Abscess
- Lymphocele
- Radiation change
- Fistula/sinus tract formation)

Liver disease:
- Cirrhosis
- Steatosis
- Iron deposition disease

Inflammatory processes:
- Inflammatory bowel disease
- Infectious bowel disease and its complications

Acute bowel pathology:
- **Acute appendicitis**
- **Diverticulitis**
- **Enteritis**
- **Colitis**

NOT a CTA Exam

NOT FOR: **Renal Stones**

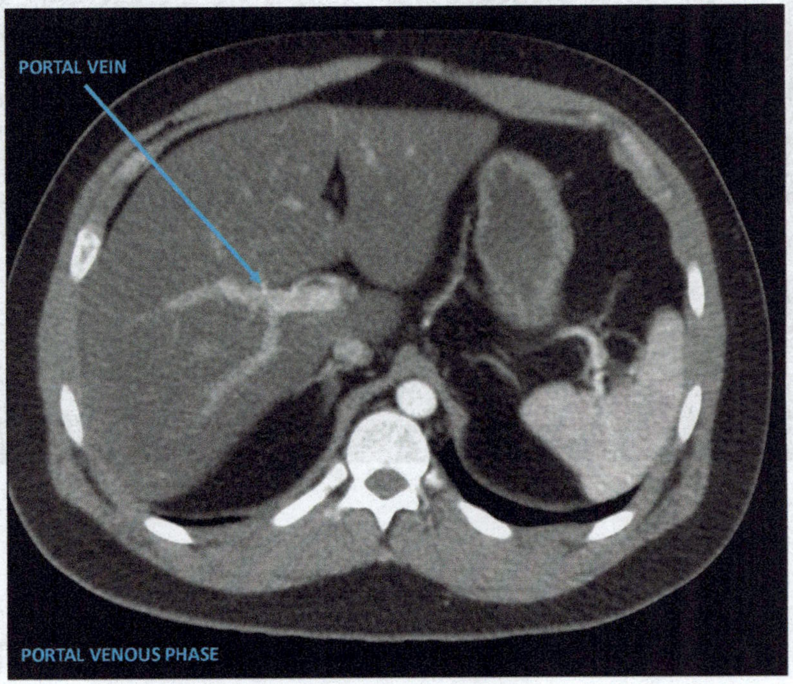

CT ABDOMEN & PELVIS WITH CONTRAST (CTA PHASE)

COMMON INDICATIONS:

Abnormalities of abdominal or pelvic vascular structures
Evaluation for abdominal **aortic aneurysm or dissection**
Evaluation of **gastrointestinal bleeding (multiphase)**
Evaluation for **mesenteric ischemia (SMA)**
Evaluation of post-traumatic or post-surgical vascular injury
Endoleak (multiphase)

NOT FOR:

Abdominal visceral trauma
Abdominal fluid collections/abscesses
Abdominal infections and inflammatory processes
Renal stones

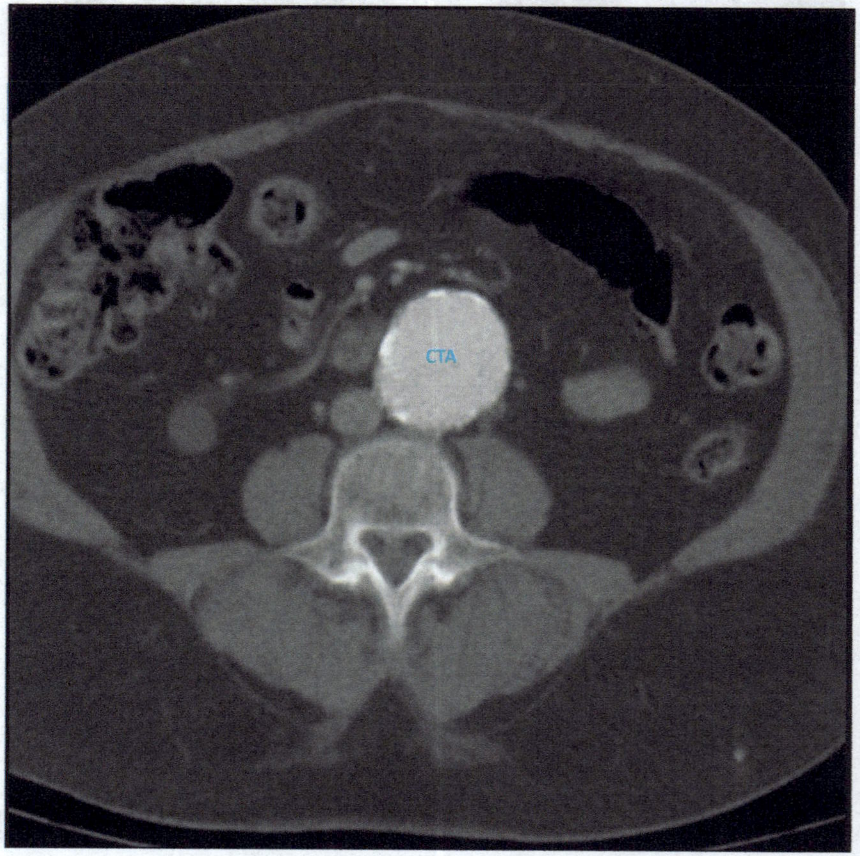

CHEST CT WITHOUT CONTRAST

CT CHEST WITHOUT CONTRAST:

Abnormalities discovered on chest radiographs
Pulmonary parenchymal and airway disease (HRCT may be better)
Acute respiratory illness such as pneumonia (unresolving)
Follow-up for solitary pulmonary nodule (SPN)
Evaluation of pneumonia, heart failure (pleural effusions / pulmonary edema)
Evaluation for pneumothorax

HRCT:

Type of Noncontrast chest CT
Detect, characterize, and determine the extent of diseases that involve the lung parenchyma and airways.
Evaluation of known or clinically suspected **diffuse lung disease**
Quantification of the extent of diffuse lung disease
Occupational lung diseases: **Silicosis, pneumoconiosis**

NOT FOR:

Chest Trauma (need contrast to see evaluate aorta)
Tumor or inflammation
Pulmonary mass/tumor (other than SPN)
Vascular pathology
HRCT not for pulmonary nodules (big slice gap)

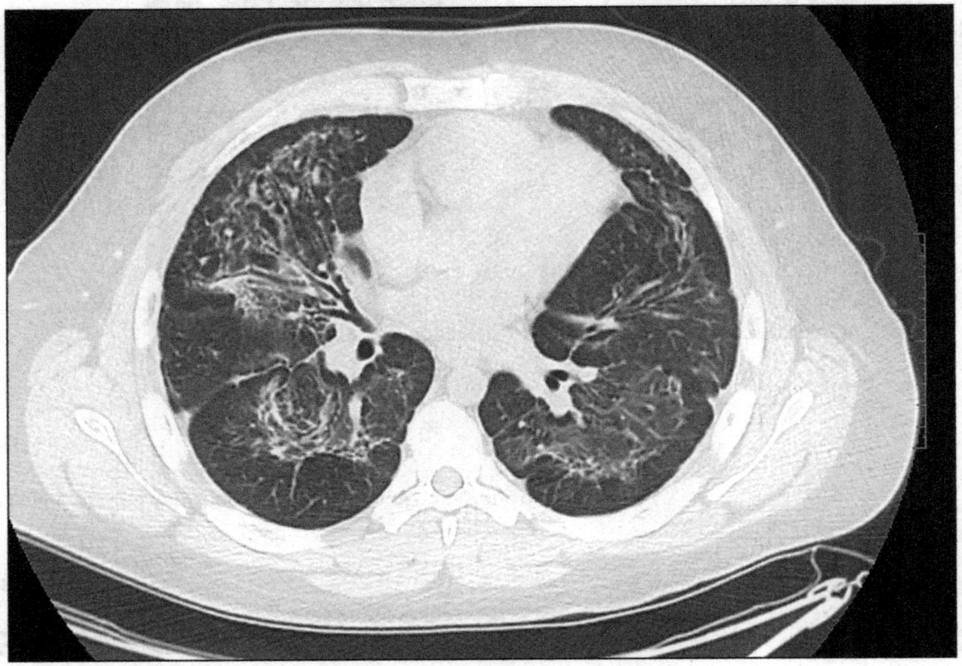

CHEST CT WITH CONTRAST (NON-CTA PHASE)

COMMON INDICATIONS:

Evaluation of abnormalities discovered on chest radiograph images
Blunt or penetrating trauma
Cancer (Lung cancer; staging; metastatic disease)
Staging and follow-up of lung cancer and other primary thoracic malignancies, and detection and evaluation of metastatic disease.
Evaluation of cardiothoracic extrathoracic diseases
Evaluation of known or suspected thoracic cardiovascular abnormalities
Evaluation of postoperative patients and surgical complications
Evaluation of the chest wall & pleural disease
Treatment planning for radiation therapy
Mediastinal pathology (adenopathy)

NOT FOR:

Pneumonia
Interstitial lung disease, IPF, UIP (HRCT)
Solitary pulmonary nodule (do noncontrast)
ICU patients (x-ray is first line imaging modality)

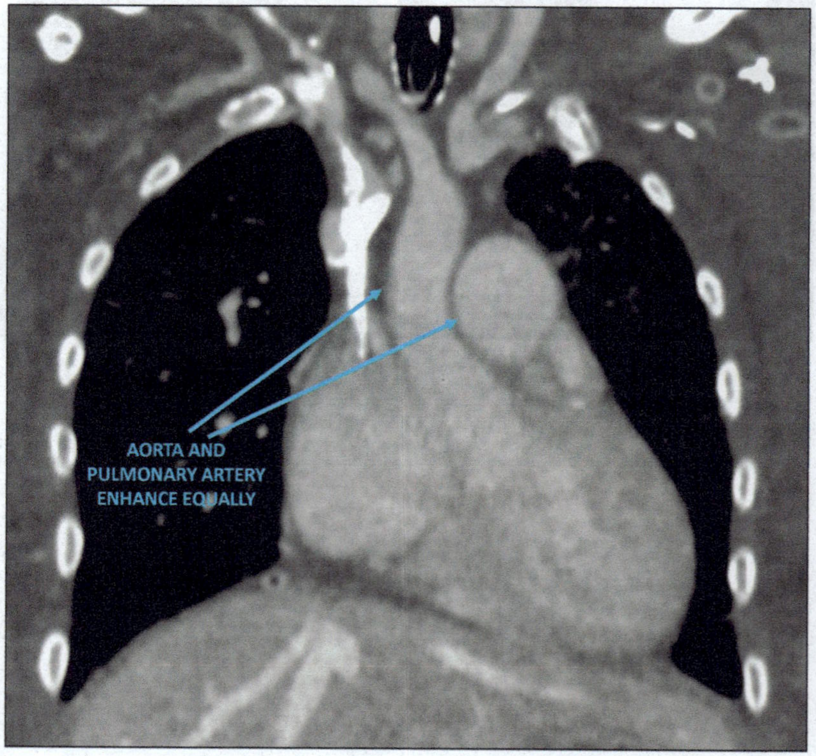

CT CHEST WITH CONTRAST (CTA PHASE)

CTA – AORTIC DISSECTION:

Aortic anatomy
Demonstrate **intimal flaps, branch vessel involvement**
Patency of the false lumen
Aortic atherosclerotic plaque

CTA – PE:

Direct visualization of intraluminal clot
Right ventricular strain
Pulmonary hypertension

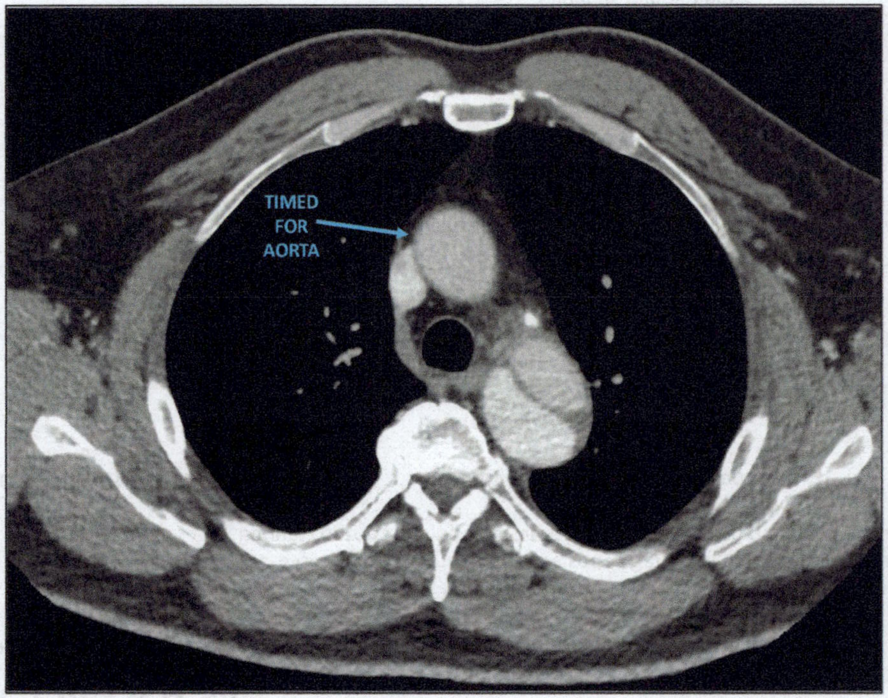

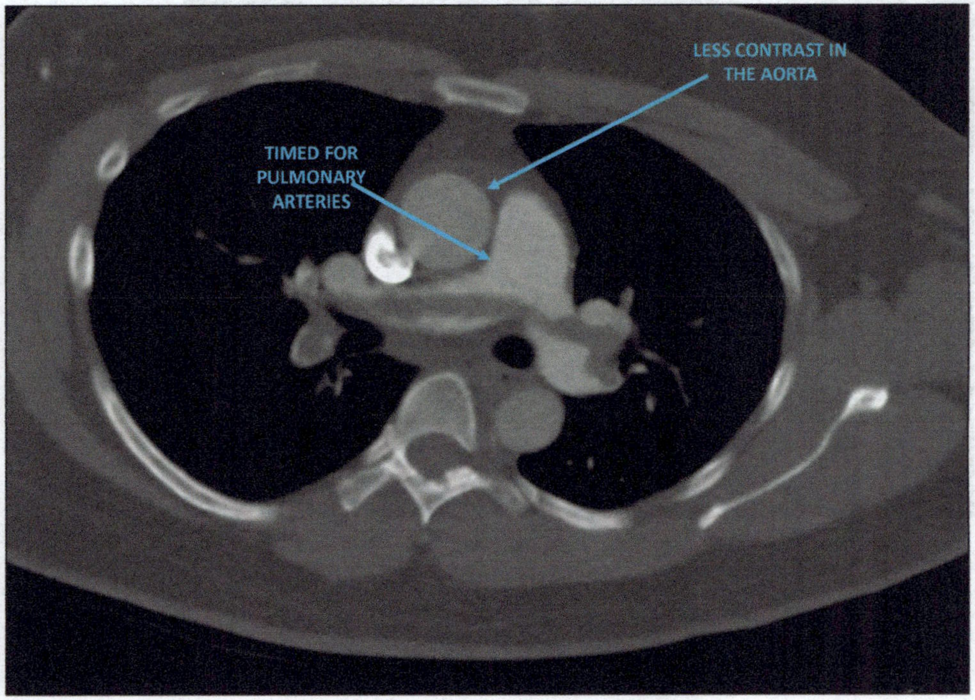

CONTRAST

HIGH-YIELD POINTS:
- **No contrast if GFR <60 → Risk of Nephrogenic Systemic Fibrosis**
- **No contrast if Creatinine > 1.5 or Multiple Myeloma (AKI)**
- **Discontinue contrast before Metformin and resume 48 hours after scan**
- Jod-Basedow phenomenon can be seen after administration of iodine IV contrast
- Barium contrast is contraindicated in toxic megacolon due to risk of perforation

CONTRAST INDUCED NEPHROPATHY:

AKI within 24 – 48 hours after contrast

Contrast causes ATN

Risk factors:
- **CKD**
- **Diabetic nephropathy**
- **MM**
- **Decreased renal perfusion**

Increased serum creatine within 1 – 2 days after contrast

UA:
- Muddy brown granular casts
- Epithelial cell casts

Prevention:
- **Decrease dose**
- **IVNS vs. Sodium bicarbonate**
- **Avoid nephrotoxic medications**
- **Avoiding hypovolemia**

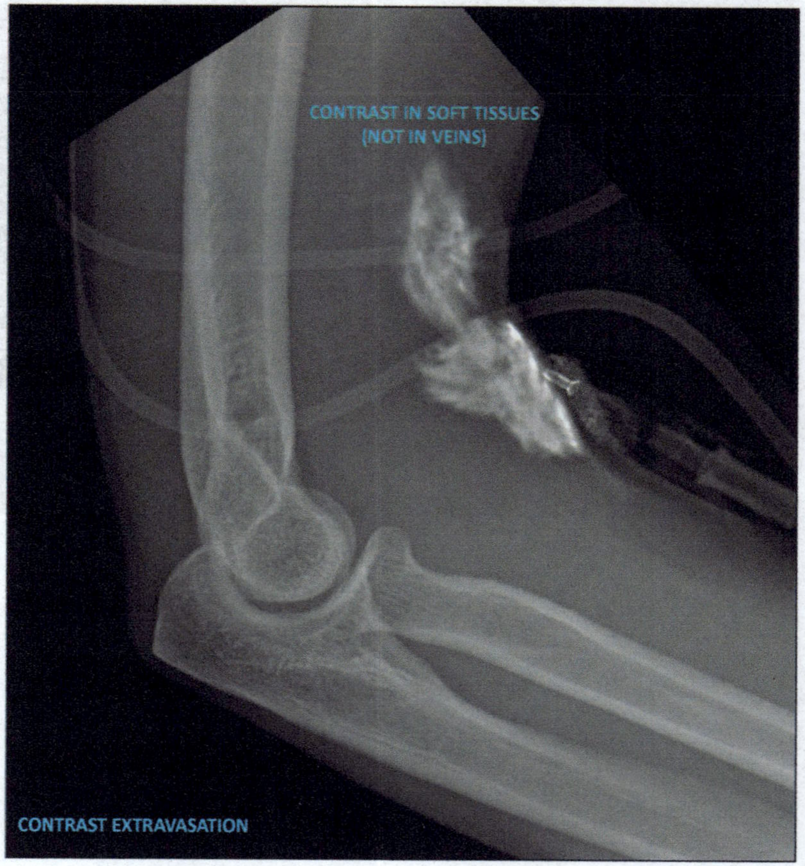

FLUOROSCOPY

VFSE

- Known or suspected **aspiration** pneumonia
- **Oral feeding assessment** for vented pts
- **Protective maneuvers to prevent aspiration**
- Coughing, choking, drooling with swallowing
- Neurologic disorders → **affect swallowing**
- Used primarily for **evaluation of function**

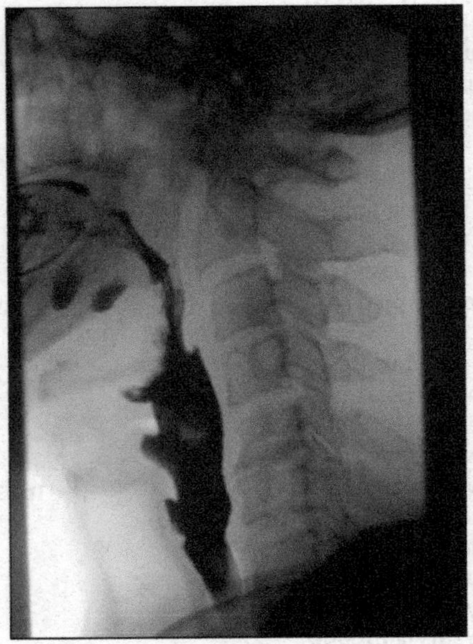

ESOPHAGRAM

- **Postoperative evaluation for leak**
- **Perforation in pneumomediastinum**
- **Esophageal obstruction**
- Dysphagia / Odynophagia
- Esophagitis / Strictures
- GERD

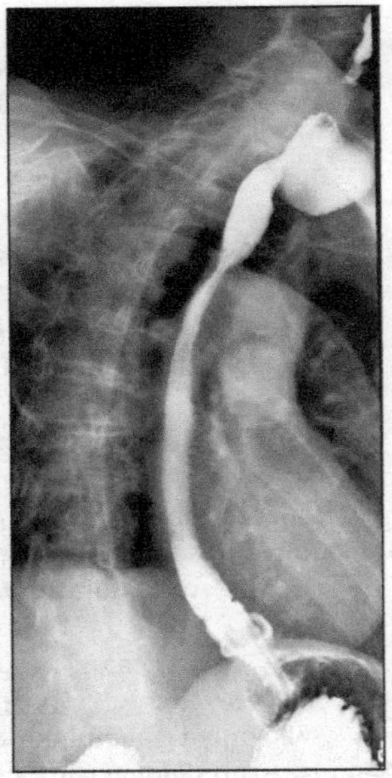

UPPER GI SERIES

- **GERD**
- **Abdominal / epigastric pain**
- Dyspepsia / **Peptic ulcer disease**
- Post-op evaluation for **leak** (water soluble)
- **Duodenal ulcer repair** (water soluble)
- *Gastric sleeve evaluation* (water soluble)
- Suspected or known gastritis or duodenitis

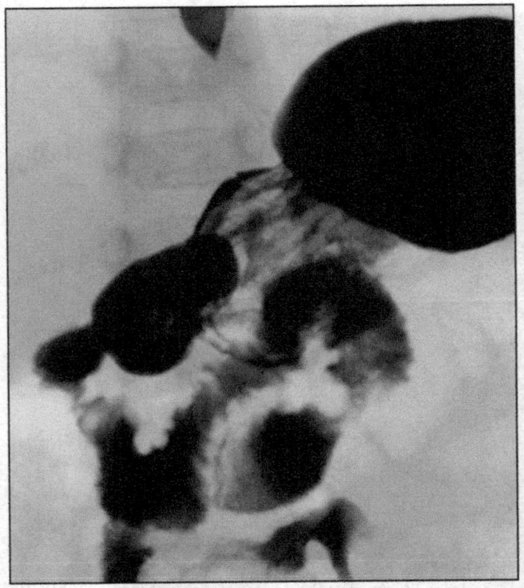

BARIUM ENEMA

- **Diverticular disease (not acute diverticulitis)**
- **Inflammatory bowel disease (not active)**
- **Colon cancer** screening (mass or stricture)
- Incomplete colonoscopy
- Distal obstruction
- Preoperative evaluation prior to anastomosis
- Abdominal pain / Diarrhea / Constipation
- **Weight loss**
- History of previous colon polyp or neoplasm
- Bowel fistulas (Chron's disease)

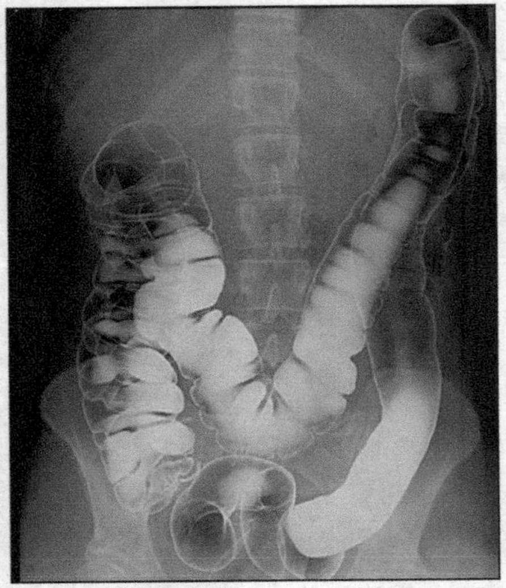

ULTRASOUND: ABDOMEN

COMMON INDICATIONS:

Abdominal pain
Palpable abnormalities such as an abdominal mass or organomegaly
Abnormal labs or abnormal findings on other imaging examinations
Abdominal and/or retroperitoneal pathology
Abdominal trauma (FAST)
Search for the presence of free

RENAL:

Evaluation of urinary tract infection
Flank and/or back pain (renal stones / hydronephrosis)
Abnormal laboratory values (echogenic kidneys)
Suspected congenital abnormalities
Transplantation evaluation (doppler)

FAST EXAM:

Free fluid / blood in peritoneal, pleural, pericardial cavities
NOT used to identify specific organ injuries
False positive in patients with ascites
Cannot be used to asses retroperitoneal space

EVALUATION OF:

Gallstones
Choledocholithiasis
Gallbladder pathology
Hepatitis & Jaundice
Splenomegaly
Hepatic steatosis
Biliary ductal dilation

COMPONENTS:

Liver
Gallbladder
CBD
Pancreas
Kidneys
Spleen
Aorta
IVC

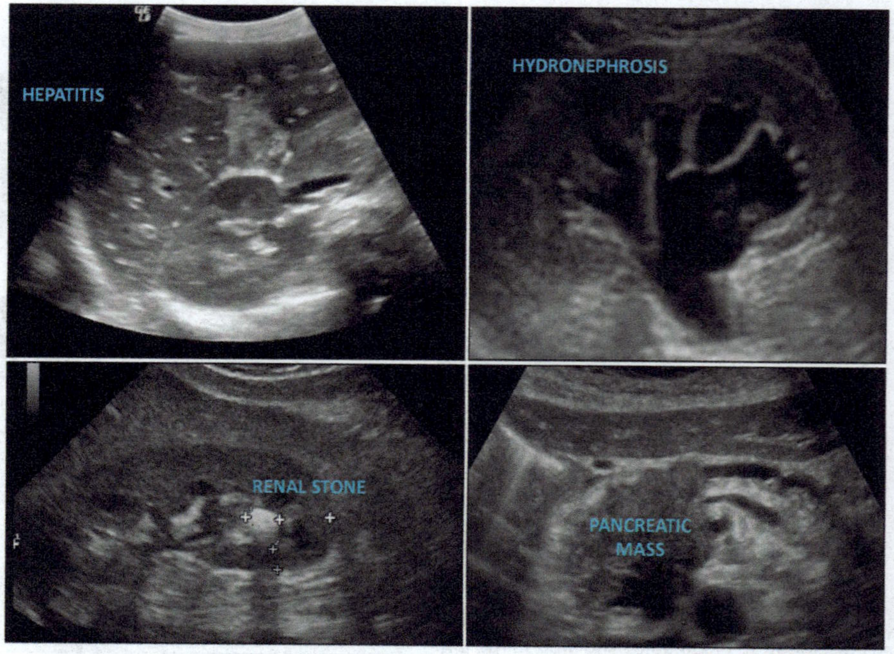

ULTRASOUND: PELVIS

COMMON INDICATIONS:

Evaluation for **pelvic pain**
Evaluation for uterine **fibroids / adenomyosis**
Evaluation for dysfunctional **uterine bleeding / menstrual abnormalities**
Evaluation for **ovarian torsion**
Evaluation for **ovarian cystic lesions +/- rupture**
Evaluation for **endometriosis**
Evaluation for **pelvic inflammatory disease / salpingitis / TOA**
Evaluation of pregnancy and/or associated complications
Evaluation for **ectopic pregnancy**

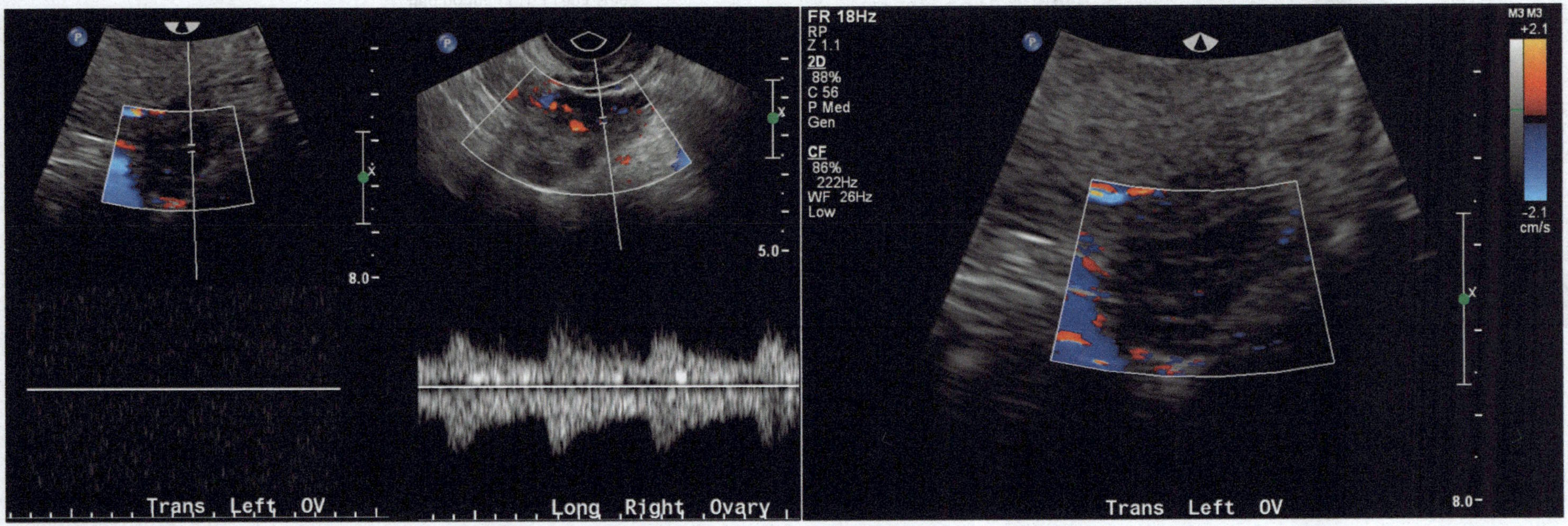

XRAY: CHEST

COMMON INDICATIONS:

Infection
Pneumothorax
Assessment of **lines and tubes**
Preoperative clearance
Evaluate for **fluid overloaded states (pleural effusion / edema)**
Chest trauma (ribs, mediastinum)
Asthma / Bronchiolitis
Inhaled foreign body
Evaluate cardiac silhouette (heart size / pericardial effusion)
Evaluate for pleural effusions
Free air (must be upright)
Assess osseous structures (ribs in trauma patient)

NOT FOR:

Evaluation of evaluation of **murmurs**
Evaluation of **hypertension**
Evaluation of pulmonary embolism
Aortic dissection / PE

CXR PROTOCOL:

No lateral:
Consolidation
Pneumothorax
Pregnant patients
Children under 16
Bed bound (ICU) / can't stand

Pneumothorax: **INSP/EXP**

Foreign Body: **INSP/EXP or UPRIGHT/LD**

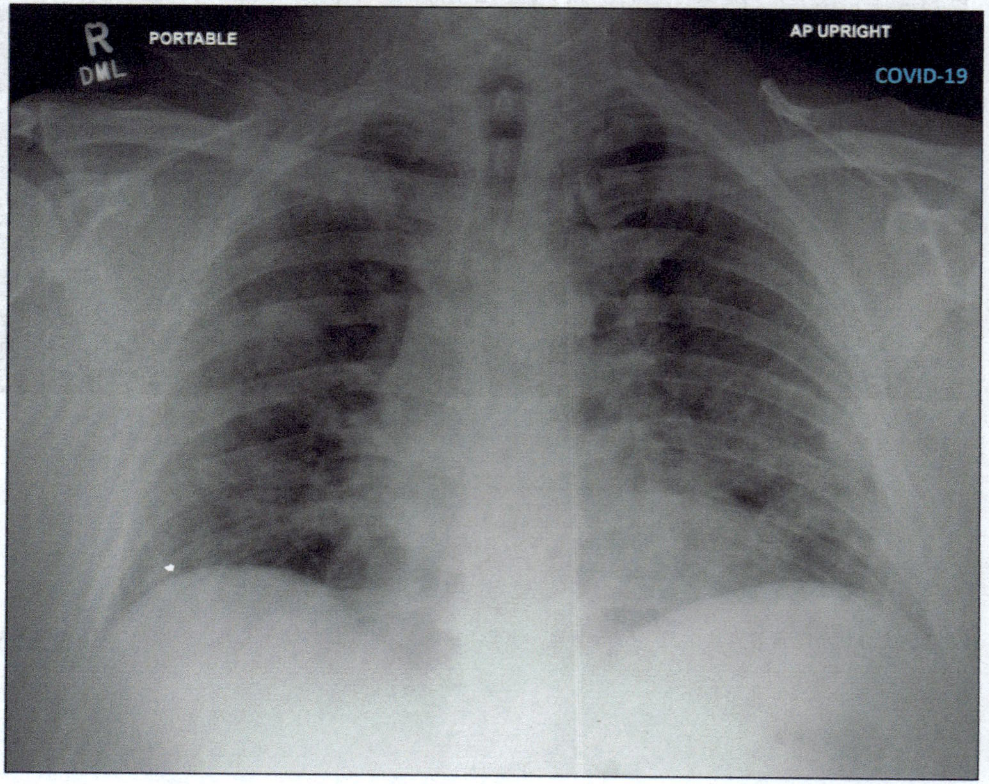

XRAY: ABDOMINAL

COMMON INDICATIONS:

- **Suspected bowel obstruction / perforation (Need "Free Air views)**
- **Suspected intussusception**
- **Foreign Bodies**
- Suspected Abdominal Mass
- Renal stones (CT noncontrast better)
- Suspected constipation in children

NOT FOR:

- **Most blunt abdominal trauma (CT with contrast PV-phase)**
- Pyloric stenosis (ultrasound)
- Vague central abdominal pain
- Gastroenteritis
- Hematemesis
- Uncomplicated appendicitis
- **Evaluation of gallstones**

FREE-AIR VIEWS:

- **Cross table lateral**
- **Erect**
- **LLD**

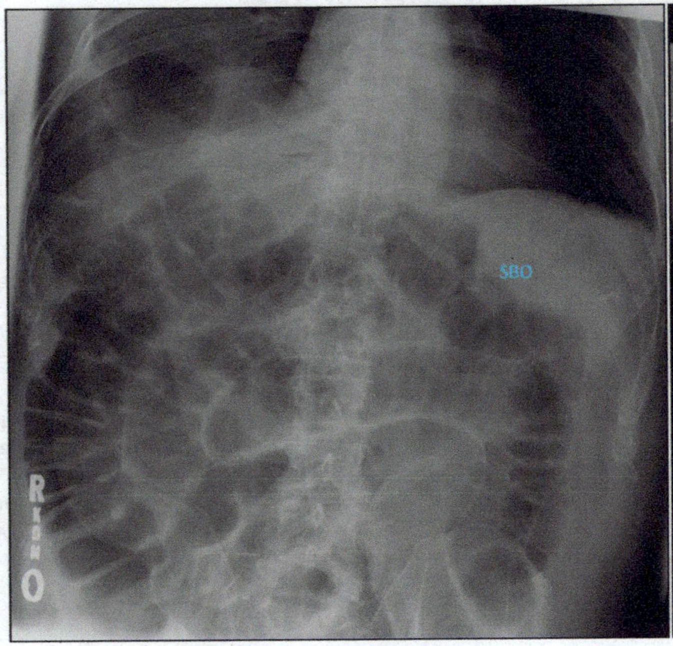

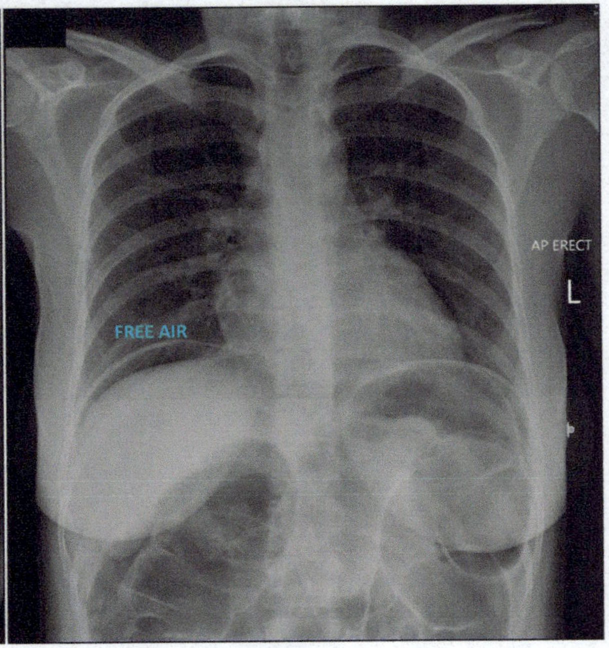

XRAY: SKELETAL

COMMON INDICATIONS:

Trauma
Multiple views: "1 view is no view"
Post-reduction films for dislocations
First line for **skeletal trauma**
Often no CT needed for further evaluation (exceptions)
Non accidental Trauma → Complete skeletal survey
Degenerative Joint Disease
Painful hip: SCFE, LCP
Osteomyelitis (MRI better)
Septic arthritis (MRI better)
Metabolic bone disorders (hyperparathyroidism)

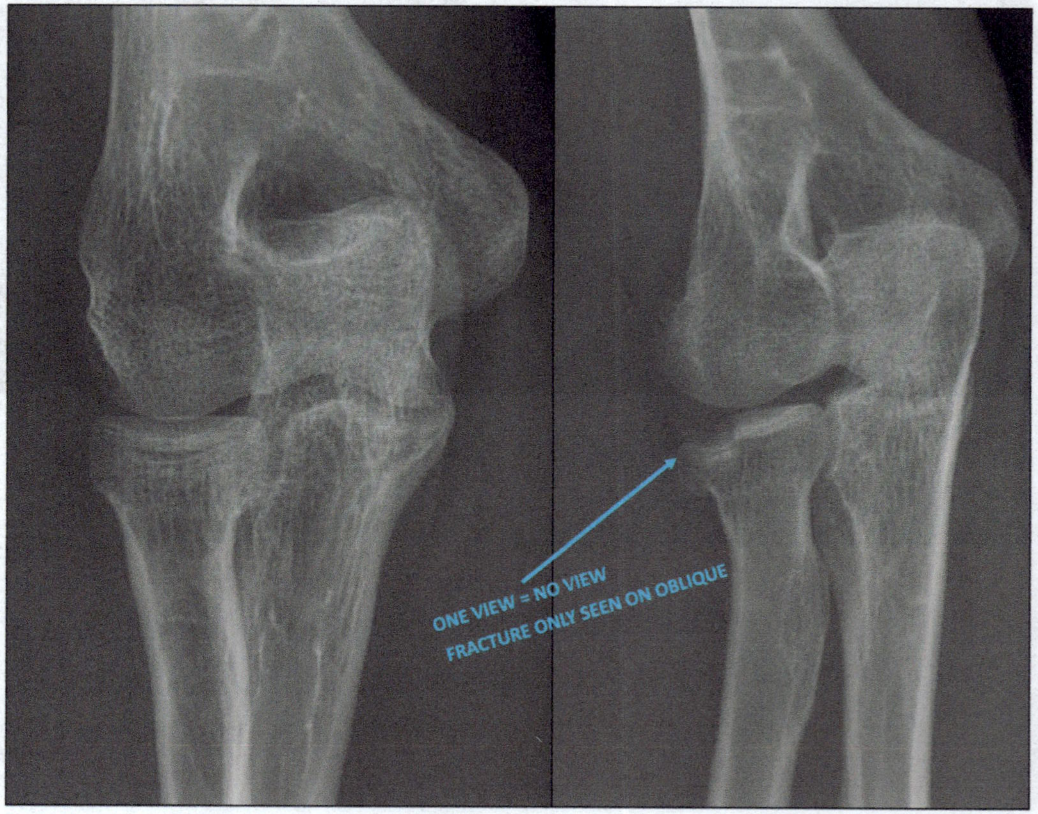

PEDIATRIC IMAGING

ULTRASOUND:
- **Intussusception (air enema to reduce)**
- **Appendicitis (do before CT)**
- Hypertrophic pyloric stenosis

FLOUROSCOPY:
- **Malrotation (UGI)**
- **Hirschsprung disease (barium enema)**
- Vesicoureteral reflux (cystourethrogram)

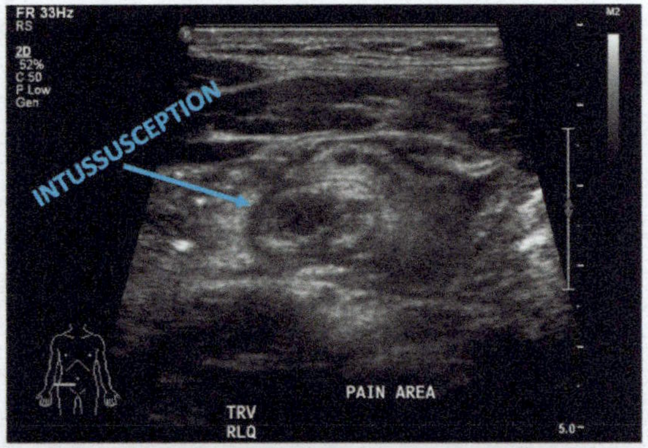

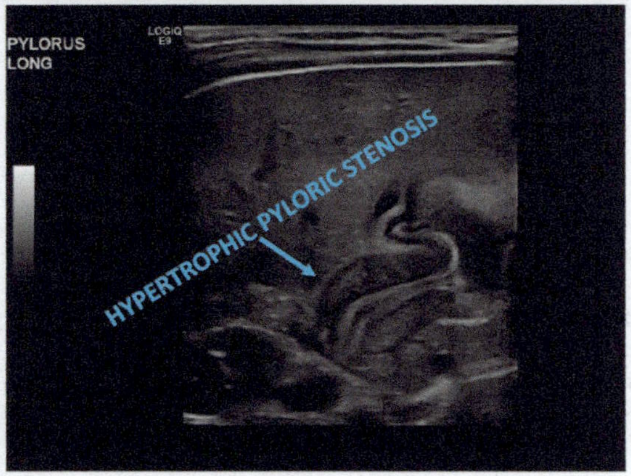

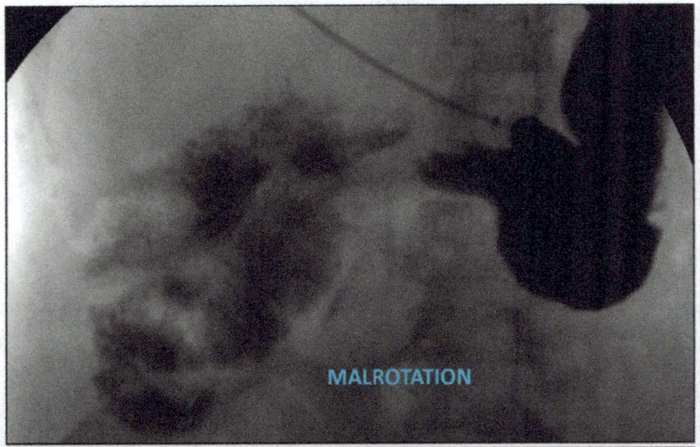

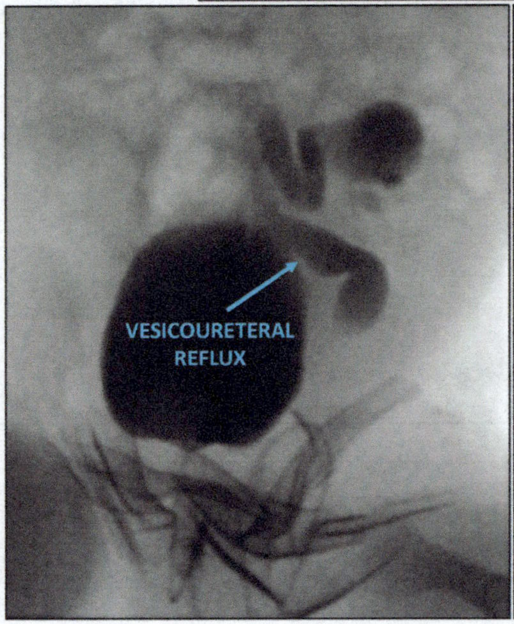

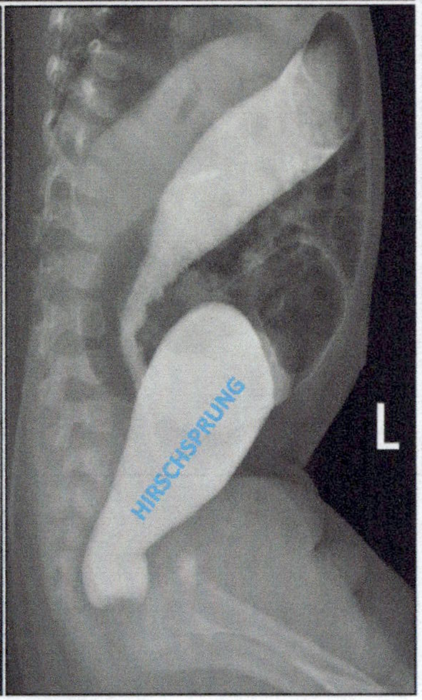

NUCLEAR MEDICINE

COMMON INDICATIONS:
- **V/Q for pregnant patients or contraindication/severe allergy to contrast**
- **HIDA scan for Biliary leak**
- **Gastrointestinal bleeding study**

BONE SCAN:
- Evaluation **metastatic bone lesions (not lytic)**
- Delayed fracture healing
- Avascular necrosis

GALLIUM SCAN:
- **Localizing Abscess**
- Staging lymphoma
- Melanoma
- **Osteomyelitis-discitis**

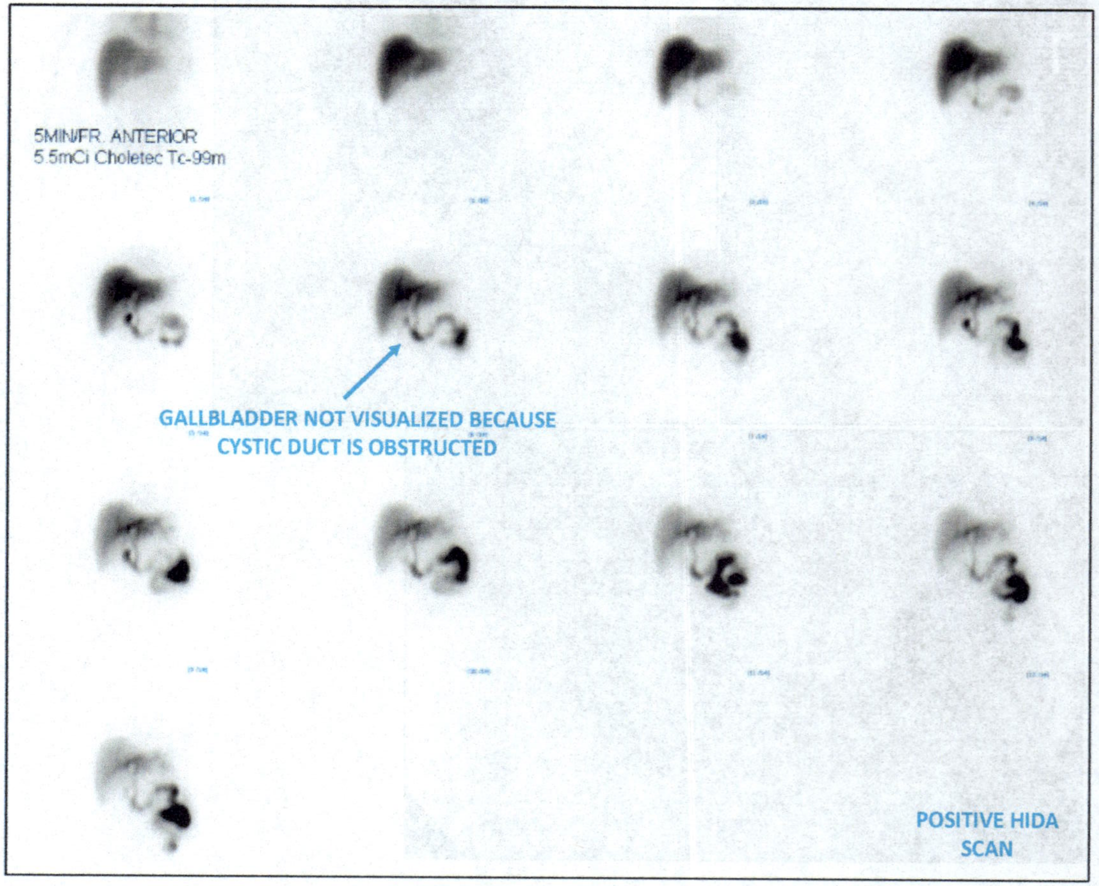

UNSTABLE PATIENTS

Radiologic and other ancillary tests, should be performed in the hemodynamically stable patient only

Hemodynamically unstable patients → OR for laparotomy

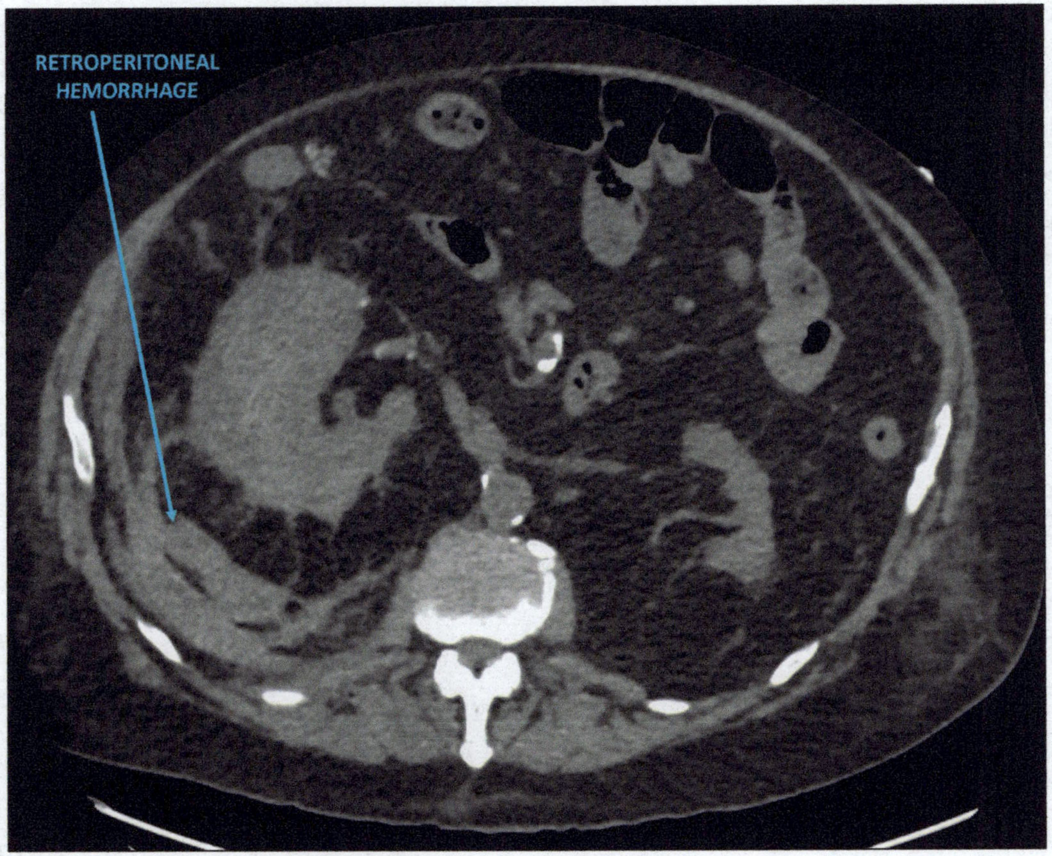

HIGH-YIELD REVIEW

XRAY

Mild ionizing radiation
Initial evaluation for fractures
Initial evaluation for chest or respiratory complaints
- Pneumonia
- Asthma
- Pneumothorax
- Heart failure ⍰ Pulmonary edema / pleural effusions
- COPD/emphysema
- Lung cancer
- NOT pulmonary emboli

Initial evaluation for cardiac complaints
Initial evaluation for joint disease / arthritis
Initial evaluation of osteomyelitis → MRI
Initial evaluation for osteoporosis → DEXA
Initial evaluation for foreign bodies
Initial evaluation for gastrointestinal complaints
- Small bowel obstruction
- Evaluation for free air
- Evaluation for renal calculi
- Pediatric constipation

MRI

No radiation
Contrast given for infectious / Inflammatory / Neoplastic concerns

Further evaluation for joint disease / trauma
- ACL tears
- Rotator Cuff tears / Labral tears (may be arthrographic contrast)
- Chondral disease
- Bone tumors

Further evaluation for Neurologic disease
- Stroke
- Brain tumors (with contrast)
- Multiple sclerosis

No contrast if GFR <60 → Risk of Nephrogenic Systemic Fibrosis

CT

Contrast given for acute abdominal pathology
CTA for PE or Dissection study
Noncontrast for stone study
Further evaluation for respiratory complaints:
- Pneumonia
- Heart failure
- Pneumothorax
- COPD/Emphysema
- Interstitial lung disease

Evaluation for trauma of the Chest, Abdomen, Pelvis, Spine
Further evaluation for abdominal complaints
- Appendicitis (after US if child)
- Diverticulitis
- Small bowel obstruction

Solid organ pathology (Cirrhosis, splenic disease, pancreatitis)
Initial evaluation of stroke / TIA / intracranial hemorrhage head trauma

No contrast if Creatinine >1.5 or Multiple Myeloma (AKI)
Discontinue contrast before Metformin and resume 48 hours after scan

FLX

Evaluation for Hirschsprung disease (pediatric enema)
Evaluation for malrotation (pediatric UGI)
Evaluation for dysphagia (Esophgram)
Evaluation for Aspiration (VSFE)
Procedures

PEDIATRIC PATIENTS

ULTRASOUND
Intussusception (air enema to reduce)
Appendicitis (do before CT)
Hypertrophic pyloric stenosis

FLOUROSCOPY
Malrotation (UGI)
Hirschsprung disease (barium enema)
Vesicoureteral reflux (cystourethrogram)

ULTRASOUND

No ionizing radiation
Initial evaluation for acute cholecystitis
Initial evaluation for liver pathology (Cirrhosis / Ascites / Jaundice)
Initial evaluation for hydronephrosis / nephrolithiasis
Initial evaluation for splenomegaly
Evaluate for DVT (LE US)
Initial evaluation for UTI
Initial evaluation for testicular / ovarian torsion
Initial evaluation for pelvis/gynecological pathology
- Uterine fibroids
- Ovarian cysts / Endometriosis
- PID / Salpingitis / TOA
- Pregnancy / Ectopic

NUCLEAR MEDICINE

V/Q scan in pregnant or contrast allergic
HIDA scan for biliary leak
Gastrointestinal bleeding study

BONE SCAN:
Evaluation metastatic bone lesions (not lytic)

GALLIUM SCAN:
Localizing Abscess
Osteomyelitis-discitis

INDEX

Made in United States
Orlando, FL
05 November 2026

90207158R00190